Challenging Concepts in Critical Care

Published and forthcoming titles in the Challenging Concepts in series

Anaesthesia (Edited by Dr Phoebe Syme, Dr Robert Jackson, and Professor Tim Cook)

Cardiovascular Medicine (Edited by Dr Aung Myat, Dr Shouvik Haldar, and Professor Simon Redwood)

Emergency Medicine (Edited by Dr Sam Thenabadu, Dr Fleur Cantle, and Dr Chris Lacy)

Infectious Disease and Clinical Microbiology (Edited by Dr Amber Arnold and Professor George Griffin)

Interventional Radiology (Edited by Dr Irfan Ahmed, Dr Miltiadis Krokidis, and Dr Tarun Sabharwal)

Neurology (Edited by Dr Krishna Chinthapalli, Dr Nadia Magdalinou, and Professor Nicholas Wood)

Neurosurgery (Edited by Mr Robin Bhatia and Mr Ian Sabin)

Obstetrics and Gynaecology (Edited by Dr Natasha Hezelgrave, Dr Danielle Abbott, and Professor Andrew Shennan)

Oncology (Edited by Dr Madhumita Bhattacharyya, Dr Sarah Payne, and Professor Iain McNeish)

Oral and Maxillofacial Surgery (Edited by Mr Matthew Idle and Mr Andrew Monaghan)

Respiratory Medicine (Edited by Dr Lucy Schomberg and Dr Elizabeth Sage)

Challenging Concepts in Critical Care

Cases with Expert Commentary

Edited by

Dr Christopher Gough

Registrar in Anaesthesia and Intensive Care Medicine,
Royal United Hospital Bath NHS Foundation, UK

Dr Justine Barnett

Consultant in Anaesthesia and Intensive Care Medicine,
Royal United Hospital Bath NHS Foundation, UK

Professor Tim Cook

Consultant in Anaesthesia and Intensive Care Medicine,
Royal United Hospital Bath NHS Foundation, UK

Professor Jerry Nolan

Consultant in Anaesthesia and Intensive Care Medicine,
Royal United Hospital Bath NHS Foundation, UK

Series editors

Dr Aung Myat

NIHR Academic Clinical Lecturer in Interventional Cardiology,
Brighton and Sussex Medical School,
Brighton, UK

Dr Shouvik Haldar

Consultant Cardiologist and Electrophysiologist, Heart Rhythm Centre,
Royal Brompton and Harefield NHS Foundation Trust,
Honorary Clinical Senior Lecturer,
Imperial College London, London, UK

Professor Simon Redwood

Professor of Interventional Cardiology and Honorary Consultant Cardiologist,
King's College London and St Thomas' Hospital, London, UK

OXFORD
UNIVERSITY PRESS

OXFORD
UNIVERSITY PRESS

Great Clarendon Street, Oxford, OX2 6DP,
United Kingdom

Oxford University Press is a department of the University of Oxford.
It furthers the University's objective of excellence in research, scholarship,
and education by publishing worldwide. Oxford is a registered trade mark of
Oxford University Press in the UK and in certain other countries

© Oxford University Press 2020

The moral rights of the authors have been asserted

First Edition published in 2020

Impression: 1

Published in the United States of America by Oxford University Press
198 Madison Avenue, New York, NY 10016, United States of America

British Library Cataloguing in Publication Data

Data available

Library of Congress Control Number: 2019938551

ISBN 978-0-19-881492-4

Printed and bound by
CPI Group (UK) Ltd, Croydon, CR0 4YY

FOREWORD

'Challenging Concepts in Critical Care' moves away from the traditional and somewhat dry format of didactic chapters. It offers a refreshing new take on educating doctors and allied healthcare practitioners working in critical care by using a detailed case-based approach for each section with a succession of key learning points, expert commentary, and lots of valuable references. This is a neat way of contextualizing everyday problems, and offers a reasonable management pathway to follow, based on current knowledge and recommended practices. A broad gamut of topics are covered from sepsis and respiratory failure through to organ donation, burns, and pandemic planning. The editors, authors, and expert commentators should be congratulated on an enjoyable, original, and highly informative read.

Mervyn Singer MB BS MD FRCP(Lon) FRCP(Edin) FFICM
Professor of Intensive Care Medicine
University College London
London, UK

ACKNOWLEDGEMENTS

With thanks to our families and colleagues for their considerable support throughout this project.

CONTENTS

CONTRIBUTORS

Justine Barnett
Consultant in Anaesthesia and ICM, Royal United Hospitals, Bath, UK

Catherine Bryant
Consultant Anaesthetist and Intensivist, Gloucestershire Hospitals NHS Foundation Trust, Great Western Road, Gloucester, UK

Jamie Cooper
Professor in Intensive Care Medicine, The Alfred Hospital, Melbourne, Australia

Ron Daniels
CEO, UK Sepsis Trust; Consultant in Critical Care and Anaesthesia, Heart of England NHS Foundation Trust, Solihull, UK

Nishita Desai
Specialty Registrar in Intensive Care Medicine, London North West Healthcare Trust, London, UK

Jeremy Farrar
Professor, Director, Wellcome Trust, London, UK

Lucinda Gabriel
Clinical Fellow in Critical Care, Guy's and St Thomas' Hospital NHS Foundation Trust, London, UK

Kim Gupta
Consultant in ICM and Anaesthesia, Royal United Hospitals, Bath, UK

Nicholas Hart
Clinical Director, Professor of Respiratory and Critical Care Medicine, Director of Research Delivery, Lane Fox Respiratory Service, St Thomas' Hospital, Guy's & St Thomas' NHS Foundation Trust, London, UK

Richard Hunt
Advanced Trainee in Intensive Care Medicine and Anaesthesia, Derriford Hospital, Plymouth, UK

Martin Huntley
Consultant in Anaesthesia and Intensive Care Medicine, Harrogate and District NHS Foundation Trust, Harrogate, UK

Matthew A. Kirkman
Specialty Registrar in Neurosurgery and Honorary Fellow in Neurocritical Care, Neurocritical Care Unit, The National Hospital for Neurology and Neurosurgery, University College London Hospitals, London, UK

Amy Krepska
Consultant Anaesthetist, Royal Brisbane and Women's Hospital, Brisbane, Australia

Clinton Lobo
Consultant in Anaesthesia and Intensive Care Medicine, Southmead Hospital, North Bristol NHS Trust, Bristol, UK

David J. Lockey
Consultant Anaesthetist and Intensivist, North Bristol NHS Trust, Hon Professor, University of Bristol, UK

Peter MacNaughton
Clinical director Critical Care, Derriford Hospital, Plymouth, UK

Laith Malhas
Consultant Anaesthetist, University Hospitals Coventry and Warwickshire NHS Trust, Coventry, UK

Alex Manara
Consultant in Anaesthesia and Intensive Care Medicine, Southmead Hospital, North Bristol NHS Trust, Bristol, UK

Ramani Moonesinghe
Consultant in Anaesthesia and ICM, University College London Hospitals, London, UK

Sian Alys Moxham
Specialty Registrar in Anaesthesia and Intensive Care Medicine, Bristol School of Anaesthesia, Bristol, UK

Deirdre Murphy
Senior Consultant Intensivist, Cabrini Health, Malvern, Melbourne, Australia

Patrick B. Murphy
Consultant Physician, Lane Fox Respiratory Unit, St Thomas' Hospital, Guy's and St Thomas' NHS Foundation Trust, London, UK

Dave Murray
Consultant Anaesthetist, James Cook University
Hospital, Middlesbrough, UK

Virginia Newcombe
Consultant in Intensive Care and Emergency Medicine,
Addenbrooke's Hospital, Cambridge, UK

Paul Nixon
Consultant Intensivist, The Alfred Hospital, Melbourne,
Australia

Jerry Nolan
Consultant in ICM and Anaesthesia, Royal United
Hospitals Bath, Bath; Professor of Resuscitation
Medicine, University of Bristol, Bristol, UK

Matt Oliver
NIHR UCL Clinical Lecturer in Anaesthesia, NELA
Research Advisor, London North Central Anaesthetic
Registrar, London, UK

Nim Pathmanathan
Consultant in ICM and Anaesthesia, Royal Devon and
Exeter NHS Foundation Trust, Exeter, UK

Tasneem Pirani
Consultant in General Intensive Care and Liver Intensive
Care, King's College Hospital, London, UK

Andrew Ray
Specialty Registrar in Anaesthesia and Intensive Care
Medicine, Bristol School of Anaesthesia, Bristol, UK

Marius Rehn
Consultant Anaesthesiologist, Division of Prehospital
Services, Air Ambulance Department, Oslo University
Hospital, Oslo; Norwegian Air Ambulance Foundation,
Oslo; University of Stavanger, Faculty of Health
Sciences, Stavanger, Norway

Sanjoy Shah
Consultant Intensivist, University Hospitals Bristol,
Bristol, UK

Martin Smith
Consultant and Honorary Professor in Neuroanaesthesia
and Neurocritical Care, Neurocritical Care Unit, The
National Hospital for Neurology and Neurosurgery,
University College London Hospitals, London, UK

Matt Thomas
Consultant in Anaesthesia and ICM, University Hospitals
Bristol, Bristol, UK

Gary Wares
Consultant in ICM and Anaesthesia, The Royal Marsden
Hospital, London, UK

Julia Wendon
Professor of Hepatology and Consultant Intensivist,
King's College London, London, UK

Amber E. Young
Consultant Paediatric Anaesthetist and Lead Children's
Burns Research Centre, University Hospitals Bristol NHS
Foundation Trust; Senior Research and NIHR Doctoral
Fellow, Bristol Centre for Surgical Research, Population
Health Sciences, Bristol Medical School, University of
Bristol, Bristol, UK

ABBREVIATIONS

ABG	arterial blood gas
ACE	angiotensin-converting enzyme
ACLF	acute-on-chronic liver failure
ACS	acute coronary syndrome
AD	acute decompensation
ADH	antidiuretic hormone
AECOPD	acute exacerbation of chronic obstructive pulmonary disease
AH	alcoholic hepatitis
AKI	acute kidney injury
ALF	acute liver failure
ALP	alkaline phosphatase
APTT	activated partial thromboplastin time
ARDS	acute respiratory distress syndrome
ASA	American Society of Anesthesiologists
AST	aspartate transaminase
BE	base excess
BIS	bispectral index
BMI	body mass index
BNP	beta-type natriuretic peptide
bpm	beats per minute
CAM	Confusion Assessment Method
CAM-ICU	Confusion Assessment Method for the Intensive Care Unit
CLD	chronic liver disease
CMV	cytomegalovirus
CO	carbon monoxide
COHb	carboxyhaemoglobin
COPD	chronic obstructive pulmonary disease
CPAP	continuous positive airway pressure
CPC	cerebral performance category
CPP	cerebral perfusion pressure
CRP	C-reactive protein
CRRT	continuous renal replacement therapy
CSF	cerebrospinal fluid
CSW	cerebral salt wasting
CTA	computed tomography angiogram
cTnI	cardiac troponin I
CVC	central venous catheter
CVP	central venous pressure
CVVHDF	continuous venovenous haemodiafiltration
CXR	chest X-ray
DBD	donation after brain death
DCD	donation after circulatory death
DCI	delayed cerebral ischaemia
DVT	deep vein thrombosis
ECG	electrocardiogram
ECMO	extracorporeal membrane oxygenation
ED	emergency department
EEG	electroencephalogram
EGDT	early goal-directed therapy
eGOS	extended Glasgow Outcome Scale
EMS	emergency medical services
EPAP	expiratory positive airway pressure
ERC	European Resuscitation Council
ERCP	endoscopic retrograde cholangiopancreatography
ESICM	European Society of Intensive Care Medicine
ETCO$_2$	end-tidal carbon dioxide
EVD	external ventricular drain
FFP	fresh frozen plasma
FiO$_2$	fraction of inspired oxygen
FLAIR	fluid-attenuated inversion recovery
GABA	gamma-aminobutyric acid
GCS	Glasgow Coma Scale
G-CSF	granulocyte-colony stimulating factor
GDFT	goal-directed fluid therapy
GMC	General Medical Council
GvHD	graft-versus-host disease
HD	haemodialysis
HE	hepatic encephalopathy
HES	hydroxyethyl starch
HF	haemofiltration
HFNO	high-flow nasal oxygenation
HLA	human leucocyte antigen
HRS	hepatorenal syndrome
HSCT	haematopoietic stem cell transplantation
IABP	intra-aortic balloon pump
ICP	intracranial pressure
ICU	intensive care unit
IMCA	Independent Mental Capacity Advocate
INR	international normalized ratio
IPAP	inspiratory positive airway pressure
LOLA	l-ornithinine l-aspartate
LPA	lasting power of attorney
MAP	mean arterial pressure
MARS	molecular adsorbent recirculating system

mcg	microgram(s)
MELD	Model for End-stage Liver Disease
MERS	Middle Eastern respiratory syndrome
MIE	mechanical insufflation–exsufflation
min	minute(s)
MMM	multimodality monitoring
MRC	Medical Research Council
MRI	magnetic resonance imaging
MTC	major trauma centre
NAI	non-accidental injury
NELA	National Emergency Laparotomy Audit
NEWS	National Early Warning Score
NG	nasogastric
NHS	National Health Service
NICE	National Institute for Health and Care Excellence
NIV	non-invasive ventilation
NMBD	neuromuscular blocking drug
NMD	neuromuscular disease
NSE	neuron-specific enolase
NSM	neurogenic stunned myocardium
OHCA	out-of-hospital cardiac arrest
OR	operating room
$PaCO_2$	partial pressure of carbon dioxide
PaO_2	partial pressure of oxygen
$PbtO_2$	brain tissue oxygen tension
PCI	percutaneous coronary intervention
PCR	polymerase chain reaction
PCT	procalcitonin
PD	peritoneal dialysis
PEEP	positive end-expiratory pressure
PICC	peripherally inserted central catheter
PIP	peak inspiratory pressure
PJP	*Pneumocystis jirovecii* pneumonia
PLR	passive leg raise
PPE	personal protective equipment
PPI	proton pump inhibitor
P-POSSUM	Portsmouth Physiological and Operative Severity Score for the Enumeration of Mortality and Morbidity

PRN	as required
PRx	pressure reactivity index
PT	prothrombin time
qSOFA	quick Sequential (Sepsis-Related) Organ Failure Assessment
RASS	Richmond Agitation–Sedation Scale
RCT	randomized controlled trial
REE	resting energy expenditure
ROSC	return of spontaneous circulation
RRT	renal replacement therapy
RSBI	rapid shallow breathing index
SAH	subarachnoid haemorrhage
SARS	severe acute respiratory syndrome
SBP	spontaneous bacterial peritonitis
SBT	spontaneous breathing trial
$ScvO_2$	central venous oxygen saturation
SIADH	syndrome of inappropriate antidiuretic hormone
SIR	systemic inflammatory response
SIRS	systemic inflammatory response syndrome
SN-OD	specialist nurse in organ donation
SOFA	Sequential [Sepsis-Related] Organ Failure Assessment
SORT	Surgical Outcomes Risk Tool
SpO_2	oxygen saturation by pulse oximetry
SSC	Surviving Sepsis Campaign
SSEP	somatosensory evoked potential
SvO_2	mixed venous blood oxygen saturation
TBI	traumatic brain injury
TBSA	total body surface area
TCD	transcranial Doppler
TTM	targeted temperature management
UK	United Kingdom
US	United States
V/Q	ventilation/perfusion
VA	venoarterial
VF	ventricular fibrillation
VOD	veno-occlusive disease
WFNS	World Federation of Neurological Societies
WLST	withdrawal of life-sustaining treatment

1 Sepsis

Laith Malhas

Expert Commentary Ron Daniels

Case history

A 68-year-old man was brought into the emergency department (ED) at 19:00 by his son, having been found at home generally unwell. The patient was not able to answer any questions himself, but the son reported that he tried to call his father in the day with no answer, and on visiting found him confused. He last spoke to him 4 days previously, when his father had seemed well. His only past medical history was recently diagnosed hypertension for which he had just started lisinopril 10 mg once daily prescribed by his general practitioner.

On initial assessment in the ED, his lungs were clear on auscultation, heart sounds normal, central capillary refill time was 4 seconds, and his peripheries were cool with no oedema. He had a soft abdomen with no palpable masses or organomegaly but grimaced on palpation of the left side. Bowel sounds were absent. He answered only direct questions and was confused, although no focal neurology was found and his pupils were equal and responsive to light.

His observations were as follows:

A. Oxygen saturation by pulse oximetry (SpO_2) 99% on room air.
B. Respiratory rate 18 breaths/min.
C. Heart rate 99 beats/min (bpm).
D. Blood pressure (BP) 96/40 mmHg.
E. Glasgow Coma Scale (GCS) score 13 (E3, V4, M6).
F. Temperature 35.8°C.

He had not passed any urine since being found. His National Early Warning Score (NEWS) was 7 (Table 1.1).

Table 1.1 National Early Warning Score (NEWS), developed by the Royal College of Physicians. Each variable is allocated a score and each of these is added to give a total NEWS score

Physiological parameters	3	2	1	0	1	2	3
Respiratory rate (breaths/min)	≤8		9–11	12–20		21–24	≥25
Oxygen saturations (%)	≤91	92–93	94–95	≥96			
Any extra oxygen		Yes		No			
Temperature (°C)	≤35.0		35.1–36.0	36.1–38.0	38.1–39.0	≥39.1	
Systolic blood pressure (mmHg)	≤90	91–100	101–110	111–219			≥220
Heart rate (bpm)	≤40		41–50	51–90	91–110	111–130	≥131
Level of consciousness				A			V, P, or U

A, alert; P, pain; U, unresponsive; V, voice.

Initial management involved placement of an 18-gauge peripheral venous cannula with venous blood samples sent for full blood count, urea and electrolytes, liver function tests, clotting studies, and gas analysis, and starting an intravenous (IV) infusion of 1 L of 0.9% sodium chloride.

His results returned at 20:00 and were as follows:

Venous blood gas		
pH	7.28	(7.35–7.45)
PaCO$_2$ (kPa)	6.6	(4.7–6)
PaO$_2$ (kPa)	3.9	(>10)
HCO^{3-} (mmol/L)	18.8	(22–28)
BE (mmol/L)	−6.7	(±2)
Lactate (mmol/L)	5.5	(0.5–2)

Full blood count		
Hb (g/L)	98	(130–180)
Plat (× 10^9/L)	118	(150–400)
WCC (× 10^9/L)	18.2	(4–11)

Urea and electrolytes		
Na (mmol/L)	148	(135–145)
K (mmol/L)	4.7	(3.5–5)
Urea (mmol/L)	22	(2.5–6.7)
Cr (µmol/L)	380	(60–110)
Alb (g/L)	22	(35–50)
CRP (mg/L)	183	(<10)
Glucose (mmol/L)	15.0	(6–10)

Liver function and clotting		
Bili (µmol/L)	8	(3–20)
Alk Phos (U/L)	131	(30–130)
ALT (U/L)	27	(10–40)
INR	1.6	

Alb, albumin; Alk Phos, alkaline phosphatase, ALT, alanine aminotransferase; BE, base excess; Bili, bilirubin; Cr, creatinine; CRP, C-reactive protein; Hb, haemoglobin; INR, international normalized ratio; K, potassium; Na, sodium; Plat, platelets; U, units; WCC, white cell count.

After being reviewed by the ED doctor, his acute kidney injury (AKI) was identified and attributed to dehydration, and his mild hypothermia was noted.

⊛ **Learning point** Defining and identifying sepsis

The first consensus definitions were determined by the American College of Chest Physicians and the Society of Critical Care Medicine in 1992, which formally defined the systemic inflammatory response syndrome (SIRS), sepsis, and other clinical classifications. This was updated in 2001 in conjunction with the European Society of Intensive Care Medicine [1], a collaboration which resulted in a widening of the original list of four SIRS criteria to over 20 signs and symptoms of infection to improve specificity. This was later condensed into a more pragmatic set of six criteria by the Surviving Sepsis Campaign (SSC) [2]. However, it was widely recognized that the consensus definitions continued to be imperfect, as the SIRS criteria as a tool for detecting sepsis tended to be oversensitive and poorly specific to either critical illness in general or sepsis in particular.

A third revision was published in 2016 by the European Society of Intensive Care Medicine and Society of Critical Care Medicine, coined Sepsis-3, which abandoned the term severe sepsis and attempted to simplify recognition [3]. Sepsis is now described as organ dysfunction secondary to infection. Organ dysfunction can be tracked with the Sequential (Sepsis-Related) Organ Failure Assessment (SOFA) score, a clinical scoring system already used for identifying organ dysfunction in intensive care units (ICUs). SIRS was still described as a useful tool to identify possible infection, but no longer formed part of the formal diagnosis of sepsis. The authors instead recommended the use of bedside clinical scoring systems to improve reliability of recognition, and proposed 'quick SOFA' (qSOFA) as a bedside test.

The qSOFA comprises:

- alteration in mental status
- systolic blood pressure less than or equal to 100 mmHg, or
- respiratory rate at least 22/min.

(continued)

with any two indicating a high risk of sepsis.

qSOFA was derived by a retrospective analysis of large (primarily US derived) datasets as a method of clinically identifying patients who were likely to have a poor outcome, defined as an ICU stay of 3 days or more, or death.

Sepsis-3: terms and definitions

- Sepsis is defined as life-threatening organ dysfunction caused by a dysregulated host response to infection.
- Organ dysfunction can be identified as an acute change in total SOFA score of 2 points or more due to the infection.
- The baseline SOFA score can be assumed to be zero in patients not known to have pre-existing organ dysfunction.
- A SOFA score of 2 or greater reflects an overall mortality risk of approximately 10% in a general hospital population with suspected infection.
- Patients with suspected infection who are likely to have a prolonged ICU stay or to die in the hospital can be promptly identified at the bedside with qSOFA.
- Septic shock is a subset of sepsis in which underlying circulatory and cellular/metabolic abnormalities are profound enough to substantially increase mortality.

Patients with septic shock can be identified by the presence of sepsis with persisting hypotension requiring vasopressors to maintain mean arterial pressure (MAP) at 65 mmHg or higher and a serum lactate level greater than 2 mmol/L despite adequate volume resuscitation. With these criteria, hospital mortality is greater than 40%.

This patient presented with an elevated white blood cell count which leads to a suspicion of infection, along with a qSOFA score of 2 which identifies him as more likely to have a poor outcome.

qSOFA has not been universally embraced. Organizations such as the Latin American Sepsis Institute and the UK National Institute for Health and Care Excellence (NICE) have gone as far as to intentionally avoid recommending its use. In 2016, a large prospective validation exercise in over 30,000 patients found qSOFA to be inferior to existing early warning scores (EWS) in identifying patients with sepsis at risk of adverse outcome [4].

Other groups have also developed diagnostic approaches to increase the reliability of suspecting sepsis and initiating treatment pathways. NICE offers guidance with age-specific risk stratification tools for anyone presenting with possible sepsis. These stratify elements of history and examination into categories indicating low, moderate–high, and high risk of severe illness/death (Table 1.2) [5].

These remain included in operational tools such as the UK Sepsis Trust's Red Flag Sepsis system (Figure 1.1) [6].

> **ⓖ Expert comment**
>
> A reliance on laboratory investigations to identify many of the organ dysfunction criteria means, in a resource-challenged busy clinical environment, that patients without obvious shock or hypoxia are missed. Patients get one opportunity to present their illness to a health professional—it is not always possible to review the patient in a timely manner with laboratory results as soon as they become available. qSOFA, and proposed alternatives such as the NEWS, move away from reliance on laboratory criteria.

Table 1.2 Risk stratification tool for adults, children, and young people aged 12 years and older with suspected sepsis

Category	High-risk criteria	Moderate- to high-risk criteria
History	Evidence of new altered mental state	History of new alteration in behaviour or mental state
		History of acute deterioration of functional ability
		Immune impairment (including oral steroids)
		Recent (within 6 weeks) history of trauma, surgery, or invasive procedure
Respiratory	Elevated respiratory rate: ≥25 breaths/min Acquired oxygen requirement >FiO$_2$ 0.4, to maintain SpO$_2$ >92% (or >88% in known COPD)	Elevated respiratory rate: 21–24 breaths/min

(continued)

Table 1.2 Continued

Category	High-risk criteria	Moderate- to high-risk criteria
Blood pressure	SBP ≤90 mmHg or at least 40 mmHg below normal	SBP 91–100 mmHg
Circulation and hydration	HR >130 bpm Not passed urine for at least 18 hours If catheterized, urine output <0.5 mL/kg/hour	HR 91–130 bpm or new arrhythmia Not passed urine for 12–18 hours For catheterized patients, urine output 0.5–1 mL/kg/hour
Temperature		Tympanic temperature <36°C
Skin	Mottled or ashen appearance Central or peripheral cyanosis Non-blanching rash	Any signs of potential infection e.g. discharge at surgical site

bpm, beats per minute, COPD, chronic obstructive pulmonary disease; HR, heart rate; SBP, systolic blood pressure.
Source: data from The National Institute for Health and Care Excellence (NICE). (2016) *Sepsis: recognition, diagnosis and early management* [NG51]. Copyright © 2016 NICE. Available at https://www.nice.org.uk

🛈 Expert comment

There are concerns that, while valid in hospital, the new definitions used in Sepsis-3 may not be sensitive enough for use outside hospital, for example, when considering hospital referral. As serum lactate has been validated as a predictor of mortality, including identifying 'cryptic shock' (hypoperfusion with normotension) [7], organizations not already using track-and-trigger EWS might usefully include qSOFA as a screening tool, adding lactate where necessary. Until there is further prospective validation of qSOFA, those already using NEWS/modified EWS can reasonably continue using a combination of a high index of suspicion of sepsis and the EWS to trigger consideration of sepsis. In the UK, NICE will be issuing a Quality Standard which is likely to reinforce the use of its risk stratification system described previously, which the UK Sepsis Trust has operationalized into Red Flag and Amber Flag Sepsis criteria (Figure 1.1).

The formal identification of sepsis using a change in SOFA score is more widely accepted, but in low- and middle-income countries needs careful interpretation, for example, to identify the criteria for septic shock.

Noting the high lactate, the ED junior doctor suspected high-risk ('Red Flag') sepsis (likely septic shock) according to NICE guidelines and initiated treatment. Supplemental oxygen was given and a further litre of 0.9% saline started. A urinary catheter was inserted, draining 280 mL of residual urine, which was clear but concentrated, with dipstick testing showing no evidence of leucocytes.

A venous blood culture sample was sent and antibiotics started according to hospital protocols (IV amoxicillin 1 g, metronidazole 500 mg, and gentamicin 320 mg for sepsis with a suspected intraabdominal cause). Although a 5-day course was anticipated, the antibiotics were prescribed for an initial 48-hour period with a plan to review the drug, indication, and duration at this point. The chest X-ray was unremarkable.

After discussion with the ED middle-grade doctor, the patient was referred to the surgical team and to the ICU team for review, due to his clinical deterioration as shown by his elevated NEWS score.

ED/AMU Sepsis Screening & Action Tool

Your logo

THE UK SEPSIS TRUST

To be applied to all non-pregnant adults and young people over 12 years **with fever** (or recent fever) symptoms, or who are clearly unwell with any abnormal observations

Patient details (affix label):

Staff member completing form:

Date (DD/MM/YY):

Name (print):

Designation:

Signature:

Important:
Is an end of life pathway in place? Yes ☐   Is escalation clinically inappropriate? Yes ☐   Initials ☐   Discontinue pathway

1. Does patient look sick?   Tick ☐ N
    OR has NEWS (or similar) triggered? ☐

↓Y

2. Could this be due to an infection?   Tick

Yes, but source unclear at present ☐ N
Pneumonia ☐
Urinary Tract Infection ☐
Abdominal pain or distension ☐
Cellulitis/septic arthritis/infected wound ☐
Device-related infection ☐
Meningitis ☐
Other (specify: ....) ☐

↓Y

3. Is any ONE Red Flag present?   Tick

Responds only to voice or pain/unresponsive ☐ N
Acute confusional state ☐
Systolic B.P ≤ 90 mmHg (or drop >40 from normal) ☐
Heart rate > 130 per minute ☐
Respiratory rate ≥ 25 per minute ☐
Needs oxygen to keep SpO$_2$ ≥ 92% ☐
Non-blanching rash, mottled/ashen/cyanotic ☐
Not passed urine in last 18 h/UO <0.5 ml/kg/hr ☐
Lactate ≥ 2 mmol/l ☐
Recent chemotherapy ☐

↓Y

Low risk of sepsis
Use standard protocols, consider discharge (approved by senior decision maker) with safety netting

↑N

4. Any Amber Flag criteria?   Tick

Relatives concerned about mental status ☐
Acute deterioration in functional ability ☐
Immunosuppressed ☐
Trauma/surgery/procedure in last 6 weeks ☐
Respiratory rate 21–24 ☐
Systolic B.P 91–100 mmHg ☐
Heart rate 91–130 OR new dysrhythmia ☐
Not passed urine in last 12–18 hours ☐
Temperature <36°C ☐
Clinical signs of wound, device or skin infection ☐

↓Y

Send bloods *If 2 criteria present, consider if 1*   Time complete   Initials
To include FBC, U&Es, CRP, LFTs, clotting
Ensure urgent senior review
Must review with results within 1 hour

Is AKI present? (tick)   YES ☐   NO ☐

Y

Clinician to make antimicrobial prescribing decision within 3h   Time complete   Initials
If senior clinician happy, may discharge with appropriate safety netting   Discharged?   Initials

Red Flag Sepsis!! Start Sepsis 6 pathway NOW (see overleaf)
This is time critical, immediate action is required.

Sepsis Six and Red Flag Sepsis are copyright to and intellectual property of the UK Sepsis Trust, registered charity no. 1158843. **sepsistrust.org**

Figure 1.1 Extract from the UK Sepsis Trust clinical toolkit for emergency departments made with formal arrangement with NICE.
Reproduced with permission from UK Sepsis Trust, registered charity no. 1158843.

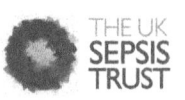

Sepsis Six Pathway

Your logo

To be applied to all adults and young people over 12 years of age with suspected or confirmed Red Flag Sepsis

Make a treatment escalation plan and decide on CPR status	Time zero	Consultant informed? (tick)	Initials
Inform consultant *(use SBAR)* patient has Red Flag Sepsis			

Action (complete ALL within 1 hour) — Reason not done/variance

1. Administer oxygen
Aim to keep saturations >94%
(88–92% if at risk of CO_2 retention e.g. COPD)

Time complete
Initials

2. Take blood cultures
At least a peripheral set. Consider e.g. CSF, urine, sputum
Think source control! Call surgeon/radiologist if needed
CXR and urinalysis for all adults

Time complete
Initials

3. Give IV antibiotics
According to Trust protocol
Consider allergies prior to administration

Time complete
Initials

4. Give IV fluids
If hypotensive/lactate >2mmol/l, 500 ml stat.
May be repeated if clinically indicated-
do not exceed 30ml/kg

Time complete
Initials

5. Check serial lactates
Corroborate high VBG lactate with arterial sample
*If lactate >4mmol/l, call Critical Care and
recheck after each 10ml/kg challenge*

Time complete
Initials

Not applicable- initial lactate ☐

6. Measure urine output
May require urinary catheter
Ensure fluid balance chart commenced
& completed hourly

Time complete
Initials

If after delivering the Sepsis Six, patient still has:
- systolic B.P <90 mmHg
- reduced level of consciousness despite resuscitation
- respiratory rate over 25 breaths per minute
- lactate not reducing
Or if patient is clearly critically ill at any time
Then call Critical Care Outreach immediately!!

Space available for local short antimicrobial guideline/escalation policy

Sepsis Six and Red Flag Sepsis are copyright to and intellectual property of the UK Sepsis Trust, registered charity no. 1158843. **sepsistrust.org**

Figure 1.1 Continued

> ★ **Learning point** Initial management
>
> Prompt early initiation of treatment has consistently been shown to reduce mortality from sepsis [8–10]. For this reason, there has been much effort to ensure that, once the diagnosis of sepsis is made, evidence-based care bundles are implemented.
>
> The SSC divides the initial management into two care bundles, the first to be completed by 3 hours from the diagnosis being made:
>
> 1. Measure serum lactate level.
> 2. Obtain blood cultures prior to administration of antibiotics.
> 3. Administer broad-spectrum antibiotics.
> 4. Administer 30 mL/kg crystalloid in divided aliquots for management of hypotension or if lactate is 4 mmol/L or greater.
>
> The ideal time of administration of antibiotics is immediately before sepsis develops from the underlying infection, but attempting to predict this risks overtreatment.
>
> Once sepsis does develop, any delay is linked to increasing progression of the septic process to multiorgan failure. Empiric antibiotics should be administered within 1 hour of the identification of sepsis. When possible, blood cultures should be obtained before administering antibiotics, but this should not delay initiation of antibiotics.
>
> As with the diagnostic criteria, keeping therapeutic protocols simple improves uptake and ultimately patient outcomes. The value of early treatment has been shown by several care bundles which reduce the time to completion of all tasks to 1 hour. For this reason, the UK Sepsis Trust's 'Sepsis Six' has become widely popular as an effective 1-hour bundle for when sepsis is suspected and has been shown to reduce sepsis-associated mortality rates by up to 50% [11, 12]. The Sepsis Six can be remembered as 'take three, give three'.
>
> **The Sepsis Six:**
>
> **Take 3**
>
> 1. Take blood cultures.
> 2. Measure serial serum lactates.
> 3. Measure accurate hourly urine output.
>
> **Give 3**
>
> 4. Administer oxygen to maintain saturations at greater than 94% (88–92% in chronic obstructive pulmonary disease).
> 5. Give broad-spectrum antibiotics.
> 6. Give IV fluid challenges if the patient is hypotensive or their lactate is elevated.

> ❶ **Expert comment**
>
> The inclusion of high-flow oxygen was slightly contentious given that cautious oxygen therapy is recommended in other acute conditions. The harmful effects of hyperoxia have been demonstrated in healthy individuals, and growing evidence highlights the deleterious effects of high inspired oxygen concentrations in treating patients with acute myocardial infarction, ischaemic stroke, neonatal resuscitation, and adult resuscitation following cardiac arrest [13]. The recent Hyperoxia and Hypertonic Saline in Patients with Septic Shock (HYPERS2S) trial documented significantly more serious adverse events in patients with sepsis treated for 24 hours with 100% oxygen versus those treated to achieve normoxia (SpO$_2$ 88–95%) [14]. While hyperoxia is potentially harmful, significant hypoxia is undeniably harmful and must be avoided or treated.

The patient was reviewed by the surgical team who did not consider the patient to have peritonitis but arranged an abdominal computed tomography scan.

On review by the intensive care senior trainee at 20:35, an arterial line was inserted, and on examination the patient was found to have cool peripheries. Based on clinical judgement and the presence of suspected sepsis, a fluid bolus of 500 mL Hartmann's solution was infused IV.

The patient's NEWS score subsequently deteriorated to 9 with minimal urine output.

⊘ Expert comment

The value of fluid resuscitation has always been unclear, and recently the routine use of liberal fluid resuscitation has been called into question [15]. Until further evidence becomes available, even considering recent evidence, we recommend that fluid be given rapidly to correct hypovolaemia in the early stages following presentation, but relatively restricted compared with historical practice once the patient has stabilized.

✪ Learning point Fluid resuscitation

Fluid resuscitation remains one of the mainstays of early treatment for patients with sepsis and septic shock, working by increasing intravascular volume, venous return, and hence cardiac output to improve blood pressure and organ/tissue perfusion. However, the type and quantity of fluid to use is contentious and studies have produced conflicting results. Problems arise from the complex and variable pathophysiological changes in sepsis, and interpretation of trials is complicated by the inclusion of heterogeneous patients at different stages in their clinical course.

Fluid type

The two main groups are crystalloid and colloid, with further division between balanced and non-balanced solutions.

Crystalloids

Crystalloid solutions can either be balanced solutions (e.g. Hartmann's solution and Plasma-Lyte 148), which are designed to mimic plasma and buffer against pH changes, or unbalanced 0.9% sodium chloride (commonly known as normal saline). Normal saline has been used historically because it is a cheap, stable, and easily manufactured isotonic solution; however, in studies comparing it with balanced solutions [16] it has been shown to:

- increase metabolic and dilution acidosis
- decrease renal blood flow
- increase risk of renal failure [17]
- create a coagulopathy
- increase inflammation
- be associated with an increased risk of death.

Although these perceived attributes have generated a move towards use of balanced solutions and away from 'abnormal' saline, in the 0.9% Saline versus Plasma-Lyte 148 for ICU fluid Therapy (SPLIT trial), use of a buffered crystalloid compared with saline did not reduce the risk of AKI in a heterogeneous group of critically ill patients [18].

Colloids

Colloidal solutions became popular because of the theoretical physiological advantage of being retained in the intravascular space for longer than crystalloids. The three main colloids are albumin, gelatin, and hydroxyethyl starch (HES).

Research has identified side effects and worsening outcomes (including higher mortality rates) associated with the use of some colloids, particularly in the setting of sepsis. The US Food and Drug Administration and the European Medicines Agency issued warnings after a proven increased risk of renal failure and death when HES was used in septic patients in the ICU [19]. The use of HES is contraindicated in critically ill patients.

These adverse effects of HES are thought to be from the colloid molecule accumulating in the interstitial tissues, exacerbated by the endothelial dysfunction brought about by the septic process. Within the kidney, this causes an osmotic nephrosis and a renal compartment syndrome within the capsule. There are observational data suggesting that use of gelatin is also associated with an increase in AKI.

Albumin, a natural colloid, has theoretical advantages over synthetic colloids: it maintains endothelial function as well as having antioxidant and anti-inflammatory properties. A subgroup analysis of septic patients in the Saline versus Albumin Fluid Evaluation (SAFE) trial, and a larger meta-analysis [20], suggested an association with reduced mortality. However, a more recent meta-analysis that included subsequent trials from the Early Albumin Resuscitation for Sepsis and Septic Shock (EARSS) study group and the Albumin Italian Outcomes Study (ALBIOS) trial found that albumin, when included in a fluid regimen for septic patients, showed no benefit in reducing mortality, though neither did it cause harm [21].

Given the additional expense of colloids over crystalloids, there should be evidence of benefit to justify their use. The SSC guidance currently recommends crystalloids as the initial fluid of choice and recommends albumin when patients require substantial amounts of crystalloids.

(continued)

How much fluid?

The complex pathophysiology of sepsis necessitates caution: give too little fluid and circulatory function will not be restored, give too much and excess fluid quickly leads to tissue oedema increasing organ dysfunction, morbidity, and mortality. Tissue oedema manifests clinically as peripheral oedema, increased extravascular lung water and, in some patients, acute respiratory distress syndrome. Multiple studies have shown an association between mortality and excessively positive fluid balance [22–25] and increased extravascular lung water [26].

The goal is to identify those patients whose cardiac output will improve with fluid—those who are *fluid responsive*. Patients can be divided into *fluid responders*, who may benefit from more fluid, or *fluid non-responders* in whom further fluid may be detrimental: these patients will require other support. Approximately 50% of all patients—with and without sepsis—in ICU are fluid responders [27].

Several variables have been used to predict fluid responsiveness with variable success, either as static measurements or dynamically in response to a fluid challenge or passive leg raise (PLR) (Table 1.3). From a basic science perspective, this is a clinical intervention to attempt to identify the patient's position on the Frank–Starling curve.

Table 1.3 Methods of monitoring fluid responsiveness

Static monitors	Dynamic monitors
Central venous pressure (CVP)	Stroke volume variation (SVV)
Pulmonary artery occlusion pressure (PAOP)	Pulse pressure variation (PPV)
Heart rate (HR)	Pleth variability index (PVI)
Mean arterial pressure (MAP)	Doppler and ultrasound measured changes (oesophageal Doppler monitor (ODM)/ echocardiography)
Flow time corrected (FTc)	Inferior vena cava distensibility/collapsibility index on ultrasonography

Static measurements have generally been found to be unhelpful in identifying fluid responders. The central venous pressure (CVP) or CVP responsiveness is now considered to be of little or no value. In conjunction with a PLR, the pulse pressure is useful [28]. The flow time corrected has mainly been used in perioperative patients, but is determined by systemic vascular resistance as well as intravascular volume [29].

Dynamic monitors rely on measurement of haemodynamic responses to variations in cardiac filling (e.g. caused by natural variation in heart rate during respiration). In patients undergoing positive pressure ventilation, the intermittent rise and fall of intrathoracic pressure leads to alterations in venous return and reflex responses in heart rate. These affect cardiac filling and the resulting haemodynamic changes can be used to assess the likelihood of fluid responsiveness. Dynamic monitors perform better in stable situations such as a patient who is undergoing pressure control ventilation and who has a normal heart rate and rhythm. Minimally invasive monitors are grouped into uncalibrated and calibrated devices, the latter being the more accurate. Other cardiac output monitors estimate cardiac output based on detection of a change in concentration of a dye (LiDCO), cold (PICCO), thoracic bioimpedance (CCO, Edwards Lifesciences), or analysis of the arterial line waveform (LiDCO rapid, FloTrac) and may rely on fluid administration or PLR to predict fluid responsiveness [30].

Bedside echocardiography is used routinely on many ICUs and is increasingly being undertaken by intensive care clinicians. Echocardiography enables assessment of right and left cardiac function, regional wall movement abnormalities (pre-existing or new ischaemic heart disease), valvular function, and, importantly, fluid status. While static measurements give some information, dynamic measures are more useful to determine fluid volume status. Variations in vena cava diameter (distensibility index) with the respiratory cycle provide good predictive information: visualization of the superior vena cava with transoesophageal echocardiography and the inferior vena cava with transthoracic echocardiography or transabdominal ultrasonography are possible, the latter requiring less extensive training. The main advantage of these methods is that the patient does not have to be in sinus rhythm—atrial fibrillation is common in the critically ill [31].

> **⑥ Expert comment**
>
> The SSC recommends initial fluid challenges in patients with hypoperfusion with suspicion of hypovolaemia up to a maximum of 30 mL/kg; further fluid challenges are based on haemodynamic improvement of static or dynamic variables. Little controversy surrounds the rationale behind initial restoration of circulating volume; however, too much fluid beyond the initial correction of hypovolaemia will worsen tissue oedema and oxygen delivery. Adequate initial fluid resuscitation should be followed by conservative late fluid management, defined as even or negative fluid balance measured on at least two consecutive days during the first 7 days after the onset of septic shock [32].

> **➕ Clinical tip** Passive leg raise
>
> The PLR is a clinical tool to determine fluid responsiveness and is a simple, non-invasive, and accurate bedside test which can be performed by nursing staff in conjunction with monitoring of dynamic variables [33]. Leg elevation induces an autotransfusion roughly equivalent to a 500 mL fluid challenge but is in effect reversible so that the non-responder is not given fluid that could be harmful.
>
> A PLR requires positioning of the patient head up at 45° and then tilting the bed back in a Trendelenburg position until the head of the bed is horizontal (Figure 1.2). This provides a greater autotransfusion volume than simply elevating the legs with the trunk in a supine position. Any response occurs in the first minute and therefore requires a dynamic flow measurement (or flow derivation) device with sufficiently fast response time. It has been studied with a variety of minimally invasive cardiac output monitors: an increase in cardiac output or stroke volume of 10% is taken to indicate a fluid-responsive patient. Intra-abdominal hypertension may impair venous drainage and invalidate the results.
>
>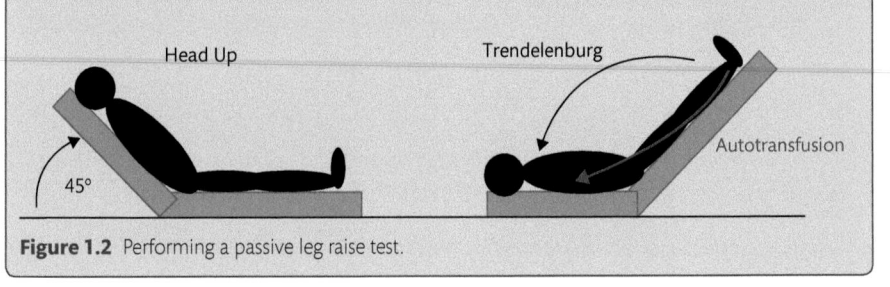
>
> **Figure 1.2** Performing a passive leg raise test.

Given the patient's lack of response to an initial 3 L of fluid resuscitation (the patient weighed approximately 80 kg), he was admitted to the ICU for invasive monitoring and early goal-directed therapy (EGDT). On arrival in the ICU at 21:30, a central venous catheter was inserted.

Vital signs at this time were:

Heart rate	92 bpm
Average BP (MAP)	99/43 (62) mmHg
SpO$_2$	99%
GCS score	14
Urine output	35 mL/hour
Central venous oxygen saturation	56%

Arterial blood gas values, breathing 80% oxygen were:

Arterial blood gas	FiO$_2$ 0.8	
pH	7.35	(7.35–7.45)
PaCO$_2$ (kPa)	7.35	(4.7–6)
PaO$_2$ (kPa)	25.6	(>10)
HCO$_3$$^-$ (mmol/L)	28.1	(22–28)
BE (mmol/L)	–4.7	(±2)
Lactate (mmol/L)	5.1	(0.5–2)
Na (mmol/L)	144	(135–145)
K (mmol/L)	3.4	(3.5–5)
Glucose (mmol/L)	15.0	(6–10)
Cl$^-$ (mmol/L)	106	(97–107)

An insulin infusion was started to normalize the blood glucose values; a nasogastric feeding tube was inserted, its position confirmed, and enteral feeding started.

> ✪ **Learning point**
>
> The second SSC care bundle, to be completed within the first 6 hours, gives physiological end points to be met as an indication of adequate organ perfusion and oxygen delivery.
>
> 1. Infuse vasopressors for hypotension that does not respond to initial fluid resuscitation to maintain a MAP of at least 65 mmHg.
> 2. In the event of persistent arterial hypotension despite volume resuscitation (septic shock) or an initial lactate level greater than or equal to 4 mmol/L (36 mg/dL):
>   o Measure central venous oxygen saturation (ScvO$_2$).
>   o Measure cardiac output if available.
>   o Consider inotropic support.
> 3. Remeasure lactate if initial lactate was elevated.
>
> Earlier recommendations with rigid physiological end points had been taken from an initial study of EGDT [34] but this approach has been overturned by three more recent studies. The US ProCESS, the Australian ARISE, and the UK ProMISe studies have all failed to show a difference in outcome when EGDT was compared with usual care [35–37]. The SSC now advises that measurement of CVP and ScvO$_2$ are not routinely necessary for patients with septic shock. The SSC is revising the haemodynamic bundle in accordance with the latest evidence [38].

> ❻ **Expert comment**
>
> In addition to source control and antimicrobial therapy, fluid resuscitation to correct hypovolaemia remains the central tenet of resuscitation in septic shock. The failure of ProCESS, ARISE and ProMISe to show treatment benefit in the intervention groups may reflect that basic care has improved so much that protocolized care has less impact. This was demonstrated recently across a group of hospitals in North America in a study identifying that early compliance with basic care elements meant illness did not progress and meant patients were subsequently ineligible for EGDT as they did not meet entry criteria [39]. A pragmatic approach, using basic physiological principles, is to fluid resuscitate using a suitable end point, such as warm peripheries, improved GCS score, and good urine output; to support persistent hypotension using vasopressors; and to assess for and address signs of inadequate cardiac output or oxygen delivery.

Despite fluid resuscitation, haemodynamic goals were not being achieved and nor-adrenaline was started to maintain the patient's MAP at greater than 70 mmHg. This goal was chosen because of the patient's previous poorly controlled hypertension. Once the blood pressure had been stabilized, an abdominal computed tomography scan was undertaken, which identified diverticulitis without evidence of perforation or abscess formation. On review, the surgical team decided on conservative management. The microbiology consultant recommended a change in antibiotic therapy to meropenem.

✪ Learning point Microbiology

Appropriate antibiotic therapy is an essential component in the management of the septic patient. To initiate appropriate antibiotics, and to subsequently narrow the spectrum in response to culture results, it is essential to investigate the patient thoroughly to identify a source of sepsis, and to take several samples for microbiology testing. Ideally, microbiology samples should be collected prior to commencement of antibiotic therapy, so long as this does not delay administration of the treatment.

Liaison with a microbiologist ensures appropriate antibiotic choice taking into account likely pathogens and local antibiotic resistance patterns. It also enables narrowing of the antibiotic therapy when culture results become available. Good antibiotic stewardship involves the use of appropriate antibiotics, for an appropriate duration, to effectively treat the underlying infection while minimizing development of antimicrobial resistance.

The patient did not improve overnight, and so a PiCCO arterial line was inserted to enable dynamic cardiac output measurement. This guided his vasopressor requirement, and further crystalloid boluses were guided by PLRs.

The vital signs at this time were:

Heart rate	89 bpm
BP (MAP)	98/43 (61) mmHg despite 0.32 mcg/kg/min noradrenaline
SpO$_2$	98%
GCS score	14 (E4 V4 M6)
Urine output	35 mL/h

Arterial blood gas on 80% oxygen		
pH	**7.37**	(7.35–7.45)
PaCO$_2$ (kPa)	**7.34**	(4.7–6)
PaO$_2$ (kPa)	**10.7**	(>10)
HCO^{3-} (mmol/L)	**28.9**	(22–28)
BE (mmol/L)	**−5.8**	(±2)
Lactate (mmol/L)	**3.5**	(0.5–2)
Na (mmol/L)	**143**	(135–145)
K (mmol/L)	**3.8**	(3.5–5)
Glucose (mmol/L)	**8.9**	(6–10)
Cl$^-$ (mmol/L)	**111**	(97–107)

A bedside focused cardiac ultrasound was undertaken, enabling specific conditions to be excluded from contributing to his increasing inotropic requirement. The focused echocardiogram showed good global cardiac function without any regional wall movement abnormalities or major valve dysfunction, no pericardial effusion, normal right-sided pressures, and a subjectively adequate volume status.

> ✪ **Learning point** Indicators of perfusion and adequacy of treatment
>
> Several variables have been studied as indicators of disease severity, adequacy of perfusion, and as a measure of response to treatment.
>
> **Lactate**
>
> A raised lactate (>2 mmol/L) has long been identified as an indicator of severity of illness, and is associated with organ dysfunction and mortality in septic patients [43]. The raised lactate reflects increased production and possibly decreased clearance. It is produced by anaerobic metabolism resulting from mitochondrial hypoxia as a result of the septic process, as well as increased sodium-potassium pump activity and ATP use through catecholamine stimulation and cytokine-mediated uptake of glucose associated with the stress response [44]. Hepatic dysfunction and inhibition of the rate-limiting enzyme pyruvate dehydrogenase reduces lactate clearance [45].
>
> A value of at least 4 mmol/L is used as the marker of severity in defining shock in septic patients [46]. In a recent analysis from the SSC database, a cut-off value of greater than 4 mmol/L, especially with hypotension, identified a significant increase in mortality. Comparing patients with a lactate greater than 4 mmol/L and hypotension, with patients with a lactate less than 2 mmol/L and no hypotension, mortality was 44.5% versus 29% [47].
>
> Lactate clearance has been used as a measure of successful resuscitation. This strategy assumes that the hyperlactataemia results from global tissue hypoxia [48]. If tissue dysfunction and increased lactate does result from a predominantly anaerobic metabolic stress response, then its early decrease indicates a reversal of this stress response. However, further use of lactate clearance as a goal beyond this initial decrease would not be beneficial and possibly harmful if used as an exclusive target [49].

> 🍎 **Expert comment**
>
> Lactate is an adaptive, endogenous compound used by organs including the heart as a metabolic substrate in stress situations. Hyperlactataemia is associated with an adverse outcome, but the presence of lactate per se may not be harmful. Lactate clearance as a therapeutic target is reasonable in the immediate period following presentation, but a failure to achieve a reduction in lactate levels after administration of 30 mL/kg of crystalloid (or equivalent) should be considered as indicative of microcirculatory (rather than macrocirculatory) failure and prompt urgent critical care admission for invasive monitoring and organ support rather than more fluids.

> **Venous blood oxygen saturation**
>
> If the mixed venous blood oxygen saturation (SvO_2) is reduced in the context of normal oxygen content of arterial blood, it represents either decreased oxygen delivery or increased consumption and, theoretically, is a determinant of the severity of shock. With the declining use of the pulmonary artery catheter, the $ScvO_2$ has been used in its place but its values do not correlate with those of the SvO_2 in critically ill patients because of altered perfusion and metabolic patterns. Normalization of both was included in Rivers' EGDT protocol as a goal indicating adequate tissue oxygenation, with apparent success in previous studies [50]. However, recent studies suggest these end points (and lactate clearance) do not affect survival [51–53].
>
> In most patients with sepsis, the $ScvO_2$ is normal or even high—indicating either a problem of oxygen consumption by tissues or an anaerobic metabolic stress response [54, 55]. The SCC no longer recommends the routine use of $ScvO_2$.
>
> **Measures of the microcirculation**
>
> The disruption to the macrocirculation caused by sepsis, and mediated by vasodilatation and increased capillary permeability, has been the main focus of sepsis identification and management because it provides systemic variables which can be measured easily even outside critical care environments. However, sepsis also disrupts the regulation of microcirculatory perfusion, which is responsible for the maintenance of the blood–tissue interface. This disruption can persist after the correction of the macrocirculation, leading to tissue hypoxia, mitochondrial stress, and organ dysfunction [56]. This may manifest as persistent hyperlactataemia, or worsening organ dysfunction or metabolic status, despite apparently acceptable macrocirculatory indices and adequate fluid resuscitation and perfusion.

(continued)

Despite technological developments enabling assessment of microcirculatory function, they are not used clinically because they are expensive and there is no consensus on how to interpret the results [57].

Methods available include:

- Video microscopic techniques [58]:
  - Nailfold videocapillaroscopy
  - Sublingual videocapillaroscopy
- Laser Doppler
- Near-infrared spectroscopy.

Currently, sublingual videocapillaroscopy and near-infrared spectroscopy appear to show the greatest promise.

Despite a lack of evidence of outcome benefit, vasopressin was added as a second-line therapy once the noradrenaline infusion rate had increased to 0.60 mcg/kg/min, in an attempt to achieve a MAP of 70 mmHg [40, 41]. Hydrocortisone was added at a physiological dose of 50 mg hydrocortisone four times a day, despite scant evidence in support [42]. This combination led to achievement of the target MAP and within 12 hours the noradrenaline infusion rate had been decreased to 0.45 mcg/kg/min. The patient's oxygen requirement continued to increase.

> ✪ **Learning point Vasopressors and inotropes**
>
> In patients with sepsis-induced hypotension, vasopressors and/or inotropes may be required to restore circulatory function. Ideally, they are started once patients have been identified as fluid unresponsive; however, they are often required to maintain an adequate MAP and to improve tissue perfusion while fluid resuscitation continues. If the perfusion pressure to organs decreases below a certain threshold (60 mmHg in animal studies [59]), regional autoregulatory mechanisms are lost and tissue perfusion decreases linearly with further reductions in perfusion pressure. Regional autoregulation is further disrupted by the pathophysiological changes in sepsis and by microcirculatory dysfunction.
>
> A target MAP of 65 mmHg has been recommended by the SSC, but individualized target pressures are more rational, for example, a higher pressure for those with chronic hypertension whose autoregulatory window may have shifted.
>
> Patients with sepsis may have a high, normal, or low cardiac output depending on previous reserves and the severity of sepsis. Initially, a reduced systemic vascular resistance may result in a high cardiac output and at this stage vasopressor support may be required to counteract hypotension. While this physiological response to sepsis in otherwise healthy individuals is typically seen in compensation for vasodilatory shock, sepsis can also lead to both systolic and diastolic myocardial dysfunction. No benefit has been shown in increasing a normal cardiac output to supranormal values; in fact, by increasing cardiac oxygen consumption it may be harmful [60]. Normovolaemic patients with a reduced cardiac output may require inotropic support.
>
> **Vasopressors**
>
> Noradrenaline, a mixed alpha and beta$_1$ adrenergic agonist, is the preferred vasopressor. It counteracts the vasodilation caused by sepsis and causes venoconstriction, which increases venous return and therefore cardiac output. Noradrenaline is also an inotrope, increasing cardiac output via beta$_1$ adrenoreceptors. High-dose noradrenaline may cause intense vasoconstriction and, despite increasing blood pressure, may reduce tissue perfusion.
>
> Adrenaline is a potent alpha and beta adrenergic agonist and is a second-line therapy that can be used in addition to noradrenaline, or alone, to maintain the blood pressure if noradrenaline alone is insufficient. Adrenaline provides both inotropic and vasopressor effects. It can cause hyperglycaemia and a transient increase in lactate, caused by glycolysis, lipolysis, and insulin resistance rather than hypoperfusion of tissues.
>
> *(continued)*

Vasopressin (also known as ADH, arginine vasopressin, and argipressin) acts on vasopressin receptors in the circulation and kidney to cause vasoconstriction and water retention. It may be added and can enable reduction in the dose of noradrenaline. It appears safe when used early, but it has not been shown to improve outcome from septic shock [41, 61].

In comparison with noradrenaline, dopamine (required in high doses for a vasopressor effect) is associated with increased side effects (mainly arrhythmias) and its use in sepsis is not recommended. Phenylephrine is a pure alpha agonist, which tends to reduce cardiac output and is not recommended for the treatment of sepsis. An analysis of a large US database has shown that the use of phenylephrine instead of noradrenaline to treat septic shock was associated with increased mortality [62].

Inotropes

Once intravascular volume and vascular tone have been adequately addressed, any further impairment of perfusion is likely to reflect reduced cardiac function—clinical suspicion should be confirmed where possible with appropriate cardiac output monitoring or echocardiography.

Sepsis-induced myocardial dysfunction is caused by inflammatory mediators, nitric oxide, interstitial myocarditis, coronary ischaemia, calcium channel dysfunction, endothelin receptor antagonism, and apoptosis [63]. The myocardial dysfunction can be treated with inotropes, which improve cardiac contractility and perfusion, although this may be at the expense of tachycardia. An increase in myocardial oxygen demand relative to the cardiac output may cause or worsen ischaemia.

Targeting supranormal cardiac output is not desirable—the aim is to restore a low cardiac output state to normal. Dobutamine is typically used as the first-line inotrope: its $beta_1$ agonist properties confer inotropy while $beta_2$ properties cause mild vasodilatation, though this may be affected by pre-existing medication (e.g. beta blockers) or morbidity (e.g. cardiac failure) that alter individual patients' responsiveness. Dobutamine has a ceiling of action and further inotropic activity may then require the addition of adrenaline, though this is likely to increase myocardial oxygen demand and may also cause excessive vasoconstriction.

⓰ Expert comment

In practice, most patients with septic shock are managed using vasopressors alone—most commonly noradrenaline. It would be good practice, but is not always feasible, to assess cardiac output immediately following resuscitation in all patients with sepsis. If a patient stabilizes rapidly following low-dose noradrenaline, for example, 0.08 mcg/kg/min, and clinical indices of perfusion including mentation, urine output, and lactate levels improve, then it would be deemed reasonable to omit formal cardiac output monitoring. There is no clear guidance as to what level of vasopressor support cardiac output assessment should be undertaken. A pragmatic approach would be to institute cardiac output monitoring within the first few hours for all patients in whom indices of perfusion do not normalize with vasopressor support alone, and in any patient requiring higher dose vasopressors (e.g. >0.3 mcg/kg/min of noradrenaline). Once blood pressure is restored, attention should never deviate from the harmful effects of vasopressors and, as with IV fluids, a 'just enough is enough' approach is adopted. Early reduction of vasopressor support may help in reducing long-term complications and tachyphylaxis. Drugs such as enoximone and milrinone (phosphodiesterase-3 inhibitors, inodilators) and the calcium sensitizer levosimendan are infrequently used in sepsis, but may have a role in complex cases (see Case 2).

✪ Learning point Other supportive therapies

Several other therapies are used to treat patients with sepsis—some are considered standard care for all critically ill patients, including the following:

- Glucose control. Although initial work showed promise in maintaining tight glycaemic control in sepsis, it is now understood that the harmful effects of severe hypoglycaemia which might result outweigh any perceived benefit. The avoidance of significant hyperglycaemia is now the goal, with an appropriate target of 4–10 mmol/L [64, 65].

(continued)

- Stress ulcer prophylaxis. Feeding early and continuously and treating with a proton pump inhibitor until receiving full feed is a mainstay of avoidance of stress ulcers and gastrointestinal bleeding
- Thromboprophylaxis. See Case 13.
- Nutritional support. See Case 13.
- Lung protective ventilation strategies. See Case 3.
- Diuretics and renal replacement therapy. Initial sepsis management invariably produces a positive fluid balance; however, once stabilized, aim for a negative balance to counteract administered drug solutions and feeds. Several diuretics (e.g. furosemide combined with spironolactone and bendroflumethiazide or metolazone) may be useful in combination to improve diuresis and minimize the side effects of a single agent.
- Sedation and analgesia. See Case 10.

> **ⓐ Expert comment**
>
> The 2000s saw the rise and fall in popularity of recombinant activated protein C for sepsis. Early studies suggested significant benefit but this was not seen in subsequent studies and the drug is no longer available. This is a typical picture that has been observed with many previous sepsis-specific modulatory therapies. Failure of these therapeutic agents may not only be due to lack of efficacy of the agents, but may also reflect the enormous heterogeneity of patients included and their source of infection, pathogen and microbial load, host response characteristics, and the clinical time course of the septic episode before presentation to healthcare and subsequent recognition of sepsis.

Steroid therapy and the use of blood products are also important aspects of the treatment of sepsis.

Corticosteroids

An adequate hypothalamic–pituitary–adrenal axis response to the stress of sepsis has been linked to survival, with relative insufficiency of endogenous corticosteroids implicated in adverse outcomes and delayed reversal of shock [66]. Supplemental hydrocortisone reduces the time to shock reversal but the mechanisms involved are complex and not fully understood [67]. Steroids increase vessel sensitivity to alpha agonists, aiding restoration of MAP by catecholamine vasopressors, and they can improve vasopressor-unresponsive septic shock (hypotension despite fluid resuscitation and vasopressors for more than 60 min). Some systematic reviews have demonstrated reduced mortality, albeit only in those severely ill (expected 28-day mortality >50%); however, the more recent Corticosteroid Therapy of Septic Shock (CORTICUS) trial [42] failed to show a mortality benefit in patients without sustained shock.

Tests of hypothalamic–pituitary–adrenal axis function are difficult to interpret in the critically ill and for this reason testing for adrenocortical suppression is not recommended. In practice, hydrocortisone 50 mg 6 hourly is typically started once the dose of noradrenaline exceeds approximately 0.25–0.3 mcg/kg/min and is tapered off once vasopressors are no longer needed.

Blood products

Anaemia is common in critical illness and has multiple causes. Taking blood for tests is an important contributor to anaemia in patients who are on the ICU for prolonged periods and careful management of testing and technique can limit the impact. Avoiding unnecessary use of blood products is important. Accepting lower haemoglobin values (70–90 g/L vs 100–120 g/L) has no effect on the mortality of critically ill adults [68, 69]. The transfusion trigger should be a haemoglobin concentration of 70 g/L and the haemoglobin target of 70–90 g/L, except for patients with active coronary artery disease where the trigger is 90 g/L.

Use of erythropoietin does not improve outcome in septic patients and may cause harm because of increased rates of thrombosis. Guidance on the use of platelets and fresh frozen plasma in sepsis is the same as for any critically ill patient.

Despite the inotropic requirement starting to reduce, the patient's oxygen requirement rose further, and invasive ventilation was commenced, along with propofol and alfentanil sedation. A chest X-ray showed bilateral opacities consistent with pulmonary oedema, and a repeat bedside focused echocardiogram showed good biventricular function, with no atrial or ventricular dilation. In the face of reducing inotropic requirement, and little response to bolus diuretics, a furosemide infusion was commenced to achieve a significant negative fluid balance. This had no adverse effect on the inotropic dosing, which continued to improve.

> **ⓘ Expert comment**
>
> All patients with sepsis and septic shock are at risk of acute respiratory failure. The fluid volumes used in the initial resuscitation, combined with endothelial leakage, predispose these patients to pulmonary oedema, but sepsis is also a common trigger for acute respiratory distress syndrome (see Case 3), which can make differentiating between them difficult. A key principle in these patients, particularly in the face of improving haemodynamic state, is to ensure a negative fluid balance. This can be achieved by bolus diuretic use, by diuretic infusion, or through haemofiltration.

After 48 hours of invasive ventilation, using a lung protective strategy, combined with 2 days of negative fluid balance of 2000 mL each, the patient had progressed to a spontaneous breathing mode, and the oxygen requirement significantly improved. He was extubated onto nasal high-flow oxygen (see Case 16), which was gradually weaned off over the following 24 hours. By this time, the vasopressin was stopped and the noradrenaline weaned off over a further 36 hours. He was able to give a history of having diarrhoea and vomiting for the week preceding admission. He was discharged from ICU on day 9.

Discussion

Epidemiology and pathogenesis

The incidence of sepsis requiring ICU admission is 0.25–0.38 per 1000 population per year, equating to approximately 20,000 cases per year in the UK and more than 20 million cases per year globally. Despite improvements in medicine, the incidence of sepsis is increasing. Data from the UK Intensive Care National Audit & Research Centre identified that hypotensive sepsis accounts for 10% of all admissions with an ICU mortality of 18.2% and hospital mortality of 28.3% [70].

The Sepsis Occurrence in Acutely ill Patients (SOAP) study described the incidence of sepsis in ICUs in Europe in 2002 [71]. It found that 37.4% of adult patients in ICU had sepsis, of whom 24.7% had sepsis on admission, with a mortality rate of 18.5% on ICU and 24.1% in hospital. The causative organism was identified in 60% of cases, being Gram positive in 40%, Gram negative in 38%, and fungal in 17%. The most common source of infection was the lung (68%) followed by the abdomen (22%).

Pathophysiology of sepsis

The immune system involves the complex interaction of cellular and humoral responses designed to eradicate pathogens and resultant infections. The inflammatory mediator process consists of a balance between a proinflammatory process, designed to eliminate the pathogens, and an anti-inflammatory process, to contain the response to the infected area.

SIRS is a disorderly activation of the inflammatory process leading to an unbalanced systemic response with resultant harm. The development of SIRS and sepsis involves dysfunction of both the innate and adaptive immune systems. Endothelial cells play an important role in the immune response by altering vascular tone, permeability, adhesion molecule expression, and coagulation function to facilitate an effective immune response. The coagulation and fibrinolytic systems are closely linked to both the immune system and endothelial function, and are also affected by sepsis. Altered bleeding times and decreased platelet counts are seen clinically.

Arterial vasodilation reduces perfusion pressure and venous vasodilation causes a relative hypovolaemia and reduced cardiac output. The resultant hypotension is worsened by any cardiac dysfunction and causes tissue hypoperfusion. It is this reduced perfusion which decreases global oxygen delivery.

The microvascular effects caused by systemic endothelial dysfunction lead to capillary vasodilation, loss of the endothelial glycocalyx layer, and increased endothelial permeability. Capillary beds lose their autoregulation ability, which further compromises tissue perfusion already affected by the poor perfusion pressure from the microvascular dysfunction. This is also exacerbated by coagulation dysfunction causing microthrombus formation in the capillaries where blood flow has become disorganized and stagnant. A combination of tissue hypoperfusion and shunt results. As well as the vascular effects, mitochondrial dysfunction occurs during sepsis, ultimately resulting in apoptosis and cell death.

The combination of reduced oxygen delivery (from macrovascular dysfunction) and the reduced capillary flow and blood/tissue gas exchange (from microvascular dysfunction), together with impaired utilization of oxygen at a cellular level (from mitochondrial dysfunction), mean tissues are no longer able to function. Organ systems begin to shut down in a protective mechanism to prevent widespread cell death and multiple organ dysfunction syndrome ensues. If not reversed, this process leads to vital organ system failure and death.

Difficulties in the treatment of sepsis

Challenges remain around antimicrobial treatment with source control, and fluid therapy.

The use of IV fluids, while being the foundation of supportive management, is an area which generates controversy. The balance between restoring cardiovascular function and fluid overloading is delicate. The physiology is more complex than it initially appears. IV fluid therapy does not generate the volumes of distribution expected from Starling's original model of semipermeable capillaries, leading to a revised equation which includes the effect of the endothelial glycocalyx layer. This is further influenced by the capillary pressure at the time of infusion, as well as the patient and their pathology (e.g. damage to the glycocalyx layer caused by inflammation).

The most effective therapy for sepsis is adequate, early antimicrobial therapy and source control. Management is then supportive to maintain organ function and prevent death until sepsis subsides. Targeted broad-spectrum antibiotics are commenced initially, but the choice of antibiotic should be narrowed as soon as possible. Emerging antibiotic resistance is an increasing clinical problem, and with limited new antibiotics coming to market, effective antibiotic stewardship is an essential component of good clinical care.

A final word from the expert

Strategies toward the recognition and management of sepsis are continually evolving as our understanding of the condition develops. In time, our knowledge of both individual pathogenic profiles and host response, coupled with more rapid pathogen and biomarker profile identification, is likely to advance such that therapies can be tailored to the disease profile. For now, however, a broad brush and a culture of awareness are our best weapons.

References

1. Levy M, Fink M, Marshall J, et al. 2001 SCCM/ESICM/ACCP/ATS/SIS International sepsis definitions conference. *Intensive Care Med.* 2003;29:530–8.
2. Surviving Sepsis Campaign. Surviving Sepsis Campaign [Internet]. Available from: http://www.survivingsepsis.org/ (accessed November 2016).
3. Singer M, Deutschman C, Seymour C, et al. The third international consensus definitions for sepsis and septic shock (sepsis-3). *JAMA.* 2016;23:801–10.
4. Churpek M, Snyder A, Han X, et al. qSOFA, SIRS, and early warning scores for detecting clinical deterioration in infected patients outside the ICU. *Am J Respir Crit Care Med.* 2016;195:906–11.
5. National Institute for Health and Care Excellence (NICE). *Sepsis: Recognition, Diagnosis and Early Management.* NICE Guideline [NG51]. London: NICE; 2016. Available from: https://www.nice.org.uk/guidance/ng51.
6. Nutbeam T, Daniels R, Keep J. The UK Sepsis Trust. ED/AMU Sepsis Screening & Action Tool [Internet]. sepsistrust.org. Available from: http://sepsistrust.org/ (accessed November 2016).
7. Mikkelsen M, Miltiades A, Gaieski D, et al. Serum lactate is associated with mortality in severe sepsis independent of organ failure and shock. *Crit Care Med.* 2009;37:1670–7.
8. Levy M, Dellinger R, Townsend S, et al. The Surviving Sepsis Campaign: results of an international guideline-based performance improvement program targeting severe sepsis. *Intensive Care Med.* 2010;36:222–31.
9. Kumar A, Roberts D, Wood K, et al. Duration of hypotension before initiation of effective antimicrobial therapy is the critical determinant of survival in human septic shock. *Crit Care Med.* 2006;34:1589–96.
10. Daniels R, Nutbeam T, McNamara G, et al. The sepsis six and the severe sepsis resuscitation bundle: a prospective observational cohort study. *Emerg Med.* 2011;28:507–12.
11. Daniels R, Nutbeam T, Laver K. *Survive Sepsis Manual,* 1st edn. The official training programme of the Surviving Sepsis Campaign. Birmingham: Good Hope Hospital, Heart of England Foundation Trust; 2007.
12. Robson WP, Daniels R. The Sepsis Six: helping patients to survive sepsis. *Br J Nurs.* 2008;17:16–21.
13. Martin DS, Grocott MP. Oxygen therapy in critical illness: precise control of arterial oxygenation and permissive hypoxemia. *Crit Care Med.* 2013;41:423–32.
14. Asfar P, Schortgen F, Boisrame-Helms J, et al. Hyperoxia and hypertonic saline in patients with septic shock (HYPERS2S): a two-by-two factorial, multicentre, randomised, clinical trial. *Lancet.* 2017;5:180–90.
15. Marik PE. Fluid responsiveness and the six guiding principles of fluid resuscitation. *Crit Care Med.* 2016;44:1920–2.

16. Shaw AD, Bagshaw SM, Goldstein SL, et al. Major complications, mortality, and resource utilization after open abdominal surgery: 0.9% saline compared to Plasma-Lyte. *Ann Surg.* 2012;255:821–9.

17. Bellomo R, Hegarty C, Story D, et al. Association between a chloride-liberal vs chloride-restrictive intravenous fluid administration strategy and kidney injury in critically ill adults. *JAMA.* 2012;308:1566–72.

18. Young P, Bailey M, Beasley R, et al. Effect of a buffered crystalloid solution vs saline on acute kidney injury among patients in the intensive care unit: the SPLIT randomized clinical trial. *JAMA.* 2015;314:1701–10.

19. Myburgh JA, Finfer S, Bellomo R, et al. Hydroxyethyl starch or saline for fluid resuscitation in intensive care. *N Engl J Med.* 2012;367:1901–11.

20. Delaney AP, Dan A, McCaffrey J, et al. The role of albumin as a resuscitation fluid for patients with sepsis: a systematic review and meta-analysis. *Crit Care Med.* 2011;39:386–91.

21. Patel A, Laffan MA, Waheed U, et al. Randomised trials of human albumin for adults with sepsis: systematic review and meta-analysis with trial sequential analysis of all-cause mortality. *BMJ.* 2014;349:4561.

22. Murphy CV, Schramm GE, Doherty JA, et al. The importance of fluid management in acute lung injury secondary to septic shock. *Chest.* 2009;136:102–9.

23. Payen D, de Pont AC, Sakr Y, et al. A positive fluid balance is associated with a worse outcome in patients with acute renal failure. *Crit Care.* 2008;12:R74.

24. Boyd JH, Forbes J, Nakada TA, et al. Fluid resuscitation in septic shock: a positive fluid balance and elevated central venous pressure are associated with increased mortality. *Crit Care Med.* 2011;39:259–65.

25. Silva JM, de Oliveira AM, Nogueira FA, et al. The effect of excess fluid balance on the mortality rate of surgical patients: a multicenter prospective study. *Crit. Care.* 2013;17:R288.

26. Chung FT, Lin SM, Lin SY, et al. Impact of extravascular lung water index on outcomes of severe sepsis patients in a medical intensive care unit. *Respir Med.* 2008;102:956–61.

27. Marik PE, Cavallazzi R. Does the central venous pressure predict fluid responsiveness? An updated meta-analysis and a plea for some common sense. *Crit Care Med.* 2013;41:1774–81.

28. Monnet X, Marik P, Teboul JL. Passive leg raising for predicting fluid responsiveness: a systematic review and meta-analysis. *Intensive Care Med.* 2016;42:1935–47.

29. Lee JH, Kim JT, Yoon SZ, et al. Evaluation of corrected flow time in oesophageal Doppler as a predictor of fluid responsiveness. *Br J Anaesth.* 2007;99:343–8.

30. Hett DA, Jonas MM. Non-invasive cardiac output monitoring. *Intensive Crit Care Nurs.* 2004;20:103–8.

31. Charron C, Caille V, Jardin F, et al. Echocardiographic measurement of fluid responsiveness. *Curr Opin Critical Care.* 2006;12:249–54.

32. Marik PE. Surviving sepsis: going beyond the guidelines. *Ann Intensive Care.* 2011;1:17.

33. Marik PE. Hemodynamic parameters to guide fluid therapy. *Transfus Altern Transfus Med.* 2010;11:102–12.

34. Rivers E, Nguyen B, Havstad S, et al. Early goal-directed therapy in the treatment of severe sepsis and septic shock. *N Engl J Med.* 2001;345:1368–77.

35. ProCESS Investigators. A randomized trial of protocol-based care for early septic shock. *N Engl J Med.* 2014;2014:1683–93.

36. Arise Investigators, ANZICS Clinical Trials Group. Goal-directed resuscitation for patients with early septic shock. *N Engl J Med.* 2014;2014:1496–506.

37. Mouncey PR, Osborn TM, Power GS, et al. Trial of early, goal-directed resuscitation for septic shock. *N Engl J Med.* 2015;372:1301–11.

38. Surviving Sepsis Campaign. Updated Bundles in Response to New Evidence [Internet]. Available from: http://www.survivingsepsis.org/SiteCollectionDocuments/SSC_Bundle.pdf (accessed 24 April 2015).

39. Miller III RR, Dong L, Nelson NC, et al. Multicentre implementation of a severe sepsis and septic shock treatment bundle. *Am J Respir Crit Care Med.* 2013;188:77–82.

40. Russell JA, Walley KR, Singer J, et al. Vasopressin versus norepinephrine infusion in patients with septic shock. *N Engl J Med.* 2008;358:877–87.

41. Gordon AC, Mason AJ, Thirunavukkarasu N, et al. Effect of early vasopressin vs norepinephrine on kidney failure in patients with septic shock: the VANISH randomized clinical trial. *JAMA.* 2016;316:509–18.

42. Sprung CL, Annane D, Keh D, et al. Hydrocortisone therapy for patients with septic shock. *N Engl J Med.* 2008;358:111–24.

43. Gattinoni L, Vasques F, Camporota L, et al. Understanding Lactatemia in Human Sepsis. Potential Impact for Early Management. *Am J Respir Crit Care Med.* 2019;200:582–9.

44. Bakker J, Nijsten MW, Jansen TC. Clinical use of lactate monitoring in critically ill patients. *Ann Intensive Care.* 2013;3:12.

45. Vary TC. Sepsis-induced alterations in pyruvate dehydrogenase complex activity in rat skeletal muscle: effects on plasma lactate. *Shock.* 1996;6:89–94.

46. Trzeciak S, Dellinger RP, Chansky ME, et al. Serum lactate as a predictor of mortality in patients with infection. *Intensive Care Med.* 2007;33:970–7.

47. Casserly B, Phillips GS, Schorr C, et al. Lactate measurements in sepsis-induced tissue hypoperfusion: results from the Surviving Sepsis Campaign database. *Crit Care Med.* 2015;43:567–73.

48. Nguyen HB, Rivers EP, Knoblich BP, et al. Early lactate clearance is associated with improved outcome in severe sepsis and septic shock. *Crit Care Med.* 2004;32:1637–42.

49. Marik PE, Bellomo R. Lactate clearance as a target of therapy in sepsis: a flawed paradigm. *OA Crit Care.* 2013;1:3.

50. Castellanos-Ortega Á, Suberviola B, García-Astudillo LA, et al. Impact of the Surviving Sepsis Campaign protocols on hospital length of stay and mortality in septic shock patients: results of a three-year follow-up quasi-experimental study. *Crit Care Med.* 2010;38:1036–43.

51. Gao F, Melody T, Daniels DF, et al. The impact of compliance with 6-hour and 24-hour sepsis bundles on hospital mortality in patients with severe sepsis: a prospective observational study. *Crit Care.* 2005;9:R764.

52. Sebat F, Johnson D, Musthafa AA, et al. A multidisciplinary community hospital program for early and rapid resuscitation of shock in nontrauma patients. *Chest* 2005;127:1729–43.

53. Lin SM, Huang CD, Lin HC, et al. A modified goal-directed protocol improves clinical outcomes in intensive care unit patients with septic shock: a randomized controlled trial. *Shock.* 2006;26:551–7.

54. Ince C, Sinaasappel M. Microcirculatory oxygenation and shunting in sepsis and shock. *Crit Care Med.* 1999;27:1369–77.

55. Pope JV, Jones AE, Gaieski DF, et al. Multicenter study of central venous oxygen saturation (ScvO2) as a predictor of mortality in patients with sepsis. *Ann Emerg Med.* 2010;55:40–6.

56. Ince C. The microcirculation is the motor of sepsis. *Crit Care.* 2005;9:S13.

57. De Backer D, Hollenberg S, Boerma C, et al. How to evaluate the microcirculation: report of a round table conference. *Crit Care.* 2007;11:R101.

58. Romagnoli S, Tujjar O, De Gaudio AR. Microcirculation in clinical practice. *OA Anaesthetics.* 2013;1:16.

59. Bersten AD, Holt AW. Vasoactive drugs and the importance of renal perfusion pressure. *New Horiz.* 1995;3:650–61.

60. Sharma VK, Dellinger R. The International Sepsis Forum's frontiers in sepsis: high cardiac output should not be maintained in severe sepsis. *Crit Care.* 2003;7:272–5.

61. Russell JA, Cooper DJ, Walley KR, et al. Vasopressin and septic shock trial (VASST): baseline characteristics and organ dysfunction in vasopressor dependent patients with septic shock. *Am J Respir Crit Care Med.* 2003;167:A548.

62. Vail E, Gershengorn HB, Hua M, et al. Association between US norepinephrine shortage and mortality among patients with septic shock. *JAMA*. 2017;317:1433–42.
63. Fernandes Jr CJ, Akamine N, Knobel E. Myocardial depression in sepsis. *Shock*. 2008;30:14–17.
64. Finfer S, Chittock DR, Su SY, et al. Intensive versus conventional glucose control in critically ill patients. *N Engl J Med*. 2009;360:1283–97.
65. Griesdale DE, de Souza RJ, van Dam, et al. Intensive insulin therapy and mortality among critically ill patients: a meta-analysis including NICE-SUGAR study data. *CMAJ*. 2009;180:821–7.
66. Schroeder S, Wichers M, Lehmann LE, et al. The hypothalamic-pituitary-adrenal (HPA) axis of patients with severe sepsis: altered response to corticotropin-releasing hormone. *Crit Care Med*. 2001;29:310–16.
67. Annane D, Sébille V, Charpentier C, et al. Effect of treatment with low doses of hydrocortisone and fludrocortisone on mortality in patients with septic shock. *JAMA*. 2002;288:862–71.
68. Hébert PC, Wells G, Blajchman MA, et al. A multicenter, randomized, controlled clinical trial of transfusion requirements in critical care. *N Engl J Med*. 1999;340:409–17.
69. Holst LB, Haase N, Wetterslev J, et al. Lower versus higher hemoglobin threshold for transfusion in septic shock. *N Engl J Med*. 2014;371:1381–91.
70. Intensive Care National Audit & Research Centre. Sepsis [Internet]. Icnarc.org. Available from: https://www.icnarc.org/Our-Audit/Audits/Cmp/Our-National-Analyses/Sepsis (accessed 24 January 2015).
71. Vincent JL, Sakr Y, Sprung CL, et al. Sepsis in European intensive care units: results of the SOAP study. *Crit Care Med*. 2006;342:344–53.

2 Acute heart failure

Amy Krepska

Expert Commentary Deirdre Murphy

Case history

A 38-year-old female, who was previously fully active with no significant past medical history, presented with a 4-week history of a viral prodromal illness including fevers and chills. In the last 2 weeks, she had developed orthopnoea, shortness of breath on minimal exertion, lethargy, and abdominal discomfort.

On examination, she was warm and well perfused, with a heart rate of 170 beats per minute (bpm), blood pressure of 90/50 mmHg, and a raised jugular venous pressure. She had normal heart sounds with no murmurs. She had a tachypnoea of 28 breaths/min and on examination of her chest had crackles up to the mid zones. Oxygen saturation by pulse oximetry (SpO_2) was 94% breathing 6 L/min via a Hudson mask.

Her electrocardiogram (ECG) showed a narrow complex supraventricular tachycardia with widespread T-wave inversion. Initial blood tests are shown in Table 2.1.

Table 2.1 Initial blood tests (normal range in brackets)

Hb (g/L)	135 (130–165)
MCV (fL)	92 (77–95)
Plt (×10⁹/L)	345 (150–450)
WCC (×10⁹/L)	12.2 (4.0–11.0)
Na (mmol/L)	135 (135–145)
K (mmol/L)	3.6 (3.5–5.0)
Urea (mmol/L)	7.2 (3.3–6.7)
Cr (μmol/L)	105 (45–120)
Glucose (mmol/L)	6.3 (3.5–8.5)
Bili (μmol/L)	12 (3–20)
ALT (IU/L)	135 (10–50)
ALP (IU/L)	140 (30–130)
Albumin (g/L)	38 (35–50)
Corrected Ca (mmol/L)	2.1 (2.15–2.6)
Troponin (ng/mL)	0.7 (0–0.4)
INR	1.4 (0.9–1.4)
TSH (mIU/L)	3.8 (0.5–5)
Arterial blood gas	
pH	7.29 (7.35–7.45)
PO_2 (kPa)	7.6 (>10)
PCO_2 (kPa)	3.5 (4.4–6.1)
HCO_3^- (mmol/L)	22.4 (22–26)
BE (mmol/L)	−5.1 (±2)
Lactate (mmol/L)	3.6 (≤2)

ALP, alkaline phosphatase; ALT, alanine aminotransferase; BE, base excess; Bili, bilirubin; Ca, calcium; Cr, creatinine; Hb, haemoglobin; HCO_3^-, bicarbonate; INR, international normalized ratio; K, potassium; MCV, mean cell volume; Na, sodium; PCO_2, partial pressure of carbon dioxide; PO_2, partial pressure of oxygen; Plt, platelets; TSH, thyroid-stimulating hormone; WCC, white cell count.

An urgent chest X-ray showed pulmonary oedema and a large heart and a diagnosis of acute heart failure was made. She was treated with diuretics (furosemide 80 mg) and opiates (diamorphine 5 mg). However, despite this therapy, she continued to be hypoxaemic with a SpO$_2$ of 87% breathing 15 L/min supplementary oxygen via a non-rebreather mask. She was therefore admitted to the intensive care unit (ICU) for non-invasive ventilation (NIV).

✪ Learning point Acute heart failure pathophysiology

The European Society of Cardiology defines acute heart failure as the rapid onset of symptoms and signs secondary to abnormal cardiac function [1]. Although the most common presentation of acute heart failure seen in the ICU is a patient with decompensated chronic heart failure with underlying coronary artery disease, acute heart failure is a very heterogeneous condition with a constellation of signs and symptoms [2–4]. These have been classified by the European Society of Cardiology (Table 2.2) and impact prognosis and management.

Pulmonary oedema and congestive heart failure are the most common presentations [5]. Only a minority of patients present with cardiogenic shock, with *de novo* presentations of acute heart failure being particularly prevalent in this group. Some patients have reversible causes for their heart failure and it is especially important to identify these rarer aetiologies. It is also important to differentiate the presentation—that is, whether there is predominantly forward failure (low output and cardiogenic shock) or pulmonary congestion and/or right heart failure, as the treatment for these conditions will be significantly different.

Table 2.2 Classification of different types of acute heart failure by the European Society of Cardiology

Type of heart failure	Criterion 1	Criterion 2	Criterion 3
Heart failure with reduced ejection fraction (HFrEF)	Symptoms and signs	LVEF <40%	
Heart failure with mid-range ejection fraction (HFmrEF)	Symptoms and signs	LVEF 40–49%	Elevated natriuretic peptide At least one additional criterion: relevant structural heart disease, e.g. LVH ± left atrial enlargement. Diastolic enlargement
Heart failure with preserved ejection fraction (HFpEF)	Symptoms and signs	LVEF ≥50%	Elevated natriuretic peptide At least one additional criterion: relevant structural heart disease, e.g. LVH ± left atrial enlargement. Diastolic enlargement

LVEF, left ventricular ejection fraction; LVH, left ventricular hypertrophy.
Source: data from 2016 ESC Guidelines for the diagnosis and treatment of acute and chronic heart failure. The Task Force for the diagnosis and treatment of acute and chronic heart failure of the European Society of Cardiology (ESC). *European Heart Journal*, 37(27), 2129–2200. Copyright © 2016 ESC and Oxford University Press.

> **① Expert comment**
>
> The seemingly normal systolic function on echocardiography can be misleading as there tends to be non-uniform systolic contraction, longitudinal contraction being compensated for by radial contraction [6]. Furthermore, diastolic dysfunction is significant with abnormal ventricular compliance and impaired relaxation so that high filling pressures are necessary to maintain stroke volume. The TOPCAT trial showed some benefit in giving spironolactone [7]. However, the use of beta blockade is controversial [8]. As renal dysfunction often accompanies heart failure with reduced (HFrEF) or preserved ejection fraction (HFpEF), it is a significant health problem with potentially a poor prognosis [9].

> **✪ Learning point Role of non-invasive ventilation**
>
> There is a consensus to use NIV and, where possible, to avoid intubation and ventilation in the treatment of pulmonary oedema [10, 11]. The National Institute for Health and Care Excellence (NICE) guidelines recommend NIV if there is severe dyspnoea and acidaemia [12]. Continuous positive airway pressure (CPAP) can be used alone or with inspiratory support but the latter is not proven to be superior to CPAP alone [13]. CPAP reduces both preload and left ventricular afterload and therefore reduces myocardial oxygen consumption and inhibits sympathetic tone. Increasingly, high-flow nasal oxygen is also used. This provides heated and humidified gas with a higher and more constant oxygen concentration with improved comfort and tolerance, although the evidence for its benefit in this setting is still limited [14, 15].

In the ICU, an urgent transthoracic echocardiograph showed normal left ventricular size but increased left ventricular wall thickness and severe global systolic impairment with an ejection fraction of approximately 10%. The heart valves were normal. Spontaneous echocardiographic contrast was seen within the left ventricular cavity with no definite thrombus. There was normal right ventricular size and wall thickness with severe systolic impairment and very high atrial filling pressures. The features were highly suggestive of myocarditis. The patient was referred for a subendocardial biopsy. Table 2.3 details blood testing in heart failure.

Table 2.3 Description of key laboratory tests in acute heart failure

Test	Key result
Full blood count	Anaemia, raised white cell count, macrocytosis (alcohol, thyroid dysfunction), eosinophilia
Urinary tests	Beta human chorionic gonadotropin Drug screen, e.g. amphetamines, cocaine
Liver function tests	Alcohol toxicity Rapid rise in serum aminotransferases and moderate bilirubin, suggestive of hepatic hepatitis Moderate rise in alkaline phosphatase and raised bilirubin, suggestive of hepatic congestion secondary to right heart failure
Urea and electrolytes	Renal impairment due to poor perfusion
Thyroid function	Hyperthyroidism
Cardiac biomarkers	Beta-type natriuretic peptide (BNP) Troponin

✪ Learning point The role of echocardiography in acute heart failure

Echocardiography is recommended as part of the workup for acute heart failure presentations by all of the major cardiology societies [2, 10, 16]. Echocardiography is used to determine left and right ventricular systolic function for diagnosis of HFrEF or HFpEF. Increasingly, intensivists are becoming skilled in bedside echocardiography and its role is expanding in the ICU so that it is now a quasi-monitor with repeated echocardiography being used to evaluate and guide the response to therapy in critically ill patients.

The following are just some of the features that can be identified with echocardiography and used to assess patients with heart failure:

- Left ventricular function: left ventricular size, evidence of regional wall motion abnormalities, ejection fraction, and features to suggest acute inflammation or chronicity (i.e. thinning of the myocardium and structural heart disease, e.g. hypertrophic cardiomyopathy).
- Right ventricular function: right ventricular ejection fraction and right ventricular size and systolic function; tricuspid annular plane systolic excursion (TAPSE) is a simple and reliable measure of right ventricular function.
- Valvular function: congenital or acquired (degenerative) valvular pathologies and endocarditis.
- Pericardial disease: constrictive or restrictive cardiomyopathies.
- Non-invasive haemodynamics: severity of valvular lesions, cardiac output estimation, non-invasive estimation of pulmonary pressures, left atrial filling pressures, diastolic left and right ventricular function, and shunt fractions.

✪ Learning point History taking

Careful history taking is especially vital in acute decompensated heart failure to try to identify and exclude rare but reversible causes of *de novo* heart failure. In the critical care setting this is often overlooked and a collaborative history from the family can be especially useful. Vital points are length of prodromal illness, comorbidities, especially chronic inflammatory syndromes, family history, medications including chemotherapeutic drugs, alcohol, and illicit drug use, and recent pregnancy, as well as extracardiac symptoms and signs of rare infections such as Lyme and Chagas diseases. Symptoms such as palpitations, chest pain, dyspnoea, and orthopnoea indicate the extent of the failure; abdominal discomfort and nausea may indicate right heart failure.

✚ Clinical tip Dilated cardiomyopathy

With chronic processes, patients have time to adapt to their symptoms. Patients with a new diagnosis of dilated cardiomyopathy commonly give a short symptom history, often citing a viral precipitant. Careful exploration may reveal details they have discounted because of habituation, such as they now need to sleep semi-recumbent and wake up if they have fallen off the pillows or they no longer play sport as they feel tired all the time. One memorable young patient had to pause several times as she walked up the aisle at her own wedding. Her family did not think this unusual. She had thyrotoxicosis-induced heart failure with an ejection fraction at presentation of less than 10%.

✪ Learning point Clinical examination

Essential elements of a clinical examination are to assess for end-organ perfusion (e.g. mentation, peripheral perfusion, and urinary output) and to look for evidence of left, right, or biventricular failure (basal crackles, raised jugular venous pressure, and ankle oedema). Evidence of sepsis, rash, chronic liver disease, and joint involvement should also be sought.

✪ Learning point Investigations to identify aetiology and assess severity

Blood tests including renal function, eosinophil count, inflammatory markers, and liver and thyroid function should be performed. A urinary drug and pregnancy screen could also be included. Serial ECG and echocardiography also form an important part of management.

Beta-type natriuretic peptide (BNP) and troponin biomarkers can also be helpful. BNP can be a useful tool in the diagnosis and risk stratification of patients with heart failure. However, there is considerable controversy about interpretations of values especially in the setting of renal insufficiency and in the perioperative period [6].

⭐ **Learning point Myocarditis**

Myocarditis, although relatively uncommon, is a very important diagnosis to make as it can present with fulminant heart failure in previously healthy young patients. It has a very good prognosis when identified and treated early [6, 17]. It is a heterogeneous disease with a variable presentation, pathophysiology, and prognosis, and no standardized diagnostic criteria. It is caused commonly by a virus including Coxsackie B, cytomegalovirus, echovirus, Epstein–Barr virus, and human immunodeficiency virus infection. Other causes include other infectious agents such as *Mycoplasma* or *Corynebacterium diphtheriae*, autoimmune disease (e.g. systemic lupus erythematosus, giant cell myocarditis), or drugs such as anthracyclines (e.g. doxorubicin, daunorubicin, etc.) [6].

Diagnosis is based on several factors. Clinical presentation with evidence of myocardial dysfunction and laboratory abnormalities, including leucocytosis, eosinophilia, and a high erythrocyte sedimentation rate, is important. Troponin values tend to be elevated, with a reasonable specificity and positive predictive value [6]. The presentation can mimic sepsis and other conditions, so a high degree of clinical suspicion is needed. Investigations such as ECG, echocardiography, endocardial biopsy, and gadolinium-enhanced magnetic resonance imaging (MRI) can be more specific. ECG most commonly shows T-wave inversion and ST-segment depression. A biopsy can be particularly helpful as it can guide treatment, with some subtypes such as giant cell myocarditis being amenable to immunosuppression.

Intensive care patients may be too unstable to undergo an MRI and biopsy results take time to be processed. Therefore echocardiography is increasingly useful to diagnose and quantify the extent of the pathology, assessing for regional or global left ventricular wall motion abnormalities, left ventricular wall thickness, left ventricular and right ventricular size and function, and valvular regurgitation.

Further blood tests were undertaken in the ICU including cardiac biomarkers. She was administered a loading dose of intravenous amiodarone (5 mg/kg over 1 hour) and her heart rate reduced to 96 bpm. A repeat ECG showed sinus tachycardia with widespread ST-segment depression and T-wave inversion. Amiodarone was continued for another 24 hours.

❝ **Expert comment**

Myocarditis is a frequent cause of ventricular and atrial arrhythmias. Inappropriate use of rate control and negative inotropic agents (beta blockers) can precipitate the need for mechanical circulatory support. Fulminant myocarditis such as this patient had (i.e. presentation with acute heart failure and significant haemodynamic compromise) paradoxically can have a more favourable prognosis for full recovery as long as the patient can be supported during the acute phase of the illness. With fulminant myocarditis, the ejection fraction is often severely limited and the heart has not dilated as it is an acute process. The only way in which patients can maintain their cardiac output is by maintaining a rapid heart rate as they cannot increase the stroke volume. By comparison, patients with chronic dilated cardiomyopathies can have a larger stroke volume simply due to the degree of ventricular dilatation as the ventricle dilates over time in response to the heart failure in an effort to preserve stroke volume despite a low ejection fraction.

❝ **Expert comment**

Another important and increasingly recognized condition to consider in young patients presenting with new heart failure, arrhythmia, or out-of-hospital cardiac arrest is arrhythmogenic right ventricular cardiomyopathy. This is a form of cardiomyopathy which is familial in origin in a third of cases and has probably been underreported. It causes fibrofatty replacement of right ventricular tissue with a characteristic appearance of right ventricular impairment on echocardiography and cardiac MRI. It is

---

⭐ **Learning point
Rate control in acute heart failure**

American and European guidelines recommend that beta blockade should only be started at a low dose and in stable patients presenting with acute decompensated heart failure [10, 16]. Be particularly careful when using beta blockers in patients who required inotropes during their hospital course [10, 18]. If possible, avoid acute withdrawal of beta blockade.

present in between 1 in 2000 and 1 in 5000 people [19]. Presentation varies from sudden cardiac death to syncope and arrhythmias. Heart failure presentations typically are with right heart failure but left ventricular involvement is also possible.

Over the next few hours, the patient became more hypotensive (systolic blood pressure of 90–100 mmHg) and developed oliguria. Inotropic support was started with adrenaline at 0.1 mcg/kg/min and milrinone at 15 mcg/min and preparations were made to establish renal replacement therapy.

> **✪ Learning point** Inotropic therapy
>
> The best drug for the treatment of acute decompensated heart failure is unclear. The key issue is to maintain sufficient perfusion pressure and minimize myocardial oxygen demand. The choice of drug is influenced by the systolic blood pressure, the presence of coronary artery disease, and the underlying pathophysiology, such as peripartum cardiomyopathy or post cardiotomy. Large trials that have studied the use of inotropes in acute heart failure, such as OPTIME CHF and SURVIVE [20, 21], focus on exacerbations of chronic heart failure. Even in this group, no definitive benefit has been described with the use of milrinone, levosimendan, and dobutamine. If cardiogenic shock is not resolving, mechanical support should be considered early.

The patient became agitated and her arterial blood gas results showed a pH of 7.15, a $PaCO_2$ of 15 kPa, and a lactate concentration of 10 mmol/L. An intra-aortic balloon pump (IABP) was considered but it was decided that more support was needed and emergency percutaneous venoarterial extracorporeal membrane oxygenation (VA ECMO) support via the common femoral vein and artery was chosen. Minimal sedation was provided during the procedure and particular care was taken with placement of the venous wire to avoid provoking arrhythmia. VA ECMO flow was established at 3.6 L/min. A back-perfusion cannula was also inserted into the superficial femoral artery to provide adequate perfusion of the limb (Figure 2.1). Subsequently she was intubated and her lungs ventilated.

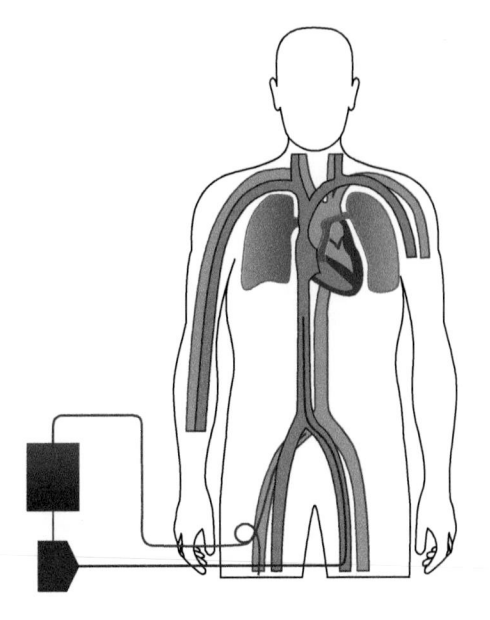

Figure 2.1 An example of a peripheral VA ECMO circuit.
Courtesy of Vin Pellegrino, The Alfred Hospital, Melbourne.

After starting VA ECMO, urine output, peripheral circulation, and mentation improved. Inotropes were provided to maintain pulsatility of her native circulation and avoid complications such as intracardiac clot.

> ⭐ **Learning point** The role of an intra-aortic balloon pump
>
> An IABP is placed in the thoracic aorta via the femoral artery, with balloon inflation in diastole and deflation in early systole. The diastolic inflation improves coronary blood flow proximally and improves systemic perfusion distally. The systolic deflation decreases afterload thus unloading the left ventricle. It can be used in many settings including cardiogenic shock not responding to fluids and inotropic support, or for haemodynamic support while awaiting myocardial recovery after intervention. Absolute contraindications include aortic regurgitation and aortic dissection; relative contraindications include severe peripheral vascular disease and an abdominal aortic aneurysm [22].
>
> There has been debate about its use in patients awaiting revascularization because the Intraaortic Balloon Pump in Cardiogenic Shock II (IABP-SHOCK II) trial showed no significant improvement in mortality with its use in this setting [23].

> ✅ **Evidence base** The IABP-SHOCK II trial
>
> In the IABP-SHOCK II trial, 600 patients with acute myocardial infarction complicated by cardiogenic shock were assigned randomly to IABP support or no IABP support. All these patients were expected to have early revascularization, either percutaneous coronary intervention or coronary artery bypass surgery. The primary end point was 30-day all-cause mortality with secondary outcomes including time to haemodynamic stabilization, ICU length of stay, and serum lactate level. There was no significant difference in any of these primary or secondary outcomes. Another important finding was that there were no significant differences in complication rates between the groups. The key conclusion was that the use of IABP did not benefit mortality or other secondary outcomes in patients who are intended for revascularization. Notably, it has been argued that this trial may have been underpowered because the expected mortality rate in both groups was lower than expected [24].

> 🔖 **Expert comment**
>
> Since the IABP-SHOCK II trial results, the use of IABP for acute heart failure seems to have decreased. One of the main limitations of IABP support in cardiogenic shock is the relatively small amount of circulatory support that it can provide, equivalent to an increase in cardiac output of approximately 0.3–0.5 L/min (i.e. 6–10% of normal resting cardiac output). The use of IABP support prophylactically in high-risk percutaneous procedures is now being superseded by VA ECMO and other forms of mechanical circulatory support (e.g. Impella, TandemHeart).

> ⭐ **Learning point** Early referral to an ECMO or ventricular assist device centre
>
> VA ECMO is indicated for cardiac failure that is potentially reversible but is unresponsive to conventional therapy. Myocarditis is an excellent example of this: patients tend to respond well in the limited time frame that VA ECMO can offer support. VA ECMO can therefore be used either as a bridge to recovery or to transplant. It is therefore vital that any such patients are referred early. Patients with myocarditis can have a very good prognosis and hence it is important to have an aggressive therapeutic approach, including using mechanical devices when appropriate [27]. Any patient with suspected myocarditis should be referred urgently to a transplant/ventricular assist device centre.
>
> *(continued)*

> ⭐ **Learning point**
> **Ultrafiltration in acute heart failure**
>
> Volume overload is a significant problem in acute heart failure. Diuretic resistance is common, possibly as a result of upregulation of neuroendocrine pathways combined with decreased renal function. Patients with chronic heart failure may be considered for ultrafiltration to remove fluid and correct hyponatraemia [25]. Removal of fluid may improve the patient's haemodynamic state by shifting them to a more favourable part of their Starling curve. In contrast to high-dose diuretic therapy, ultrafiltration may induce less neurohormonal activation and vasoconstriction [26].

Patients are unlikely to be suitable if they are over 65 years of age or have malignancy or other severe organ failure. Figure 2.2 shows the inclusion and exclusion criteria used by The Alfred Hospital, Melbourne, Australia.

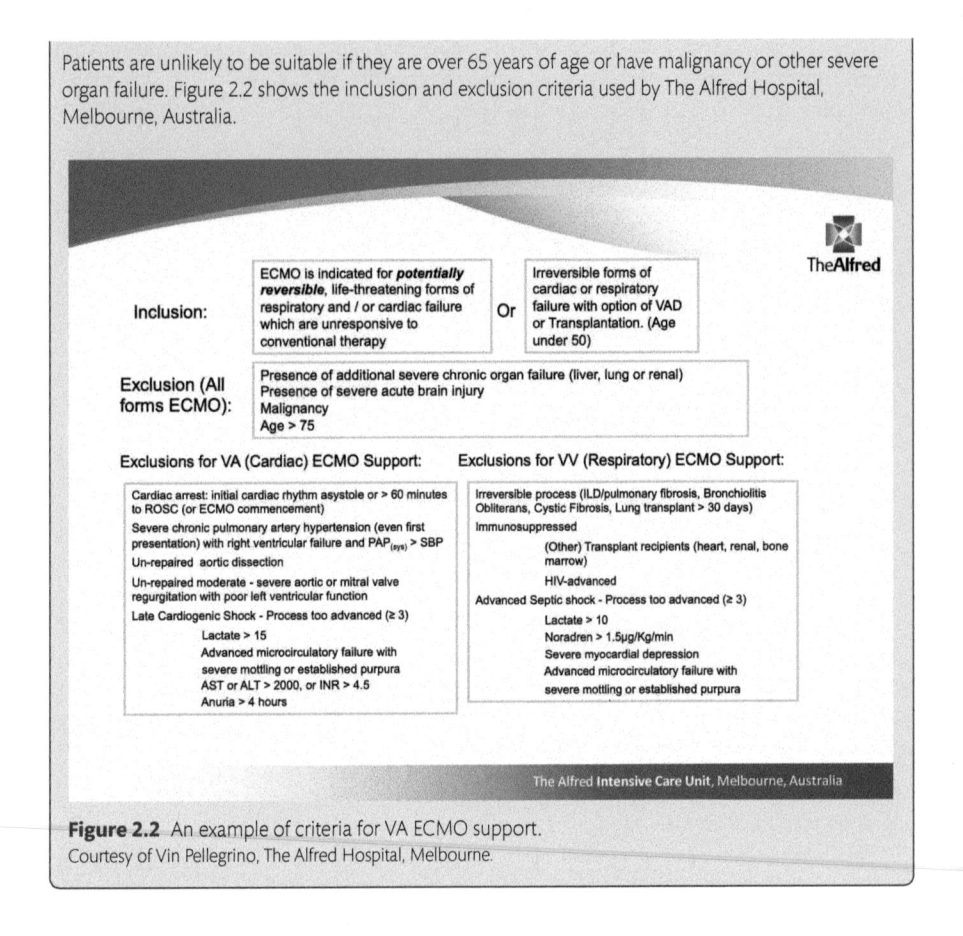

Figure 2.2 An example of criteria for VA ECMO support.
Courtesy of Vin Pellegrino, The Alfred Hospital, Melbourne.

Over the next week, repeat echocardiograms showed persistently poor function and the patient was discussed at a multidisciplinary meeting for consideration for a ventricular assist device as a bridge to transplantation. The endocardial biopsy was consistent with giant cell myocarditis. The patient was started on a combination of immunosuppression including prednisolone.

✪ Learning point Role of other mechanical devices and transplantation

ECMO support is a time-limited therapy so all patients on ECMO support should have multidisciplinary input early to enable bridges to other therapies to be considered. Both European and NICE guidelines [1, 28] recommend that mechanical assist devices be used only as a bridge to transplantation or recovery. Workup for mechanical devices and transplantation is complex. In addition to the patient's comorbidities, organ functions, and the pathophysiology of their heart failure, psychosocial factors are also fundamental.

NICE recommends that there should be a discussion with a centre that provides mechanical circulatory support for all patients with potentially reversible, severe acute heart failure and those who are potential candidates for transplantation [12].

Over the subsequent week, there was gradual normalization of left ventricular function on echocardiography with her ejection fraction improving. She continued to have arrhythmias and an automated implantable cardioverter defibrillator was inserted. An ECMO weaning study was undertaken, whereby ECMO flows are reduced electively, and haemodynamic and echocardiography variables were assessed to determine if support could be withdrawn. As there was sufficient myocardial recovery to successfully separate from ECMO, it was agreed that a left ventricular assist device and transplantation were not required. Her left ventricular function continued to improve and she was weaned from ECMO, ventilation, renal replacement therapy, and inotropic support. Once extubated and stable she was transferred from the ICU to the coronary care unit.

In the subsequent week, a cardiac MRI showed an increased early relative enhancement and delayed enhancement pattern typical of recent myocarditis. She tolerated the introduction of beta blockade and angiotensin-converting enzyme inhibitor. At outpatient follow-up, 8 weeks after presentation, she was symptomatically almost back to her pre-illness state and her left ventricular ejection fraction had improved to 40%.

Discussion

Heart failure represents a considerable economic and social burden and affects up to 2% of the adult population in developed countries [1]. It leads to more than 67,000 hospital admissions each year in England and Wales, with 50% being readmitted within 12 months. There is a wide variation in management with one-third of patients dying within a year of their first hospital admission. There is therefore a need for ongoing review of practice [2].

It is critical that efforts are made early in the patient's admission to define the type of cardiac failure and also to seek out and treat any treatable causes. This requires a logical and structured approach. This is likely to require collaboration between ICU, cardiology, radiology, and possibly other medical teams. As end-organ failure may be a contraindication to specialist support and advanced treatments, all efforts should be made to preserve organ function and an early assessment should be made as to whether the patient can be best treated in the hospital they presented to or whether referral to a specialist centre is required.

A final word from the expert

Many district general hospitals will not have the resources described in this chapter (endocardial biopsy, IABP, rapid access to cardiac MRI) and only in specialist centres will ECMO, ventricular assist devices, and access to transplantation be available. Early discussion with a specialist centre is likely to be of benefit for the majority of patients presenting with acute heart failure and will enable the specialist centre, where necessary, to advise the clinicians in the district general hospital and facilitate timely transfer for specialist services if this becomes necessary.

References

1. Ponikowski P, Voors AA, Anker SD, et al. 2016 ESC Guidelines for the diagnosis and treatment of acute and chronic heart failure: the Task Force for the diagnosis and treatment of acute and chronic heart failure of the European Society of Cardiology (ESC). *Eur Heart J.* 2016;37:2129–200.

2. Dworzynski K, Roberts E, Ludman A, et al. Diagnosing and managing acute heart failure in adults: summary of NICE guidance. *Br Med J.* 2014;5695:g5695.

3. Mosterd A, Hoes A. Clinical epidemiology of heart failure. *Heart.* 2007;93:1137–46.

4. Nieminen M, Bohm M, Cowie M, et al. Guidelines on the diagnosis and treatment of acute heart failure. Endorsed by the European Society of Intensive Care Medicine (ESICM). *Eur Heart J.* 2005;26:384–416.

5. Rudiger A, Streit M, Businger F, Schmid E, Follath F, Maggiorini M. Presentation and outcome of critically ill medical and cardiac-surgery patients with acute heart failure. *Swiss Med Wkly.* 2009;139:110–16.

6. Mebazaa A, Gheorghiade M, Zannad F, Parrillo J (eds). *Acute Heart Failure.* London: Springer; 2008.

7. Pitt B, Pfeffer M, Assmann S, et al. Spironolactone for heart failure with preserved ejection fraction. *N Engl J Med.* 2014;370:1383–92.

8. Bergstrom A, Andersson B, Edner M, et al. Effect of carvedilol on diastolic function in patients with diastolic heart failure and preserved systolic function. Results of the Swedish Doppler-echocardiographic study (SWEDIC). *Eur J Heart Fail.* 2004;6:453–61.

9. Bhatia R, Tu J, Lee D, et al. Outcome of heart failure with preserved ejection fraction in a population-based study. *N Engl J Med.* 2006;355:260–9.

10. The Task Force for the Diagnosis and Treatment of Acute and Chronic Heart Failure 2012 of the European Society of Cardiology. ESC Guidelines for the diagnosis and treatment of acute and chronic heart failure 2012. *Eur Heart J.* 2012;33:1787–847.

11. Gray A, Goodacre S, Newby D, et al. Noninvasive ventilation in acute cardiogenic pulmonary edema. *N Engl J Med.* 2008;359:142–51.

12. National Institute for Health and Care Excellence. *Acute Heart Failure: Diagnosing and Managing Acute Heart Failure in Adults.* London: National Institute for Health and Care Excellence; 2014.

13. Weng CL, Zhao YT, Liu QH, et al. Noninvasive ventilation in acute cardiogenic pulmonary edema. *Ann Intern Med.* 2010;152:590–600.

14. Papazian L, Corley A, Hess D, et al. Use of high-flow nasal cannula oxygenation in ICU adults: a narrative review. *Intensive Care Med.* 2016;42:1336–49.

15. Nishimura M. High-flow nasal cannula oxygen therapy in adults. *J Intensive Care.* 2015;3:15.

16. Yancy C, Jessop M, Bozkurt B, et al. 2013 ACCF/AHA guideline for the management of heart failure: a report of the American College of Cardiology Foundation/American Heart Association Task Force on Practice Guidelines. *Circulation.* 2013;128:e240–32.

17. Schultz JC, Hillard A, Cooper L, et al. Diagnosis and treatment of viral myocarditis. *Mayo Clin Proc.* 2009;84:1001–9.

18. Jessup M, Abraham W, Casey D, et al. 2009 focused update: ACCF/AHA Guidelines for the Diagnosis and Management of Heart Failure in Adults: a report of the American College of Cardiology Foundation/American Heart Association Task Force on Practice Guidelines. *Circulation.* 2009;119:1977–2016.

19. Marcus F, McKenna W, Sherrill D, et al. Diagnosis of arrhythmogenic right ventricular cardiomyopathy/dysplasia. *Circulation* 2010;121:1533–41.

20. Felker GM, Benza R, Chandler A, et al. Heart failure etiology and response to milrinone in decompensated heart failure: results from the OPTIME-CHF study. *J Am Coll Cardiol.* 2003;41:997–1003.

21. Mebazaa A, Nieminen M, Packer M, et al. Levosimendan vs dobutamine for patients with acute decompensated heart failure: the SURVIVE randomized trial. *JAMA.* 2007;297:1883–91.

22. Krishna M, Zacharowski K. Principles of intra-aortic balloon pump counterpulsation. *Contin Educ Anaesthesia Crit Care Pain.* 2008;9:24–8.

23. Thiele H, Zeymer U, Neumann FJ, et al. Intraaortic balloon support for myocardial infarction with cardiogenic shock. *N Engl J Med.* 2012;367:1287–96.

24. Perera D, Lumley M, Pijis N, et al. Intra-aortic balloon pump trials: questions, answers, and unresolved issues. *Circ Cardiovasc Interv.* 2013;6:317–21.

25. National Institute for Health and Care Excellence. *Acute Heart Failure: Diagnosing and Managing Acute Heart Failure in Adults, Draft Guidelines.* London: National Institute for Health and Care Excellence; 2014.

26. Valchanov K, Parameshwar J. Inpatient management of advanced heart failure. *Contin Educ Anaesthesia Crit Care Pain.* 2008;8:167–71.

27. Senderek T, Malecka B, Zabek A, et al. Fulminant heart failure due to giant cell myocarditis affecting the left ventricle. *Adv Interv Cardiol.* 2015;11:351–3.

28. National Institute for Health and Care Excellence. *Extracorporeal Membrane Oxygenation (ECMO) for Acute Heart Failure in Adults.* London: National Institute for Health and Care Excellence; 2014.

3 Acute respiratory failure

Catherine Bryant

⊕ Expert Commentary Sanjoy Shah

Case history

A 32-year-old woman presented to the emergency department with a 3-day history of a cough productive of yellow sputum, fever, and worsening shortness of breath. She had a past medical history of asthma, depression, and alcohol dependence and was previously an intravenous (IV) drug user.

Her observations and examination were as follows:

A. Oxygen saturation by pulse oximetry (SpO_2) 90% on 15 L/min via a non-rebreathe face mask.
B. Respiratory rate 30 breaths/min. She was using accessory muscles of respiration. Auscultation identified bronchial breathing and coarse crepitations over the right mid zone.
C. Heart rate was 120 beats per minute (bpm) with a thready pulse and cool peripheries. Capillary refill time was 4 seconds. Blood pressure was 90/50 mmHg.
D. Glasgow Coma Scale score 14 (E3, V5, M6).
E. Temperature 38.5°C.

Two 16-gauge peripheral venous cannulae were inserted and venous blood samples sent for full blood count, urea and electrolytes, liver function tests, lactate, C-reactive protein (CRP), clotting, and blood cultures. A fluid challenge was undertaken with 500 mL of a balanced crystalloid solution. A urinary catheter was inserted to monitor urine output and urinalysis performed. The patient was commenced on IV co-amoxiclav 1.2 g three times daily and clarithromycin 500 mg twice daily.

> **✪ Learning point**
> **Definition of pneumonia**
>
> Features of pneumonia include the symptoms of cough, purulent sputum, increasing breathlessness, and haemoptysis, with signs of fever, tachycardia and tachypnoea, increased vocal fremitus, and bronchial breathing. It includes laboratory features of leucocytosis with neutrophilia, raised inflammatory markers (e.g. CRP, procalcitonin), radiology showing air bronchograms or consolidation, and positive microbiology [3, 4].

> **⊕ Expert comment**
>
> The management of patients with sepsis in the emergency department follows the care bundle proposed by the Surviving Sepsis Campaign [1]. The Sepsis Six tool improves implementation of the Surviving Sepsis Campaign care bundle [2]. The Sepsis Six are as follows:
>
> **Take 3**
>
> 1. Take blood cultures.
> 2. Measure serial serum lactates.
> 3. Measure accurate hourly urine output.
>
> **Give 3**
>
> 4. Administer oxygen to maintain saturations at greater than 94% (88–92% in patients with chronic lung disease).
> 5. Give broad-spectrum antibiotics.
> 6. Give IV fluid challenges if the patient is hypotensive or their lactate is elevated.
>
> For more detail, see Case 1.

Her blood results and arterial blood gas values are shown in Table 3.1.

Table 3.1 Blood results and arterial blood gas values

Full blood count		
Hb (g/L)	150	(130–180)
Plat (× 10⁹/L)	300	(150–400)
WCC (× 10⁹/L)	18.5	(4–11)
CRP (mg/L)	258	(<10)
Urea and electrolytes		
Na (mmol/L)	130	(135–145)
K (mmol/L)	4.8	(3.5–5)
Urea (mmol/L)	7.8	(2.5–6.7)
Cr (μmol/L)	90	(60–110)
Arterial blood gas on 15 L/min		
pH	7.24	(7.35–7.45)
$PaCO_2$ (kPa)	7.2	(4.7–6.0)
PaO_2 (kPa)	8.0	(>10)
HCO_3^- (mmol/L)	21.0	(22–28)
Base excess (mmol/L)	−2.3	(± 2)
Lactate (mmol/L)	2.0	(0.5–2.0)

Cr, creatinine; CRP, C-reactive protein; Hb, haemoglobin; K, potassium; Na, sodium; WCC, white cell count.

Her chest X-ray (CXR) (Figure 3.1) showed right upper lobe consolidation.

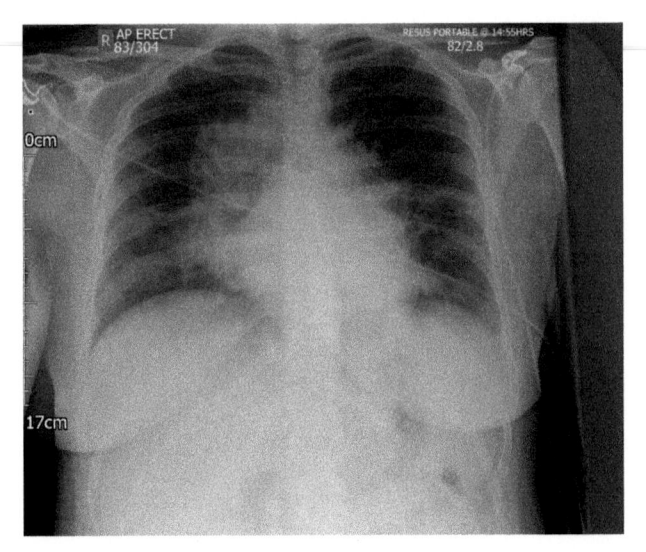

Figure 3.1 Chest X-ray on admission.

> ⭐ **Learning point**
> **Differential diagnosis of consolidation on chest X-ray**
>
> The causes of consolidation can be categorized by the type of matter that is displacing air in the alveoli:
>
> 1. Pus—pneumonia (typical and atypical)
> 2. Fluid—pulmonary oedema (cariogenic and non-cardiogenic)
> 3. Food or gastric contents—aspiration pneumonia/pneumonitis
> 4. Blood—pulmonary haemorrhage
> 5. Specific cell types—bronchogenic carcinoma, eosinophilic pneumonia

The patient was moved into a resuscitation bay for continued management, and an urgent intensive care referral was sought for her acute respiratory failure. Her cardio-vascular status improved following the initial fluid bolus, with heart rate decreasing to 110 bpm and blood pressure improving to 95/55 mmHg, and a second fluid challenge was performed with 500 mL crystalloid which resulted in a further improvement of her cardiovascular parameters.

✪ Learning point Acute respiratory failure

Acute respiratory failure is defined as impaired pulmonary gas exchange leading to hypoxaemia and/or hypercapnia. It comprises two main subtypes:

Type I—hypoxaemic, often parenchymal in origin:

- Alveolar pathology
- Interstitial or diffusion pathology
- Impairment in oxygen-carrying capacity:
  o Impaired circulation:
    ▪ Low cardiac output
    ▪ Low circulation volume
  o Impaired oxygen carriage:
    ▪ Haemoglobinopathy or low haemoglobin concentration or high-affinity haemoglobinopathy

Type II—hypercapnic, often mechanical in origin:

- Reduction in respiratory rate
- Reduction in ventilation

Common causes

Acute respiratory failure has a variety of causes, including primary pulmonary pathology or an extrapulmonary cause, although it is often multifactorial. Causes are categorized as shown in Table 3.2.

Table 3.2 Causes of respiratory failure

Location	Examples
Lung parenchyma[a]	Pneumonia, acute interstitial pneumonitis
Pleural[a]	Pneumothorax, pleural effusion, haemothorax
Pulmonary vascular[a]	Pulmonary embolism, pulmonary haemorrhage
Chest wall[b]	Flail chest
Upper airways	Upper airway obstruction, asthma, anaphylaxis
Cardiovascular[a]	Acute pulmonary oedema associated with acute coronary syndrome, valvular heard disease, myocardial infarction
Central	Cerebrovascular accident, raised intracranial pressure
Brainstem/spinal cord	Infarction, vertebral artery dissection, trauma
Neuromuscular	Myasthenia gravis, Guillain–Barré syndrome, poliomyelitis
Miscellaneous	Poisoning (intentional[b], accidental)

[a] Common cause of type I respiratory failure.
[b] Common cause of mixed type I and II respiratory failure.

✪ Learning point Approach to investigating pneumonia

Appropriate investigations for pneumonia [3, 5, 6] include the following:

Haematology:

- Full blood count
- Coagulation profile

Biochemistry:

- Liver and renal function
- Urine analysis/dipstick
- Acute phase reactants: CRP, procalcitonin
- Cardiac enzymes if associated/underlying cardiac disease

(continued)

Microbiology:

- Blood culture
- Sputum culture
- Nasopharyngeal swabs for virology
- Urinary antigen for *Streptococcus pneumoniae* and *Legionella pneumoniae*
- Atypical serology for *Mycoplasma pneumoniae*

Radiology:

- CXR
- Computed tomography (CT) scan of the chest with consideration for a pulmonary angiogram
- Ultrasonography of chest
- Two-dimensional echocardiography

The patient was reviewed by the intensive care physician in the emergency department. The patient was increasingly agitated and non-compliant with medical intervention, pulling at her face mask. She was transferred to the intensive care unit (ICU) to enable provision of ventilation and multiorgan support. She was preoxygenated using a tight-fitting facemask delivering as close to 100% oxygen as possible, and manually applied positive end-expiratory pressure (PEEP). Nasal high-flow oxygen was applied at 50 L/min of 100% oxygen to provide apnoeic oxygenation during laryngoscopy. Her trachea was intubated with a 7.5 mm tracheal tube following a rapid sequence induction with ketamine 2 mg/kg and rocuronium 1 mg/kg and sedation was maintained with infusions of propofol and alfentanil.

> **ⓕ Expert comment**
>
> Preoxygenation can be difficult to optimize in the critical care setting, especially when the patient is agitated. This, combined with a higher incidence of difficult intubation, makes a profound hypoxaemia more likely after induction of anaesthesia. This risk is reduced by optimal patient positioning and the use of rapid sequence induction checklists. The use of nasal cannulae, or ideally high-flow nasal oxygen, can eliminate or minimize hypoxaemia by providing apnoeic oxygenation during laryngoscopy. Nasal cannulae may need to be removed if intubation fails because they prevent a good seal between the mask and the face.
>
> Ketamine is a first-line induction drug in those with cardiovascular instability. Induction with propofol can cause profound hypotension, particularly if the patient is hypovolaemic, because it reduces systemic vascular resistance.

The patient's lungs were ventilated with a respiratory rate of 26 breaths/min and a tidal volume of 6 mL/kg of ideal body weight and oxygenated with a fraction of inspired oxygen (FiO_2) of 0.6 and PEEP of 12 cmH$_2$O.

Monitoring was instituted with central venous and arterial access with a pulse contour cardiac output (PiCCO) system. A passive leg raise test was performed to access fluid responsiveness (see Case 1) [7, 8]. This confirmed the need for further fluid resuscitation, which was continued with crystalloid boluses. A noradrenaline infusion was commenced targeting a mean arterial pressure of 65 mmHg, urine output of greater than 0.5 mL/kg/min, and haemoglobin value higher than 70 g/L [9–11].

> **ⓕ Expert comment**
>
> In the initial stages of sepsis, it is vital to achieve cardiovascular stability; this is usually achieved with a combination of fluid resuscitation and vasopressor and inotropic support. If substantial quantities
>
> *(continued)*

of crystalloid are required, the Surviving Sepsis Campaign guidelines collaborators suggest also using albumin [1, 12, 13]. Excessive fluid resuscitation may impair respiratory function and gas exchange and once cardiovascular stability has been achieved, close attention is paid to fluid balance. Consider aiming for a negative fluid balance as early as after the first 48 hours and consider the early use of renal replacement therapy to achieve this [14–18]. For more detail, see Case 1.

✪ Learning point Principles of management

The principles of management of acute respiratory failure are those of resuscitation, with diagnosis and treatment of the specific underlying cause, while also providing supportive care to maintain oxygenation and prevent further harm:

1. Resuscitate, diagnose, and treat as clinically relevant:
   a. Resuscitate. Administer oxygen to treat hypoxaemia. Implement sepsis bundle [19].
   b. Diagnosis. Targeted history and examination and specific investigations including arterial blood gas analysis, blood tests, microbiological assessment, and imaging (CXR/CT) to identify the cause.
   c. Treat. Treat the underlying cause where appropriate, for example:
      i. Antibiotics for pneumonia
      ii. Analgesia/fixation of a flail chest
      iii. Intercostal drain insertion for pneumothorax or pleural effusion
2. Good supportive care:
   a. Early nutrition: enteral whenever possible
   b. Attention to fluid and electrolyte balance
   c. Glycaemic control
   d. Minimize use of sedation
   e. Regular assessment and management of pain, agitation, and delirium (PAD guidelines) [20]
   f. Skin and pressure area care
3. Minimize harm:
   a. Lung protective ventilation
   b. Sedation break and spontaneous breathing trial [21, 22]
   c. Early mobilization
   d. Deep vein thrombosis and stress ulcer prophylaxis
   e. Prevent ventilator-associated pneumonia and catheter-related bloodstream infections

⊕ Clinical tip How to establish a patient with acute respiratory failure on a ventilator

Principles include the following [23, 24]:

1. Maintain adequate oxygenation:
   a. Partial pressure of oxygen (PaO_2) = 8–9 kPa or arterial blood oxygen saturation of 88–95%.
   b. Titrate PEEP according to the PEEP and FiO_2 algorithm that was used by the National Institutes of Health Acute Respiratory Distress Syndrome (ARDS) Network tidal volume trial (Table 3.3) [25, 26].

Table 3.3 Lower and higher PEEP/FiO₂ combination tables

Lower PEEP/FiO₂ combination

FiO_2	0.3	0.4	0.4	0.5	0.5	0.6	0.7	0.7	0.7	0.8	0.9	0.9	0.9	1.0
PEEP	5	5	8	8	10	10	10	12	14	14	14	16	18	18–24

Higher PEEP/FiO2 combination

FiO_2	0.3	0.3	0.4	0.4	0.5	0.5	0.5	0.6	0.7	0.8	0.8	0.9	1.0
PEEP	12	14	14	16	16	18	20	20	20	20	22	22	22–24

PEEP, positive end-expiratory pressure in cmH_2O.
Source: data from Sahetya SK., et al. Fifty Years of Research in ARDS. Setting Positive End-Expiratory Pressure in Acute Respiratory Distress Syndrome. *American Journal of Respiratory Critical Care Medicine*. 195:1429–1438. Copyright © 2017 American Thoracic Society.

(continued)

2. Accept permissive hypercapnia but maintain pH at 7.20 or higher (excluding patients with raised intracranial pressure).
3. Avoid ventilator-induced lung injury by adopting lung protective ventilation strategies.

⭐ **Learning point Lung trauma**

In acute respiratory failure, use a lung protective ventilation strategy as demonstrated in the ARDS Network tidal volume trial [27]. This ventilation strategy is based on the principle that traditional mechanical ventilation injures the diseased lung by one or more of five mechanisms [24, 28]:

1. *Volutrauma*—alveolar damage caused by excessive tidal volumes.
2. *Barotrauma*—alveolar damage caused by excessive inflation pressures.
3. *Atelectrauma*—alveolar damage caused by cyclical opening and closing, causing a sheering effect and subsequent damage.
4. *Oxygen toxicity*—damage caused by high FiO_2 concentration and resulting free oxygen radicals.
5. *Biotrauma*—worsening lung injury and distant organ dysfunction caused by inflammatory mediators and the translocation of pathogens from ventilator-induced lung injury.

💬 **Expert comment Determinants of oxygenation**

Oxygenation is a product of the FiO_2 and the functional residual capacity (FRC) of the lung. The FRC is the volume of lung open at the end of expiration; this is determined partly by PEEP and reflected in the mean airway pressure. Mean airway pressure and FiO_2 determine oxygenation and minute ventilation determines carbon dioxide (CO_2) clearance. Use of inverse ratio ventilation will increase mean airway pressure and therefore oxygenation. Volutrauma is minimized by setting a low tidal volume (6 mL/kg predicted body weight) and offsetting it with a relatively high respiratory rate (up to 35 breaths/min) while accepting a high partial pressure of CO_2 and relatively low pH so long as it does not cause cardiovascular instability.

⭐ **Learning point Key studies**

A lung protective ventilation strategy using a low tidal volume (4–8 mL/kg predicted body weight) and plateau airway pressure less than 30 cmH$_2$O is consistent with the clinical practice guidelines of the American Thoracic Society/European Society of Intensive Care Medicine/Society of Critical Care Medicine [23].

Ventilation with lower tidal volumes as compared with traditional tidal volumes for acute lung injury and the acute respiratory distress syndrome (ARDS Network study)

- Multicentre randomized controlled trial (RCT) [27], n = 861.
- Acute lung injury entry criteria.
- Tidal volume of 6 mL/kg (peak inspiratory pressure (PIP) <30 cmH$_2$O) versus 12 mL/kg (PIP <50 cmH$_2$O).
- PEEP algorithm same for both groups (shown in the upper section of Table 3.3).
- The lower tidal volume group had:
  o a lower rate of death before discharge home (31.0% vs 39.8%; P = 0.007)
  o higher rates of breathing without assistance by day 28 (65.7% vs 55.0%; P <0.001)
  o more ventilator-free days (over days 1–28) (12 ± 11 vs 10 ± 11; P = 0.007)
  o more days without failure of non-pulmonary organs or systems (during days 1–28) (15 ± 11 vs 12 ± 11; P = 0.006).
- In patients with acute lung injury and ARDS, mechanical ventilation with lower tidal volumes results in decreased mortality and an increased number of ventilator-free days.

(continued)

Expert comment

There have been many criticisms made of the ARDS Network study, but most importantly that the control arm included a target tidal volume that was higher than the standard of care at the time. Thus, a safe tidal volume (6 mL/kg) was compared with an unsafe tidal volume (10–12mL/kg); instead, the study should have compared tidal volumes of 6 mL/kg with 8 mL/kg.

Nevertheless, the study demonstrated a low mortality rate when patients with ARDS are ventilated with a lower tidal volume and patients ventilated with lower tidal volume had less non-pulmonary organ failure.

Higher versus lower positive end-expiratory pressures in patients with the acute respiratory distress syndrome (ALVEOLI study)

- Multicentre RCT [25], n = 549.
- Acute lung injury and ARDS entry criteria.
- Assigned to receive mechanical ventilation at a tidal volume of 6 mL/kg and PIP less than 30 cmH$_2$O with lower or higher PEEP values, set according to different tables of combinations of PEEP and FiO$_2$.
- PEEP values (days 1–4): 8.3 ± 3.2 cmH$_2$O (lower PEEP) versus 13.2 ± 3.5 cmH$_2$O (higher PEEP) (P <0.001).
- No difference in rate of death before hospital discharge (24.9% (lower PEEP) vs 27.5% (higher PEEP); P = 0.48) or number of days of unassisted breathing (14.5 ± 10.4 days (lower PEEP) vs 13.8 ± 10.6 days (higher PEEP); P = 0.50).
- In this study of patients with acute lung injury and ARDS who received lung protective mechanical ventilation, clinical outcomes are similar whether lower or higher PEEP values were used.

Two other studies, the Lung Open Ventilation (LOV) study and Expiratory Pressure (Express) study, which compared different PEEP strategies also failed to demonstrate any difference in mortality among patients with ARDS [29, 30]. These three studies may have failed to show any difference in mortality because they recruited heterogeneous cohorts with ARDS ranging from mild to severe based on the recent Berlin criteria (see later discussion) [31]. A subsequent individual patient meta-analysis found that higher PEEP values improved survival among those with moderate or severe ARDS (PaO$_2$/FiO$_2$ (P/F) ≤200 mmHg) but might increase mortality among those with mild ARDS [26, 32].

Over the next 12 hours, there was a further deterioration in respiratory function and the FiO$_2$ was increased to 0.8 aiming for arterial blood oxygen saturation of at least 92% (Table 3.4).

Table 3.4 Arterial blood gas results

FiO$_2$	0.8	
pH	7.39	(7.35–7.45)
PaCO$_2$ (kPa)	6.5	(4.7–6)
PaO$_2$ (kPa)	8.0	(>10)
P/F ratio (kPa)	10	(<13.3 is severe ARDS)

In light of the deteriorating gas exchange, a CT chest was undertaken to evaluate the pulmonary infiltrates, and to exclude pleural pathology such as a large effusion, pneumothorax, or pulmonary embolism. The CT scan showed bilateral extensive ground-glass infiltrates with bibasal consolidation and bilateral small pleural effusions (Figure 3.2). There was no evidence of pneumothorax.

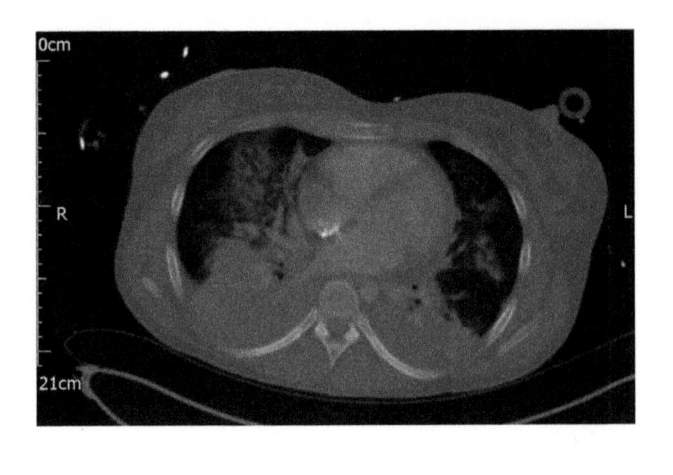

Figure 3.2 CT chest, showing bilateral extensive infiltrates (ground glass) with bibasal consolidation and bilateral small pleural effusions.

The patient was turned prone at this stage, and prone ventilation was continued for 16-hour periods (16:00–08:00) for 5 days.

⭐ Learning point Acute respiratory distress syndrome

ARDS is an acute, diffuse, inflammatory lung condition causing injury to the lung parenchyma, increased pulmonary vascular permeability, and subsequent acute severe hypoxaemia [33]. Despite advances in understanding of the pathophysiology and management of ARDS, there are few specific treatment options and it remains associated with a high mortality rate [33].

Diagnosis

The most recently updated definition of ARDS was generated by a panel of experts in 2011 and is termed the Berlin definition. It describes four key features required to diagnose ARDS [31]:

1. Acute onset, over 1 week or less.
2. Presence of bilateral opacities consistent with pulmonary oedema on CXR or CT.
3. P/F ratio less than 300 mmHg (<40 kPa) with a minimum of 5 cmH$_2$O PEEP.
4. Must not be fully explained by cardiac failure or fluid overload.

A 1994 consensus conference previously defined acute lung injury as a P/F ratio of 26.6–40 kPa, ARDS as a P/F ratio less than 26.6 kPa, and severe ARDS as a P/F ratio less than 13.3 kPa [34]. The Berlin definition replaces these terms with mild, moderate, or severe ARDS (Table 3.5).

Table 3.5 The Berlin definition

	P/F ratio (mmHg) with PEEP ≥ 5 cmH$_2$O	P/F ratio (kPa) with PEEP ≥ 5 cmH$_2$O	Mortality (%)
Mild	200–300	26.6–40	27
Moderate	100–200	13.3–26.6	32
Severe	<100	<13.3	45

P/F, PaO$_2$/FiO$_2$.

Aetiology

The causes of ARDS are considered in two broad categories—direct/pulmonary causes (direct injury to the lung) and indirect/extrapulmonary causes (secondary to systemic injuries). Examples include:

Direct/pulmonary causes	Pneumonia
	Aspiration of gastric contents
	Pulmonary contusion
	Inhalational injury
	Fat embolism

(continued)

Indirect/extrapulmonary causes	Sepsis Severe trauma Acute pancreatitis Burns Acute drug reactions Transfusion reactions/transfusion related acute lung injury (TRALI)

Pathophysiology

Generally, ARDS follows four phases, irrespective of the cause [33]:

1. The *acute* or *exudative* phase—starts early and lasts for up to 7 days. It involves disruption of the alveolar capillary membrane, infiltration by inflammatory cells, haemorrhage, and leakage of protein-rich fluid into the alveoli. This causes hypoxaemia and pulmonary infiltrates on the CXR.
2. The *subacute* or *proliferative* phase—occurring from day 5. Proliferation of inflammatory cells and type 2 alveolar cells leads to interstitial fibrosis, ongoing hypoxaemia, and reduced lung compliance.
3. The *chronic* or *fibrotic* phase—infiltration with fibroblasts and subsequent fibrosis, causes loss of the normal lung structure and worsening lung compliance.
4. The *resolution* phase—may take up to several weeks to start but results in slow repair and restoration of the normal lung architecture.

These pathophysiological changes do not occur homogeneously in the lungs, with different alveoli in different phases of injury at the same time. There may also be inflammation in other areas of the body, causing shock and injury or dysfunction of other organs, resulting in multiorgan failure. Mortality associated with severe ARDS is up to 45% in some studies and is invariably due to multiorgan failure.

The patient continued to receive infusions of propofol and alfentanil and was commenced on an infusion of atracurium (a neuromuscular blocking drug (NMBD)) for the first 48 hours. Once the infusion of atracurium was discontinued, she received a sedation hold in the morning when she was turned supine. Sedation was recommenced to facilitate safe turning from the prone position.

The patient's inflammatory markers (temperature, white blood count, and CRP) increased over the next 3 days. On day 2 of her ICU stay, her urinary antigen was positive for pneumococcal pneumonia. She was maintained on dual antibiotic therapy with IV co-amoxiclav and clarithromycin for the first 72 hours. This spectrum of this therapy was later narrowed to IV benzyl penicillin 2.4 g 6-hourly. She received antibiotics for a total of 7 days.

> ✪ **Learning point** Usual organisms
>
> Common microbiology aetiology of community-acquired pneumonia in the UK [3, 4, 35] includes:
>
> | Bacteria | Viruses |
> |---|---|
> | *Streptococcus pneumoniae* | Influenza viruses |
> | *Haemophilus influenza* | Rhinovirus |
> | *Staphylococcus aureus* | Parainfluenza viruses |
> | *Klebsiella pneumoniae* | Adenovirus |
> | *Pseudomonas aeruginosa* | Human metapneumovirus |
> | *Mycoplasma pneumoniae* | |
> | *Moraxella catarrhalis* | |
> | *Legionella pneumoniae* | |
> | *Gram-negative organisms* | |
> | *Mycobacterial tuberculosis* | |

> ✪ **Learning point** Community-acquired pneumonia: specific pathogens and epidemiological conditions and risk factors
>
> 1. Chronic obstructive pulmonary disease/smoking: *Haemophilus influenza*, *Pseudomonas aeruginosa*, *Streptococcus pneumoniae*, and *Moraxella catarrhalis*.
> 2. Alcoholism: *Streptococcus pneumoniae*, *Klebsiella pneumoniae*, oral anaerobes, and *Mycobacterium tuberculosis*.
> 3. HIV early stages: *Haemophilus influenza*, *Streptococcus pneumoniae*, and *Mycobacterium tuberculosis*.
> 4. HIV late stages: early-stage pathogens plus *Pneumocystis jirovecii* (PCP), *Cryptococcus*, atypical mycobacterial disease, *Haemophilus influenza*, and *Pseudomonas aeruginosa*.
> 5. IV drug abuse: *Staphylococcus aureus*, *Mycobacterium tuberculosis*, and *Streptococcus pneumoniae*.
> 6. Influenza activity in the community: influenza, *Staphylococcus aureus*, *Streptococcus pneumoniae*, and *Haemophilus influenza*.

Her vasopressor requirement peaked at 36 hours after intubation (noradrenaline requirement = 0.4 mcg/kg/min). Her cardiovascular function stabilized over the subsequent 24 hours, enabling weaning of the noradrenaline. By day 4, a daily negative fluid balance of 500–1000 mL could be achieved. Fluid input was minimized by rationalizing drug dilutions and avoiding 'maintenance fluids'. Her PaO_2 improved by day 3 of prone ventilation, with a simultaneous reduction in the FiO_2 to 0.5. The lung protective ventilation strategy was maintained, including prone ventilation for a total of 5 days.

> ✪ **Learning point** Conservative approach to fluid management
>
> IV fluid management in the patient with ARDS can be a significant challenge. While fluid infusion may increase cardiac output and improve end-organ perfusion, it may also worsen pulmonary gas exchange. Patients with ARDS have, by definition, non-cardiogenic pulmonary oedema with an altered capillary permeability. Excessive IV fluid will increase the capillary hydrostatic pressure and decrease the oncotic pressure, thereby worsening lung oedema. The benefit of adopting a conservative approach to fluid therapy was demonstrated by the Fluids and Catheters Treatment Trial (FACTT) [15], which compared a conservative fluid strategy (−136 mL cumulative balance over the first 7 days) with a liberal fluid strategy (+6992 mL cumulative balance over the first 7 days). This was achieved within the conservative group with a combination of avoidance of maintenance fluids and the administration of diuretics. Although there was no significant difference in mortality, patients in the conservative fluid group spent less time on a ventilator and had a shorter ICU stay. This was achieved without an increase in clinically significant adverse events such as non-pulmonary organ failure. It is now accepted that when treating ARDS patients, once the fluid resuscitation phase (rescue and optimization) has been completed, a conservative approach to fluid therapy can be adopted in the stabilization and de-escalation phases [17, 18].

> ✪ **Learning point** Rescue therapies in acute respiratory distress syndrome
>
> **Prone positioning**
>
> Positioning the patient prone improves alveolar ventilation/perfusion (V/Q) matching and therefore oxygenation [36, 37]. In ARDS, there is atelectasis within the posterior and basal (dependent) regions of the lungs, as demonstrated in the patient's CT scan (Figure 3.2). These regions are therefore poorly compliant and difficult to recruit during ventilation in the supine position. Pulmonary blood flow is maximal in these dependent regions. Placing the patient prone improves lung mechanics and oxygenation as well as aiding the clearance of respiratory secretions. Blood flow remains higher in the dorsal region of the lungs and as these regions are better
>
> *(continued)*

ventilated when prone, V/Q matching is improved. The prone position improves the P/F ratio, reduces the rate of ventilator-associated pneumonia, and is not associated with major adverse airway complications. Turning the patient with moderate to severe ARDS (P/F ratio <20 kPa) prone early on (within 24 hours of diagnosis) and for prolonged durations (at least 16 hours daily) can improve survival [36, 37].

Prone positioning in severe acute respiratory distress syndrome (PROSEVA study)

- Multicentre RCT [36], n = 466.
- Severe ARDS (P/F ratio <20 kPa, FiO_2 ≥0.6, PEEP ≥5 cmH_2O, and tidal volume 6 mL/kg) for less than 24 hours.
- After checking eligibility, a 12–24-hour stabilization period was observed and inclusion was confirmed only at the end of this period.
- Assigned to receive prone-positioning sessions of at least 16 hours or left in supine position.
- The proned group had:
  o a lower 28-day mortality (16.0% vs 32.8%; P <0.001)
  o a lower 90-day mortality (23.6% vs 41.0%; P <0.001)
  o no increase in complications compared to the supine group—in fact the incidence of cardiac arrests was higher in the supine group.
- In patients with severe ARDS, early prone ventilation for prolonged durations significantly decreases the 28-day and 90-day mortality.

> **ⓖ Expert comment**
>
> Many ICUs have adopted standard operating procedures for prone ventilation. It typically requires one person to control the head, ensure the airway is secure, and ensure that central lines are not pulled out during the turn. It is common practice to secure the patient with lower and upper sheets (this has several regional terms, e.g. the Cornish pasty technique) and to use a sliding sheet—it normally requires two people either side of the patient in addition to the person controlling the head. Complications of prone ventilation include displacement of the airway, intravascular catheters, and other devices during the turn, and pressure sores. If NMBDs are used to facilitate ventilation in the prone position, use of a bispectral index (BIS) monitor will help to ensure that sedation is adequate (indicated by BIS values in the range 50–70).

Neuromuscular blockade

Studies have shown that the addition of an infusion of a NMBD improves survival in patients with severe ARDS without increasing muscle weakness [38, 39]. The mechanism for this benefit is unclear; however, there are several possible advantages. Use of a NMBD may improve patient:ventilator synchrony, which may reduce ventilator-associated lung injury. It also helps reduce the excessive tidal volumes caused by an increased respiratory drive secondary to alveolar hypoxia, permissive hypercapnia, anxiety, and lung reflexes, which can also cause barotrauma and volutrauma. In a proof-of-concept study, partial neuromuscular blockade during partial ventilator support facilitated lung protective ventilation [40]. Spontaneous ventilation with excessive tidal volumes is now considered harmful in patients with severe ARDS [41]. NMBDs are also thought to have a direct anti-inflammatory effect, decreasing lung or systemic inflammation and subsequent organ dysfunction and failure—a common complication of ARDS. While NMBDs are associated with muscle weakness [42], use for short durations does not increase muscle weakness significantly and their benefits in terms of improved survival, improved lung recruitment, decreased ventilator-associated lung injury, and enabling both prone positioning, permissive hypercapnia, and non-physiological ventilation modes (e.g. inverse ratio) outweigh any risks in patients with severe ARDS.

Neuromuscular blockers in early acute respiratory distress syndrome (ACURASYS study)

- Multicentre RCT [38], n = 340.
- Severe ARDS (P/F ratio <150 mmHg, PEEP ≥5 cmH_2O, and tidal volume 6–8 mL/kg) for less than 48 hours.
- Infusion of cisatracurium versus placebo for 48 hours.

(continued)

- The cisatracurium group had:
  - a lower 28-day mortality (23.7% vs 33.3%; P = 0.05)
  - a lower 90-day mortality (31.6% vs 40.7%; P = 0.05).
- No significant difference in the rate of ICU-acquired paresis between the two groups.
- Early administration of a NMBD improved 90-day mortality in patients with severe ARDS without increasing muscle weakness.

On day 6, the patient's FiO$_2$ had decreased to 0.3 with PaO$_2$ consistently greater than 9 kPa over the preceding 18 hours. She was also weaned from a synchronized intermittent mandatory ventilation mode to pressure support ventilation. Her heart rate was less than 90 bpm, her blood pressure was stable without vasopressors, and fluid balance was negative for more than 48 hours. The patient underwent a sedation break and became agitated; Confusion Assessment Method (CAM)-ICU scoring confirmed delirium. Her sedation was recommenced at half the original rate and despite reassurance and reorientation by the nursing staff, she required nasogastric quetiapine 25 mg twice a day and IV clonidine 1.0 mcg/kg/hour. Over the course of the day, her sedation with propofol and alfentanil was weaned further and by later that evening she required minimal sedation. She was mobilized to the edge of her bed by the physiotherapist. On the evening review, she was commenced on IV dexamethasone to facilitate a trial of extubation the following morning. Dexamethasone was started to reduce cord oedema and help reduce the risk of post-extubation respiratory failure [43].

On day 7 of her stay, she remained afebrile, her inflammatory markers had decreased, she was haemodynamically stable, and breathing an FiO$_2$ of 0.25. On a further sedation hold she was found to be obeying commands and moving all four limbs appropriately but CAM-ICU scoring still confirmed delirium. The clonidine and quetiapine were continued. She was then weaned from pressure support with a trial of spontaneous breathing with continuous positive airways pressure at 5 cmH$_2$O. She tolerated this for 30 min without any signs of respiratory distress and was extubated to high-flow nasal oxygen and remained on this over the next 24 hours, before being weaned to supplemental oxygen via a nasal cannula aiming for a peripheral arterial oxygen saturation of 94–98%.

> **❻ Expert comment**
>
> The incidence of post-extubation stridor is about 5%. Patients with a reduced cuff leak are at the highest risk of post-extubation stridor and respiratory failure. Pretreatment with IV steroids, commenced 12 hours before a planned extubation, reduces the incidence of post-extubation laryngeal oedema and reintubation in this subgroup of patients [43].

> **✪ Learning point Weaning the patient from mechanical ventilation—spontaneous breathing trials**
>
> The ability to successfully wean the patient from mechanical ventilation is dependent on several factors [21, 22, 44]; these include:
>
> - resolution of the underlying cause of respiratory failure
> - adequate conscious level, without problematic delirium after discontinuation of deep sedation and NMBDs, to enable protection of the airway after extubation
> - adequate arterial oxygenation breathing a low FiO$_2$ (<0.5) and PEEP less than or equal to 5 cmH$_2$O
> - adequate respiratory muscle function and cough/clearance of secretions
> - haemodynamic stability with minimal inotropic and/or vasopressor agent.
>
> Once identified, patients should undergo a spontaneous breathing trial to simulate those respiratory conditions that would occur following extubation, and to observe their ability to cope. Successful completion of spontaneous breathing trial(s) increases the likelihood of the patient successfully separating from mechanical ventilation, and studies have shown that approximately 75% of patients who complete a spontaneous breathing trial can be extubated without the need for reintubation. The rate of successful weaning is higher with spontaneous breathing trials than with more modern ventilator weaning techniques. In a comparison of four methods of weaning patients, daily trials of spontaneous breathing resulted in extubation three times more quickly than with synchronized
>
> *(continued)*

intermittent mandatory ventilation and twice as quickly than with pressure-support ventilation [22]. Both a once-daily trial or the performance of multiple daily trials appear to be equally successful, and the trial can be completed with the patient breathing spontaneously on the ventilator (continuous positive airways pressure) with or without a low level of pressure support or removed from the ventilator and breathing on a T-piece. The spontaneous breathing trial duration can vary from 30 to 120 min, and should be discontinued if there is any evidence of respiratory distress, such as:

- respiratory rate greater than 40 breaths/min or less than 6 breaths/min for 5 min or longer
- arterial blood oxygen saturation less than 92%
- heart rate greater than 140 bpm or less than 60 bpm or greater than 25% above baseline
- systolic blood pressure greater than 40 mmHg above baseline
- agitation, anxiety, or discomfort.

The patient was reviewed by the physiotherapist and was mobilized from bed to chair. She received a total of three doses of IV dexamethasone and completed a total of 7 days of antibiotics for her pneumonia. Her arterial and central venous cannulae were removed and a new peripheral venous cannula was inserted. She was weaned from IV clonidine. Her swallow was assessed and confirmed safe; she was then encouraged to have sips of fluids. A carefully planned dietary programme was instituted by the ICU dietician before stopping nasogastric feeding.

Over the next 48 hours, quetiapine was stopped once she was no longer delirious and she continued to mobilize on the ICU with the help of the nurses and physiotherapist.

✪

Learning point Non-resolving pneumonia

Normal resolution of pneumonia is difficult to define. Hospitalized patients with community-acquired pneumonia typically show signs of improvement within 3–5 days of treatment. Normal resolution of pneumonia depends on multiple factors including host factors, comorbidities, aetiological factors, and development of complications. About 15% of patients hospitalized with pneumonia develop non-resolving pneumonia and about 20% are due to non-infectious causes.

Patients should have an improvement in tachycardia, oxygenation, and hypotension in 2–3 days, symptoms in 3–5 days, and cough and fatigue in 10–14 days.

Causes of non-resolving pneumonia
- Age: older than 50 years, about 30% have resolution of X-rays at 1 month
- Comorbidities: alcoholism, immunocompromised state (e.g. long-term steroids, diabetes mellitus, AIDS)
- Misdiagnosis: tuberculosis, fungal infections, *Nocardia*, and *Actinomyces*
- Bacterial resistance
- Complications:
  o Pulmonary complications: lung abscess and empyema
  o Non-pulmonary complications: infective endocarditis, septic arthritis, osteomyelitis, and discitis
- Non-infectious causes: bronchogenic carcinoma, inflammatory disease (vasculitis), pulmonary embolism, and drug-induced lung disease

Diagnostic approach
This includes:

- a thorough history including recent travel, lifestyle, and assessment of non-infectious causes
- assessment of risk factors: age, comorbidities, severity, and specific pathogens
- review of specific complications associated with pneumonia
- radiological assessment: CT chest with consideration of pulmonary angiogram
- repeat laboratory tests including sputum and blood cultures and urinary antigen evaluation
- bronchoalveolar lavage with or without transbronchial biopsy or CT-guided biopsy
- lung biopsy: open versus video-assisted.

Discussion

Community-acquired pneumonia can be defined as an acute infection of the lung parenchyma where the infection is acquired in the community. The overall incidence in adults is 5.1–6.1 cases per 1000 persons per year and this increases with increasing age. The rates are higher in men than for women and there are seasonal variations. *Streptococcus pneumoniae* is the most frequently identified cause for community-acquired pneumonia.

Streptococcal pneumonia is a classic cause of lobar consolidation. The classic presentation is that of fever, chills, cough with rusty sputum, and pleuritic chest pain with clinical signs of consolidation (increased vocal fremitus and bronchial breathing). The diagnosis is often confirmed by blood cultures or a positive urinary antigen. The optimum antibiotic regimen depends upon the presence of comorbidities, need for hospitalization, and presence of antibiotic resistance. In the UK, most empiric antibiotic regimens contain beta lactams and are often effective against streptococcal pneumonia (consult your microbiologist for local susceptibility patterns). A typical duration of antibiotics is 5–7 days in mild–moderate cases and up to 10–14 days in severe cases. Pulmonary complications of streptococcal pneumonia include empyema, necrotizing pneumonia, lung abscess, and ARDS.

Acute respiratory distress syndrome manifests as acute-onset (< 7 days), hypoxic respiratory failure with bilateral lung infiltrates often due to a clear precipitating factor. The alveolar injury and inflammation can be of alveolar origin (e.g. pneumonia) or endothelial/systemic in origin (e.g. acute pancreatitis). Over the past three decades there have been numerous attempts to define ARDS. The 2012 Berlin definition was validated based on hypoxaemia and bilateral pulmonary infiltrates in over 4000 patients. The Berlin definition stipulates an onset of less than 7 days, that the patient is ventilated with PEEP at least at 5 cmH$_2$O, and that it can be diagnosed in the presence of cardiac failure. It also includes, for the first time, chest CT as an alternative form of imaging for lung infiltrates.

The principles of management of acute respiratory failure include resuscitation, diagnosis, and treatment of the underlying disease. Lung protective mechanical ventilation and the avoidance of fluid overload are fundamental to the successful management of ARDS. Patients with severe hypoxaemia can be managed with early short-term use of neuromuscular blockade, prone position ventilation, or extracorporeal membrane oxygenation. The use of inhaled nitric oxide is rarely indicated and both beta$_2$ agonists and late corticosteroids should be avoided. A detailed discussion of extracorporeal membrane oxygenation and other rescue therapies is covered in a recent review [33]. Despite the recent advances, mortality from ARDS remains greater than 30%.

A final word from the expert

It is vital to have a sound working knowledge of the common causes of community-acquired pneumonia, and the local and national recommendations for its treatment. It is important to have a strategy for the management of acute respiratory failure which includes initial resuscitation, a structured approach to investigations and treatment of the underlying disease, and measures to provide organ support and to minimize healthcare associated complications.

References

1. Rhodes A, Evans LE, Alhazzani W, et al. Surviving Sepsis Campaign: international guidelines for management of sepsis and septic shock: 2016. *Intensive Care Med*. 2017;43:304–77.
2. Daniels R, Nutbeam T, McNamara G, Galvin C. The sepsis six and the severe sepsis resuscitation bundle: a prospective observational cohort study. *Emerg Med J*. 2011;28:507–12.
3. Prina E, Ranzani OT, Torres A. Community-acquired pneumonia. *Lancet*. 2015;386:1097–108.
4. Musher DM, Thorner AR. Community-acquired pneumonia. *N Engl J Med*. 2014;371:1619–28.
5. Baron EJ, Miller JM, Weinstein MP, et al. A guide to utilization of the microbiology laboratory for diagnosis of infectious diseases: 2013 recommendations by the Infectious Diseases Society of America (IDSA) and the American Society for Microbiology (ASM). *Clin Infect Dis*. 2013;57:e22–121.
6. Metlay JP, Fine MJ. Testing strategies in the initial management of patients with community-acquired pneumonia. *Ann Intern Med*. 2003;138:109–18.
7. Monnet X, Teboul JL. Passive leg raising. *Intensive Care Med*. 2008;34:659–63.
8. Monnet X, Marik P, Teboul JL. Passive leg raising for predicting fluid responsiveness: a systematic review and meta-analysis. *Intensive Care Med*. 2016;42:1935–47.
9. Pro CI, Yealy DM, Kellum JA, et al. A randomized trial of protocol-based care for early septic shock. *N Engl J Med*. 2014;370:1683–93.
10. Mouncey PR, Osborn TM, Power GS, et al. Trial of early, goal-directed resuscitation for septic shock. *N Engl J Med*. 2015;372:1301–11.
11. ARISE Investigators, ANZICS Clinical Trials Group, Peake SL, et al. Goal-directed resuscitation for patients with early septic shock. *N Engl J Med*. 2014;371:1496–506.
12. Caironi P, Tognoni G, Masson S, et al. Albumin replacement in patients with severe sepsis or septic shock. *N Engl J Med*. 2014;370:1412–21.
13. Delaney AP, Dan A, McCaffrey J, Finfer S. The role of albumin as a resuscitation fluid for patients with sepsis: a systematic review and meta-analysis. *Crit Care Med*. 2011;39:386–91.
14. Martin GS, Mangialardi RJ, Wheeler AP, Dupont WD, Morris JA, Bernard GR. Albumin and furosemide therapy in hypoproteinemic patients with acute lung injury. *Crit Care Med*. 2002;30:2175–82.
15. National Heart, Lung, and Blood Institute Acute Respiratory Distress Syndrome Clinical Trials Network. Comparison of two fluid-management strategies in acute lung injury. *N Engl J Med*. 2006;354:2564–75.
16. Semler MW, Wheeler AP, Thompson BT, et al. Impact of initial central venous pressure on outcomes of conservative versus liberal fluid management in acute respiratory distress syndrome. *Crit Care Med*. 2016;44:782–9.
17. Silversides JA, Major E, Ferguson AJ, et al. Conservative fluid management or deresuscitation for patients with sepsis or acute respiratory distress syndrome following the resuscitation phase of critical illness: a systematic review and meta-analysis. *Intensive Care Med*. 2017;43:155–70.
18. Hoste EA, Maitland K, Brudney CS, et al. Four phases of intravenous fluid therapy: a conceptual model. *Br J Anaesth*. 2014;113:740–7.
19. Seymour CW, Gesten F, Prescott HC, et al. Time to treatment and mortality during mandated emergency care for sepsis. *N Engl J Med*. 2017;376:2235–44.
20. Barr J, Fraser GL, Puntillo K, et al. Clinical practice guidelines for the management of pain, agitation, and delirium in adult patients in the intensive care unit. *Crit Care Med*. 2013;41:263–306.
21. Girard TD, Alhazzani W, Kress JP, et al. An official American Thoracic Society/American College of Chest Physicians clinical practice guideline: liberation from mechanical ventilation in critically ill adults. Rehabilitation protocols, ventilator liberation protocols, and cuff leak tests. *Am J Respir Crit Care Med*. 2017;195:120–33.

22. Esteban A, Frutos F, Tobin MJ, et al. A comparison of four methods of weaning patients from mechanical ventilation. Spanish Lung Failure Collaborative Group. *N Engl J Med*. 1995;332:345–50.

23. Fan E, Del Sorbo L, Goligher EC, et al. An official American Thoracic Society/European Society of Intensive Care Medicine/Society of Critical Care Medicine clinical practice guideline: mechanical ventilation in adult patients with acute respiratory distress syndrome. *Am J Respir Crit Care Med*. 2017;195:1253–63.

24. Goligher EC, Ferguson ND, Brochard LJ. Clinical challenges in mechanical ventilation. *Lancet*. 2016;387:1856–66.

25. Brower RG, Lanken PN, MacIntyre N, et al. Higher versus lower positive end-expiratory pressures in patients with the acute respiratory distress syndrome. *N Engl J Med*. 2004;351:327–36.

26. Sahetya SK, Goligher EC, Brower RG. Fifty years of research in ARDS. Setting positive end-expiratory pressure in acute respiratory distress syndrome. *Am J Respir Crit Care Med*. 2017;195:1429–38.

27. The Acute Respiratory Distress Syndrome Network. Ventilation with lower tidal volumes as compared with traditional tidal volumes for acute lung injury and the acute respiratory distress syndrome. *N Engl J Med*. 2000;342:1301–8.

28. Pinhu L, Whitehead T, Evans T, Griffiths M. Ventilator-associated lung injury. *Lancet*. 2003;361:332–40.

29. Meade MO, Cook DJ, Guyatt GH, et al. Ventilation strategy using low tidal volumes, recruitment maneuvers, and high positive end-expiratory pressure for acute lung injury and acute respiratory distress syndrome: a randomized controlled trial. *JAMA*. 2008;299:637–45.

30. Mercat A, Richard JC, Vielle B, et al. Positive end-expiratory pressure setting in adults with acute lung injury and acute respiratory distress syndrome: a randomized controlled trial. *JAMA*. 2008;299:646–55.

31. Force ADT, Ranieri VM, Rubenfeld GD, et al. Acute respiratory distress syndrome: the Berlin Definition. *JAMA*. 2012;307:2526–33.

32. Briel M, Meade M, Mercat A, et al. Higher vs lower positive end-expiratory pressure in patients with acute lung injury and acute respiratory distress syndrome: systematic review and meta-analysis. *JAMA*. 2010;303:865–73.

33. Sweeney RM, McAuley DF. Acute respiratory distress syndrome. *Lancet*. 2016;388:2416–30.

34. Bernard GR, Artigas A, Brigham KL, et al. The American-European Consensus Conference on ARDS. Definitions, mechanisms, relevant outcomes, and clinical trial coordination. *Am J Respir Crit Care Med*. 1994;149:818–24.

35. Lim WS, Baudouin SV, George RC, et al. BTS guidelines for the management of community acquired pneumonia in adults: update 2009. *Thorax*. 2009;64 Suppl. 3:iii1–55.

36. Guerin C, Reignier J, Richard JC, et al. Prone positioning in severe acute respiratory distress syndrome. *N Engl J Med*. 2013;368:2159–68.

37. Beitler JR, Shaefi S, Montesi SB, et al. Prone positioning reduces mortality from acute respiratory distress syndrome in the low tidal volume era: a meta-analysis. *Intensive Care Med*. 2014;40:332–41.

38. Papazian L, Forel JM, Gacouin A, et al. Neuromuscular blockers in early acute respiratory distress syndrome. *N Engl J Med*. 2010;363:1107–16.

39. Alhazzani W, Alshahrani M, Jaeschke R, et al. Neuromuscular blocking agents in acute respiratory distress syndrome: a systematic review and meta-analysis of randomized controlled trials. *Crit Care*. 2013;17:R43.

40. Doorduin J, Nollet JL, Roesthuis LH, et al. Partial neuromuscular blockade during partial ventilatory support in sedated patients with high tidal volumes. *Am J Respir Crit Care Med*. 2017;195:1033–42.

41. Yoshida T, Fujino Y, Amato MB, Kavanagh BP. Fifty years of research in ARDS. Spontaneous breathing during mechanical ventilation. Risks, mechanisms, and management. *Am J Respir Crit Care Med*. 2017;195:985–92.

42. Kress JP, Hall JB. ICU-acquired weakness and recovery from critical illness. *N Engl J Med.* 2014;370:1626–35.

43. Francois B, Bellissant E, Gissot V, et al. 12-h pretreatment with methylprednisolone versus placebo for prevention of postextubation laryngeal oedema: a randomised double-blind trial. *Lancet.* 2007;369:1083–9.

44. McConville JF, Kress JP. Weaning patients from the ventilator. *N Engl J Med.* 2012;367:2233–9.

CASE
4

Early management of multi-trauma

Marius Rehn

Expert Commentary David J. Lockey

Case history

A 22-year-old male cyclist was hit from the right side by a lorry while crossing a busy road junction. The cyclist was trapped underneath the lorry and could not be reached by bystanders. Paramedic-staffed ground emergency medical services (EMS) and a doctor-staffed helicopter EMS were immediately dispatched to the scene. On arrival, the patient was found to be clammy and agitated with a Glasgow Coma Scale (GCS) score of 12 (E3, V4, M5).

> ## Learning point Epidemiology of multi-trauma
>
> Globally, over 15,000 people die daily as a consequence of injuries, and many more become permanently or temporarily disabled [1–3]. The global trauma burden represents 10% of the world's deaths and is an increasing health problem that causes incalculable suffering for individuals, families, and societies [4]. Almost twice as many men as women die from injuries, which are the leading cause of death among those aged 5–44 years. Approximately one-quarter of these deaths result from road traffic collisions and almost one-quarter from suicide and homicide. Other main causes of fatal injury include falls, drowning, and war, with considerable geographical variation. Road traffic injuries are the most common cause of death between the ages of 15 and 29, whereas falls are a leading cause of fatal injury in the elderly. More than 90% of injury deaths occur in low- and middle-income countries, where the healthcare systems are often less resourced to cope with the challenges [5]. Although the death toll is largest among the poor, injuries also constitute a major public health problem in high-income European countries with an annual injury mortality rate approaching 50 per 100,000.

> ## Expert comment
>
> Cyclists are very vulnerable at junctions and several road safety campaigns have attempted to introduce initiatives to improve safety. These include awareness campaigns, alteration of road junction layouts, and modifications to large vehicles. Despite this, accidents still occur and cyclists are vulnerable particularly to large vehicles which can transfer huge energy and devastating injury at low speeds.

The patient was extricated by fire service personnel using hydraulic jacks 18 min after helicopter EMS arrival. The patient had partial airway obstruction and noisy breathing and two nasopharyngeal airways were placed together with nasal oxygen cannulae with integrated capnography and a reservoir oxygen mask delivering 15 L/min of oxygen. A 16-gauge intravenous (IV) cannula was placed in the patient's right antecubital fossa. The patient became more alert and complained of difficulty in breathing and of severe pain in the abdomen, pelvis, and both legs. Two 20 mg IV boluses of ketamine were administered. In-line immobilization of the neck was maintained during extrication.

> **ⓕ Expert comment**
>
> Cervical spine immobilization has long been a key component of early trauma management. Guidelines still emphasize immobilization but other factors may influence outcome (e.g. airway obstruction or rapid extrication) and take priority over immobilization [6, 7]. Patients who have been intubated can be safely transported in the supine position. Where intubation cannot be carried out before transfer to hospital and patients have a decreased level of consciousness, there is a potential conflict between cervical spine immobilization in the supine position and airway patency. Removal of the front component of a collar prior to intubation (with manual in-line stabilization) is standard practice. In the unconscious or sedated patient on the intensive care unit (ICU), cervical spine immobilization can be safely removed once computed tomography (CT) scanning has excluded unstable injury and this should be done to reduce the risk of collar-related venous compression and pressure injuries.

> **✪ Learning point Analgesia and sedation**
>
> Trauma patients should have their analgesic needs promptly assessed and addressed at all stages of the trauma pathway. Potential masking of clinical signs is not a reason to withhold pain relief. Effective use of analgesia enables clinicians to meet essential clinical end points, such as reducing blood loss by facilitating fracture manipulation. Judicious use of analgesics will also facilitate extrication and thereby reduce time to critical interventions and definitive care. When feasible, analgesia should be delivered intravenously and titrated to effect. In circumstances where IV access is difficult, intramuscular injection is an alternative for some drugs. Continuous waveform capnography, pulse oximetry, and clinical assessment should be used to detect airway obstruction, hypoventilation, or bradypnoea in both spontaneously breathing and ventilated patients. Analgesic and anxiolytic drugs used in the early phases of multi-trauma care should ideally have relative haemodynamic stability and acceptable risk profiles for adverse effects. Drugs with a relatively wide therapeutic margin are beneficial since patient weight is usually estimated.
>
> **Commonly used drugs**
>
> *Ketamine*
>
> An NMDA receptor antagonist classified as a dissociative agent and known to produce a state resembling general anaesthesia without cardiorespiratory depression. Ketamine is effective for analgesia, sedation, and as an induction drug for rapid sequence induction. It can be used for painful interventions on-scene, in the emergency department (ED), or on the ICU. Recovery agitation occurs in 10–20% of patients, but may be minimized with co-administration of benzodiazepines [8].
>
> *Midazolam*
>
> A rapid-onset, short-acting benzodiazepine with potent anxiolytic and hypnotic properties that also reduces skeletal muscle spasticity. It is reversible and is often used with ketamine to reduce dysphoric reactions [8]. Side effects include paradoxical reactions and cardiorespiratory depression.
>
> *Morphine*
>
> An opioid analgesic with rapid onset, long-lasting analgesic effect, well-known pharmacokinetics, and reversibility. Side effects include cardiorespiratory depression and nausea and vomiting. It should be given with an antiemetic. Incremental IV morphine is the analgesic of choice in recent UK National Institute for Health and Care Excellence (NICE) trauma guidelines [9].
>
> *Fentanyl*
>
> A potent, synthetic opioid analgesic with rapid onset, short duration of action, and reversibility. Although fentanyl is associated with cardiorespiratory depression, studies support its safety for analgesia in normotensive trauma patients [10, 11]. It is equally as effective and safe as morphine in treating acute pain and is increasingly used as a first-line drug in trauma analgesia.

The patient's clothing was completely removed and he was placed directly on to an orthopaedic scoop stretcher. A pelvic binder was applied at the level of the greater trochanters as the mechanism of injury and initial examination raised the possibility of a significant pelvic fracture.

✪ **Learning point** Pelvic injuries

In patients with major blunt trauma, the incidence of pelvic fractures is around 10%, with a 7–37% mortality rate that is influenced by type of fracture and the associated injuries [12–14]. High-energy trauma from road traffic collisions and falls are the most common mechanisms for pelvic fracture [13, 15]. The vascular anatomy of the pelvis predisposes to a risk of exsanguinating haemorrhage after fractures. Therapeutic options include endovascular control (usually by interventional radiologists although temporary control techniques have been reported in the ED and prehospital care carried out by non-radiologists [16, 17]) and extraperitoneal packing. Endovascular haemorrhage control is effective in arterial bleeding (approximately 75% of significant pelvic bleeds are of venous origin) and angiography is recommended unless immediate open surgery is required to manage bleeding from other organs. The mechanism of injury together with clinical and radiological examination are used to assess the pelvis for instability. Non-invasive pelvic circumferential compression devices (pelvic binders) should be applied if active bleeding is suspected [9]. Pelvic binders have been widely integrated into early resuscitation guidelines and aim to decrease the volume of the disrupted pelvis and promote haemostasis by splinting fractures. The presence of a binder also prompts providers to avoid unnecessary movement of the patient as this may dislodge blood clots and promote bleeding. The splint is applied directly to skin over the greater trochanter and is tightened until the alignment appears normal. Pelvic binders enable laparotomy, but restrict complete assessment of the perineum. To avoid skin necrosis at bony prominences the splint is removed, but only after radiological examination excludes instability or other means of stabilization are initiated. The effect of pelvic binders on outcome is debated and their role in pelvic vertical shear fractures remains undefined [18–20].

✪ **Learning point** Packaging and spinal precautions

Patient handling (also known as packaging) is an important part of the therapeutic process and is relevant in both the pre- and in-hospital resuscitation phases of care. Gentle patient handling minimizes spinal movement and reduces the risk of clot disturbance and further bleeding. It may also reduce heat loss and minimize cytokine release. Cervical spinal injuries occur in approximately 2% of all patients with blunt trauma and are more common in the presence of head injury [21]. Although a thorough log roll is a well-established part of trauma care, multi-trauma patients undergo extensive imaging, and an early clinical examination of the back must be weighed against the risks of clot disturbance in the very unstable patient. Inserting the two halves of an orthopaedic scoop stretcher on scene and careful removal through counter-traction after arrival in the ED enables transportation and transfer with minimal movement [22, 23]. For head-injured patients with head blocks and tape in place, the cervical collar can be loosened but left *in situ* to prevent increases in intracranial pressure caused by venous obstruction [24]. If the patient is to be moved, the collar is resecured. If possible, these patients are positioned with a slight head-up tilt (20°) to assist venous drainage.

The stretcher was then put into a thermal bag to avoid hypothermia.

The vital signs monitor revealed a non-invasive blood pressure of 95/56 mmHg, irregular heart rate of 135 beats/min (bpm), oxygen saturation by pulse oximetry (SpO_2) of 91%, respiratory rate of 16 breaths/min, and end-tidal carbon dioxide ($ETCO_2$) value of 4.5 kPa. The primary survey identified crepitus over the left iliac crest and pelvic asymmetry that suggested a pelvic fracture. The abdomen was rigid, with a left flank abrasion. The chest had left-sided crepitus with a flail segment, surgical emphysema, and possible reduced air entry (auscultation was difficult due to background noise) suggesting a left-sided pneumothorax. The irregular sinus tachycardia and bruising on the anterior chest wall raised suspicion of a possible cardiac contusion. There were no external signs of head injury. During initial assessment, a closed left femoral fracture, a closed right tibia/fibula fracture, and partial degloving of the right arm were also noted. A further 10 mg of ketamine and 2 mg of midazolam were administered IV. The femoral fracture was reduced using a traction device.

> **⊕ Expert comment**
>
> Ketamine is the drug of choice for procedural sedation and analgesia for fracture reduction in the prehospital and ED phases of trauma care. It was historically considered to be contraindicated in patients with head injury because of concerns about elevation of intracranial pressure. A growing body of evidence demonstrates no increase in intracranial pressure when ketamine is used with controlled ventilation and in combination with other sedatives [25]. It is now frequently used as an induction drug when these patients require emergency anaesthesia. Careful prevention of hypercapnia and hypocapnia is important in sedated and anaesthetized patients with actual or potential head injury.

> **✪ Learning point Haemorrhage control**
>
> Optimal haemorrhage control involves minimizing blood loss and clot disruption while maximizing clot formation. Minimizing patient handling and use of splinting enhances natural tamponade and are fundamental parts of haemorrhage control. Compression bandages are used to control obvious external bleeding. Application of tourniquets will stop extremity bleeding and outcomes are improved when tourniquets are applied before shock occurs [26]. Nevertheless, tourniquets are a temporary measure of haemorrhage control and ischaemic time must be minimized to avoid complications [27].
>
> Where there are injuries to the vessels of the neck, axilla, perineum, and groin, compressive dressings are often ineffective and proximal control tourniquets are impossible to apply [23]. Topical agents such as factor concentrates, mucoadhesive agents, and procoagulant agents are commonly used in the battlefield and may be packed into wound cavities to control haemorrhage [29]. To reduce the soft tissue into which bleeding can occur, limb fractures are drawn out to length and splinted. A pelvic binder is applied when a pelvic fracture is suspected and may reduce the volume of open-book pelvic fractures and reduce bleeding. Cumulative blood loss from small wounds should also be attended to, for instance, by suturing bleeding scalp wounds [23, 30]. Haemorrhage that is not suitable for external compression (e.g. in the neck) can also be compressed by insertion and inflation of the balloon of a Foley catheter [31].
>
> Standard venous access for fluid replacement is a 14- or 16-gauge cannula in the antecubital fossa. Where possible, an arm that is not injured and contralateral to any chest injuries is chosen. Subclavian venous access might be appropriate particularly when the chest has been decompressed and there is a low risk of causing undetected pneumothorax. Intraosseous access is usually considered inferior to venous access, but offers a safe and simple alternative [32].

> **⊕ Expert comment**
> **Tourniquets**
>
> The use of tourniquets has been routine in recent military conflicts and has been associated with decreased mortality in patients with severe limb injuries [28]. Use has been enthusiastically replicated in civilian prehospital care, but it is unclear whether delayed application of a tourniquet (by ambulance providers) is likely to be as effective as immediate application by a military victim or 'buddy' immediately after injury.

The limb fractures were reduced and splinted; a compression bandage was applied to the degloved right arm. After the fractures were reduced, the GCS score decreased to 8 (E2, V2, M4); his vital signs were blood pressure 72/45 mmHg, heart rate 141 bpm, SpO$_2$ 94%, respiratory rate 18 breaths/min, and ETCO$_2$ 3.8 kPa. A needle decompression of the left side of the chest was performed as a bridge to formal chest decompression, but without any apparent clinical benefit. The patient was transfused with 1 unit of prewarmed red blood cells while he was anaesthetized using a rapid sequence induction, and intubated.

❝ Expert comment

A major change in trauma practice in the last 10 years has been the recognition that the optimal replacement fluid for significant blood loss is blood. If possible, major trauma patients with suspected ongoing haemorrhage should be treated with blood and blood products as soon as possible, rather than crystalloids. This has resulted in mandatory major trauma transfusion protocols in receiving trauma hospitals. Although controversial, current guidelines promote administration of a one-to-one ratio of blood and fresh frozen plasma, and early administration of tranexamic acid. Other aspects of the protocols (e.g. the threshold for platelet transfusion) are more variable and often subject to local practice [9, 33].

✪ Learning point   Transfusion and coagulopathy

Extensive tissue trauma and haemorrhagic shock drives an endogenous physiological response that causes a haemostatic disequilibrium termed acute traumatic coagulopathy [34, 35].

Acute traumatic coagulopathy, metabolic acidosis, and hypothermia constitute the 'triad of death' and this is exacerbated by aggressive fluid resuscitation with crystalloids and colloids. Acute traumatic coagulopathy develops quickly and deranged coagulation has been found in up to 25% of major trauma patients on arrival in hospital. Acute traumatic coagulopathy is associated with increased transfusion requirement, multiorgan failure, and death [36]. Although prognostic models are available, early identification of acute traumatic coagulopathy to guide therapy and improve outcome remains a challenge [37, 38]. While rotation thromboelastometry (ROTEM) and thromboelastography enable evaluation of the dynamic haemostatic equilibrium, no definitive diagnostic test for acute traumatic coagulopathy has been established [39, 40]. In the absence of a validated point-of-care diagnostic test for coagulopathy, clinicians should anticipate acute traumatic coagulopathy when trauma patients present with hypotension and extensive tissue trauma. Current 'damage control resuscitation' strategies for targeting acute traumatic coagulopathy include permissive hypotension, avoidance of acidosis, avoidance of hypothermia, and more aggressive use of blood products [41]. Administration of tranexamic acid has shown clinically relevant survival benefit during trauma haemorrhage and is part of almost all major haemorrhage protocols [9, 35, 42]. An initial dose of 1 g is injected and a further 1 g infused over the following 8 hours. The use of prehospital transfusion is associated with improved short-term outcomes; however, the effect on overall survival remains controversial [43–46].

❝ Expert comment
Acute traumatic coagulopathy

Acute traumatic coagulopathy was described in 2003 and although the mechanisms of the process are still not entirely clear, the previous concept of coagulopathy after trauma caused by consumption of clotting factors does not account for the early coagulopathy seen in this patient group.

Immediately after initiation of positive pressure ventilation, a left-sided thoracostomy was performed which relieved air and drained approximately 200 mL of blood.

✪ Learning point Chest trauma

Major objectives in chest injury management are to maximize oxygen delivery as early as possible and to avoid any ventilatory contribution to hypoxia, while aiming for normocapnia (particularly in the presence of head injury). Tension pneumothoraces may cause respiratory distress and, at a late stage, lateral shift of the mediastinum and hypotension, so should be decompressed as soon as possible after injury. Pneumothoraces may be difficult to identify and may become apparent only after a period of positive pressure ventilation. Common signs and symptoms of pneumothorax include dyspnoea, external signs of trauma with significant mechanism of injury, surgical emphysema, bony crepitus, flail chest, decreased air entry, and wheeze. The traditional supine anteroposterior trauma chest X-ray has low sensitivity, but high specificity for detecting pneumothorax. A computed tomography (CT) scan remains the standard imaging modality for haemodynamically stable adult patients with chest injuries. However, chest ultrasonography as a part of the primary survey provides an additional point-of-care test with acceptable accuracy in detecting pneumothoraces [9, 47]. Pleural decompression is required in approximately 25% of patients presenting with major trauma and management strategies include needle thoracocentesis, thoracostomy, and tube thoracocentesis [48]. Open pneumothoraces are covered with a simple occlusive dressing and observed for development of tension pneumothorax [9].

(continued)

❝ Expert comment
Needle decompression and thoracostomy

Needle decompression is an easy procedure to perform but is often ineffective. Thoracostomy—the first stage of chest drain insertion—is the creation of a communication between the pleural space and the outside and can be achieved quickly. It is increasingly used as an emergency procedure to decompress suspected tension pneumothorax in mechanically ventilated patients. It is always followed by formal chest drain insertion.

Needle thoracocentesis often fails to reach and decompress the pleural space. The cannula may also kink or puncture major vessels or even the heart [49, 50]. However, it is a quick procedure that may be indicated in peri-arrest situations or in trapped victims before progressing to thoracostomy or tube thoracocentesis.

Thoracostomy involves blunt dissection and digital decompression through the pleura and is only suitable in patients undergoing positive pressure ventilation: the open parietal pleura then prevents development of a tension pneumothorax. The technique simplifies treatment in the prehospital phase as drainage and insertion of a chest tube is a secondary priority [51]. Thoracostomy is not suitable for self-ventilating patients as it will create an open pneumothorax.

Tube thoracocentesis is used for definitive chest decompression and can also be indicated to decompress a clinically significant pneumothorax in a self-ventilating patient [9]. Complications include tube misplacements causing injury to thoracic and abdominal structures [52]. Once sutured in place, the drain and its collecting system become a closed system and have the potential to allow re-tension to occur.

> **❝ Expert comment** Tension pneumothorax
>
> Recent NICE guidelines recommend that in patients with suspected tension pneumothorax, chest decompression should be performed before imaging only if there is haemodynamic instability or severe respiratory compromise. This is a departure from previous trauma practice where a large pneumothorax present on imaging was viewed by some as bad practice. Where immediate decompression is required, open thoracostomy followed by a chest drain is indicated. Drains should be sufficiently large to enable drainage of blood where present and should be inserted by operators trained and familiar with the chosen technique.

The patient's blood pressure increased to 92/65 mmHg. Other vital signs were heart rate 122 bpm, SpO_2 96%, and $ETCO_2$ 4.0 kPa. He was given tranexamic acid 1 g IV and two more units of blood during transfer to the nearest major trauma centre (MTC) by-passing the local hospital (transportation time 25 min). A pre-warning call was made and a full trauma team attended the patient.

> **✪ Learning point** Trauma team activation
>
> Early identification of major trauma enables EMS providers to classify patients according to injury severity and efficiently couple available resources with patients' needs. Triage remains a core component of a trauma system as inaccurate assessment of injury severity wastes resources and compromises quality of care [53]. To optimize patient outcome, EMS providers may bypass local hospitals and transport directly to a dedicated MTC where immediate resuscitation is provided by trained, experienced multidisciplinary trauma teams [54]. Accordingly, triage encompasses processes such as hospital destination decisions and trauma team activation. A well-performing triage system will have no under-triage (i.e. all patients with major trauma will be triaged as major trauma and taken to an MTC). To achieve this, there will always be an element of over-triage (i.e. patients triaged to an MTC with suspected major trauma who turn out not to be severely injured).

> **❝ Expert comment**
>
> MTCs are a well-defined and established part of trauma care in the US. The concept that low mortality and morbidity can be best achieved in centres with key specialities on site with high throughput of significantly injured patients is generally accepted and this has led to the formation of trauma networks in the UK (in 2012) and other countries. A significant reduction in trauma mortality was reported by

(continued)

NHS England only 2 years after the introduction of trauma networks in England (Figure 4.1). Transfer of patients identified as having major trauma directly to the MTC is facilitated by trauma triage tools used by ambulance services and trauma units.

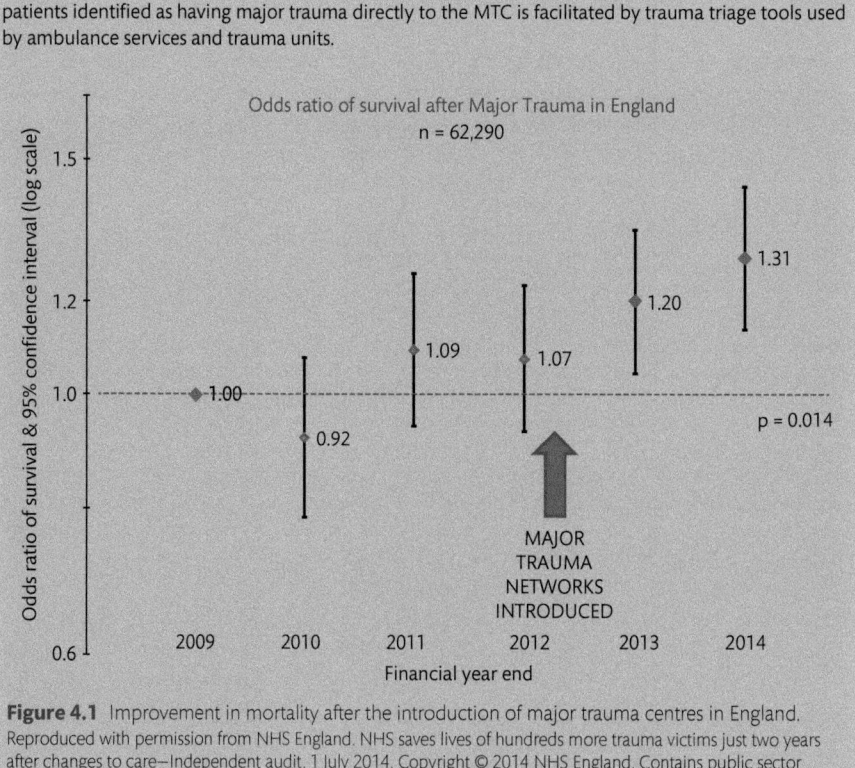

Figure 4.1 Improvement in mortality after the introduction of major trauma centres in England. Reproduced with permission from NHS England. NHS saves lives of hundreds more trauma victims just two years after changes to care—Independent audit. 1 July 2014. Copyright © 2014 NHS England. Contains public sector information licensed under the Open Government Licence v3.0. Available at https://www.england.nhs.uk/2014/07/trauma-independent-audit/.

The trauma team completed pleural drainage by inserting a chest drain into the pleural cavity. The patient remained haemodynamically unstable and was taken directly to the operating room for damage control laparotomy. A splenic laceration was identified and a splenectomy was performed. A whole-body CT confirmed an 'open-book' pelvic fracture, an L1 vertebral extension fracture without cord involvement, and bilateral lung contusions. The CT showed no head injury, suggesting that the most likely causes of the initial drop in GCS score were hypotension, administered analgesics, and/or hypoxia.

⑪ Expert comment

The spleen is a commonly injured solid abdominal organ. Historically, splenectomy was frequently performed when splenic injury was identified, but a more conservative approach is now common. Avoidance of unnecessary laparotomy and the long-term potential for infection in post-splenectomy patients are important advantages of a conservative approach. If a trauma patient is haemodynamically stable, splenic injury is assessed with contrast CT. Based on injury grade and an assessment of active bleeding, splenectomy can often be avoided with alternative approaches being interventional radiology and selective vascular embolization or a conservative non-operative approach.

⑪ Expert comment

Most adult major trauma patients with this presentation would have a whole-body CT. Recent NICE recommendations are a vertex-to-toes scanogram (i.e. scout scan before full imaging) with CT from vertex to mid thigh and further limb imaging guided by the scanogram and clinical assessment [9]. Patients with severe haemodynamic instability and suspected intra-abdominal injury may still rarely be moved directly to theatre for haemorrhage control. A whole-body CT scan would then be performed as soon as possible after surgery.

The pelvis was initially managed conservatively and had definitive surgical fixation on day 6. The femur and tibia/fibula fractures were managed with external fixation, and the spinal fracture was stabilized with internal fixation plates. The patient received a total of 12 units of red blood cells, 8 units of platelets, and 11 units of plasma. Consecutive ROTEM tests indicated an initial coagulopathy that subsequently normalized. Low-molecular-weight heparin was started on day 2 but had to be interrupted several times for planned returned to theatre.

✪ Learning point
Thromboprophylaxis

Although early mortality from trauma is often associated with haemorrhage and coagulopathy, trauma patients are also at high risk of subsequent venous thromboembolism and thromboprophylaxis is recommended as soon as it is practical. Mechanical prophylaxis can be commenced early when lower limbs are uninjured. Low-molecular-weight heparins are often commenced at 48 hours post injury although this can be controversial in the presence of intracranial bleeding which is not considered sufficiently settled [55–57].

❝ Expert comment

The timing of surgery is an important aspect of intensive care management of trauma patients with multiple injuries [61]. Historically, unstable patients spent many hours having all their injuries definitively managed. This early total management is now considered inappropriate for very unstable patients. Damage control surgery—early surgery to achieve haemostasis and control of contamination—may be more appropriate to enable correction of coagulopathy, temperature, and volume status and prevent severe systemic inflammatory response syndrome. Definitive surgery is delayed for these interventions. Fracture haemostasis can often be achieved with the use of effective splinting and external fixation techniques. In civilian practice, the need for damage control surgery is uncommon, but it is vital in the small proportion of severely injured, shocked patients received by MTCs. Most stable patients can be treated with early fracture fixation. Multidisciplinary discussion and coordination of trauma intensive care is vital to effective timing of surgery.

Enteral nutrition via a nasogastric tube was commenced on the day of admission to ICU. The patient remained in ICU sedated and his lungs ventilated with a lung protective ventilation strategy, particularly because of the presence of lung contusions [58, 59].

✪ Learning point   Lung injury and lung protective ventilation

Trauma patients are at risk of acute lung injury and acute respiratory distress syndrome for many reasons—for example, aspiration, hypoperfusion, direct lung injury, transfusion, fat embolus, systemic inflammatory response syndrome, and infection.

Lung protective ventilation with low tidal volumes (6 mL/kg predicted body weight), relatively high positive end-expiratory pressure (PEEP), and plateau pressures less than 30 cmH$_2$O is adopted early—ideally as soon as intubation has occurred to minimize risk. This can be challenging with severe chest injury (where lung contusion may necessitate use of relatively high PEEP values) or with a combination of chest injuries and head injury where lung protective ventilation strategies can conflict with ideal oxygenation and carbon dioxide management for head injury. There has been considerable recent interest in the potential benefits of non-invasive ventilation and newer modes of ventilation such as airway pressure release ventilation in trauma patients [59, 60].

❝ Expert comment

The management of severe lung injury can be difficult particularly in the presence of other pathologies with conflicting management requirements (particularly severe head injury). Non-invasive ventilation or high-flow nasal cannula oxygen are acceptable modes of support in non-intubated patients with respiratory compromise. Intubated patients with pulmonary contusion and/or flail chest should not be excessively fluid restricted, but fluid therapy should be titrated to achieve adequate organ perfusion. Thoracic epidurals provide analgesia and aid weaning in patients with only a few fractured ribs and no significant coagulopathy. In patients with major flail segments and compromise, evaluation by a thoracic surgeon for rib fixation should be considered. Although controversial, this procedure is increasingly performed and is associated with positive outcomes [63, 64].

After returning from initial surgery, a thorough tertiary survey was performed.

The tertiary survey in this patient revealed soft tissue injuries which were cleaned and dressed, and debrided during a subsequent trip to the operating theatre. Although the arrhythmias from the cardiac contusion quickly settled, the patient underwent echocardiography and cardiology evaluation including troponin testing.

⑮ Expert comment

Patients with cardiac rupture usually die at the scene and even if they arrive in the ED alive have a low survival rate. In patients with isolated chest injury, cardiac contusion can be excluded with a normal electrocardiogram and normal cardiac troponin values. When present, cardiac contusions are usually in the anterior heart (often the right ventricle). Most contusions resolve over days or weeks and do not usually cause long-term problems. Intensive care management of cardiac contusion is supportive with good fluid management, arrhythmia management, and inotropic support. Echocardiographic evaluation can detect the site and effect of contusions on cardiac function.

Regular multidisciplinary meetings between trauma, orthopaedic, and plastic surgeons, cardiologists, and intensivists were held. The patient's young age and the lack of pre-injury comorbidity were considered pivotal for his rapid recovery. Frequent complications such as haematomas, infections, and ventilatory problems did not occur. The patient was successfully extubated on day 5. At day 14 he was discharged for rehabilitation.

⑮ Expert comment

Effective rehabilitation is essential to return trauma patients to maximum functional status. This aspect of care has frequently been neglected. When the need for specialist rehabilitation is identified very early, referral is good practice—this includes spinal cord injury, brain injury, and prosthetics. In MTCs with well-functioning rehabilitation services, assessment of need and identification of likely complex rehabilitation needs are ideally assessed in the first few days after admission. This early assessment and commencement of rehabilitation has been termed acute or hyperacute rehabilitation. This may well occur on the ICU.

⑮ Expert comment

Trauma patients are particularly susceptible to gut hypoperfusion, sepsis, and multiorgan impairment. Early enteral nutrition has been associated with improved gut perfusion, lower rates of sepsis, lower rates of bacterial translocation, and improved mortality. Other therapies, including glutamine feed supplementation, lipid-rich enteral feeds, and protease inhibitors, have been suggested to improve outcomes, but are unproven [62].

✪ Learning point
Tertiary survey and missed injuries

Standardized trauma documentation is an important component of care after admission. It enables documentation of the fact that tertiary survey and appropriate imaging has occurred. This increases the likelihood that all injuries are detected and, where necessary, treated. Missed injuries are a particular problem in unconscious patients with multiple injuries.

Discussion

This chapter describes the patient pathway from the accident scene through to rehabilitation. This is intentional because critical care principles and interventions can be applied to improve outcomes at all points of the trauma patient pathway—not just within the confines of the ICU—this is in effect a restatement of the concept of 'critical care without walls' which stimulated the development of intensive therapy unit outreach services [65].

Optimal early management of multi-trauma is based on rapid and accurate identification of time-critical pathology. Multi-trauma is best managed with a multidisciplinary approach and careful coordination of surgical operations. Major trauma coordinators who monitor, track, and coordinate care of major trauma patients from admission to discharge are a key part of an effective trauma service.

Although in this case several aspects of intensive care have been highlighted that are specific to major trauma patients, most of the care delivered to trauma patients has much in common with the organ support and meticulous care that is required for all critically ill patients. One key difference between trauma and medical intensive care patients was often stated to be the relative youth of trauma patients. Although major trauma is still common in young adults, it is an increasingly common reason for elderly patients to be admitted to ICUs.

A final word from the expert

Most major trauma patients will spend some time in a critical care or high dependency area. However, this is only one part of the patient pathway and it is important to understand that the documented improvements in outcome for this group of patients have occurred only after implementation of inclusive trauma networks which include mandatory standards of care from incident to discharge. The monitoring and implementation of high-quality care is only possible when data are submitted to a national audit or registry. Regular dashboards and reports can then be generated to highlight areas for improvement or good practice. UK major trauma practice (in common with UK intensive care practice) has an effective system in place to achieve this in the form of the Trauma Audit and Research Network (TARN) (https://www.tarn.ac.uk).

Mortality is compared among centres and unexpected survivors and unexpected deaths are highlighted to direct quality improvement initiatives. Every hospital receiving trauma patients receives quarterly reports that document compliance with nationally defined quality indicators.

References

1. World Health Organization. *The Global Burden of Disease: 2004 update*. Geneva: World Health Organization; 2008.
2. World Health Organization. *Injuries and Violence: The Facts*. Geneva: World Health Organization; 2010.
3. Global Burden of Disease Study Collaborators. Global, regional, and national incidence, prevalence, and years lived with disability for 301 acute and chronic diseases and injuries in 188 countries, 1990–2013: a systematic analysis for the Global Burden of Disease Study 2013. *Lancet*. 2015;386:743–800.
4. Sasser S, Varghese M, Kellermann A, Lormand J. *Prehospital Trauma Care Systems*. Geneva: World Health Organization; 2005.
5. Gosselin RA, Spiegel DA, Coughlin R, Zirkle LG. Injuries: the neglected burden in developing countries. *Bull World Health Organ*. 2009;87:246.
6. Oteir AO, Smith K, Stoelwinder JU, Middleton J, Jennings PA. Should suspected cervical spinal cord injury be immobilised?: a systematic review. *Injury*. 2015;46:528–35.
7. Kreinest M, Gliwitzky B, Schuler S, Grutzner PA, Munzberg M. Development of a new Emergency Medicine Spinal Immobilization Protocol for trauma patients and a test of applicability by German emergency care providers. *Scand J Trauma Resusc Emerg Med*. 2016;24:71.

8. Strayer RJ, Nelson LS. Adverse events associated with ketamine for procedural sedation in adults. *Am J Emerg Med*. 2008;26:985–1028.

9. National Institute for Health and Care Excellence. *Major Trauma: Assessment and Initial Management*. London: National Institute for Health and Care Excellence; 2016.

10. Galinski M, Dolveck F, Borron SW, et al. A randomized, double-blind study comparing morphine with fentanyl in prehospital analgesia. *Am J Emerg Med*. 2005;23:114–19.

11. Soriya GC, McVaney KE, Liao MM, et al. Safety of prehospital intravenous fentanyl for adult trauma patients. *J Trauma Acute Care Surg*. 2012;72:755–9.

12. Arroyo W, Nelson KJ, Belmont PJ Jr, Bader JO, Schoenfeld AJ. Pelvic trauma: what are the predictors of mortality and cardiac, venous thrombo-embolic and infectious complications following injury? *Injury*. 2013;44:1745–9.

13. Croce MA, Magnotti LJ, Savage SA, Wood GW 2nd, Fabian TC. Emergent pelvic fixation in patients with exsanguinating pelvic fractures. *J Am Coll Surg*. 2007;204:935–9.

14. Demetriades D, Karaiskakis M, Toutouzas K, Alo K, Velmahos G, Chan L. Pelvic fractures: epidemiology and predictors of associated abdominal injuries and outcomes. *J Am Coll Surg*. 2002;195:1–10.

15. Gustavo Parreira J, Coimbra R, Rasslan S, Oliveira A, Fregoneze M, Mercadante M. The role of associated injuries on outcome of blunt trauma patients sustaining pelvic fractures. *Injury*. 2000;31:677–82.

16. Morrison JJ, Galgon RE, Jansen JO, Cannon JW, Rasmussen TE, Eliason JL. A systematic review of the use of resuscitative endovascular balloon occlusion of the aorta in the management of hemorrhagic shock. *J Trauma Acute Care Surg*. 2016;80:324–34.

17. Sadek S, Lockey DJ, Lendrum RA, Perkins Z, Price J, Davies GE. Resuscitative endovascular balloon occlusion of the aorta (REBOA) in the pre-hospital setting: an additional resuscitation option for uncontrolled catastrophic haemorrhage. *Resuscitation*. 2016;107:135–8.

18. Ghaemmaghami V, Sperry J, Gunst M, et al. Effects of early use of external pelvic compression on transfusion requirements and mortality in pelvic fractures. *Am J Surg*. 2007;194:720–3.

19. Pizanis A, Pohlemann T, Burkhardt M, Aghayev E, Holstein JH. Emergency stabilization of the pelvic ring: clinical comparison between three different techniques. *Injury*. 2013;44:1760–4.

20. Spanjersberg WR, Knops SP, Schep NW, van Lieshout EM, Patka P, Schipper IB. Effectiveness and complications of pelvic circumferential compression devices in patients with unstable pelvic fractures: a systematic review of literature. *Injury*. 2009;40:1031–5.

21. Crosby ET. Airway management in adults after cervical spine trauma. *Anesthesiology*. 2006;104:1293–318.

22. Krell JM, McCoy MS, Sparto PJ, Fisher GL, Stoy WA, Hostler DP. Comparison of the Ferno Scoop Stretcher with the long backboard for spinal immobilization. *Prehosp Emerg Care*. 2006;10:46–51.

23. Lockey DJ, Weaver AE, Davies GE. Practical translation of hemorrhage control techniques to the civilian trauma scene. *Transfusion*. 2013;53 Suppl. 1:17S–22S.

24. Hunt K, Hallworth S, Smith M. The effects of rigid collar placement on intracranial and cerebral perfusion pressures. *Anaesthesia*. 2001;56:511–13.

25. Chang LC, Raty SR, Ortiz J, Bailard NS, Mathew SJ. The emerging use of ketamine for anesthesia and sedation in traumatic brain injuries. *CNS Neurosci Ther*. 2013;19:390–5.

26. Kragh JF Jr, Walters TJ, Baer DG, et al. Survival with emergency tourniquet use to stop bleeding in major limb trauma. *Ann Surg*. 2009;249:1–7.

27. Lakstein D, Blumenfeld A, Sokolov T, et al. Tourniquets for hemorrhage control on the battlefield: a 4-year accumulated experience. *J Trauma Acute Care Surg*. 2003;54:S221–5.

28. Kragh JF Jr, Dubick MA, Aden JK, et al. U.S. Military use of tourniquets from 2001 to 2010. *Prehosp Emerg Care*. 2015;19:184–90.

29. Granville-Chapman J, Jacobs N, Midwinter MJ. Pre-hospital haemostatic dressings: a systematic review. *Injury*. 2011;42:447–59.

30. Geeraedts LM Jr, Kaasjager HA, van Vugt AB, Frolke JP. Exsanguination in trauma: a review of diagnostics and treatment options. *Injury*. 2009;40:11–20.

31. Ball CG, Wyrzykowski AD, Nicholas JM, Rozycki GS, Feliciano DV. A decade's experience with balloon catheter tamponade for the emergency control of hemorrhage. *J Trauma Acute Care Surg*. 2011;70:330–3.

32. Olaussen A, Williams B. Intraosseous access in the prehospital setting: literature review. *Prehosp Disaster Med*. 2012;27:468–72.

33. Etchill E, Sperry J, Zuckerbraun B, et al. The confusion continues: results from an American Association for the Surgery of Trauma survey on massive transfusion practices among United States trauma centers. *Transfusion*. 2016;56:2478–86.

34. Brohi K, Singh J, Heron M, Coats T. Acute traumatic coagulopathy. *J Trauma Acute Care Surg*. 2003;54:1127–30.

35. Frith D, Davenport R, Brohi K. Acute traumatic coagulopathy. *Curr Opin Anaesth*. 2012;25:229–34.

36. Davenport R, Manson J, De'Ath H, et al. Functional definition and characterization of acute traumatic coagulopathy. *Crit Care Med*. 2011;39:2652–8.

37. Mitra B, Cameron PA, Mori A, et al. Early prediction of acute traumatic coagulopathy. *Resuscitation*. 2011;82:1208–13.

38. McLaughlin DF, Niles SE, Salinas J, et al. A predictive model for massive transfusion in combat casualty patients. *J Trauma Acute Care Surg*. 2008;64:S57–63.

39. Rugeri L, Levrat A, David JS, et al. Diagnosis of early coagulation abnormalities in trauma patients by rotation thrombelastography. *J Thromb Haemo*. 2007;5:289–95.

40. Holcomb JB, Minei KM, Scerbo ML, et al. Admission rapid thrombelastography can replace conventional coagulation tests in the emergency department: experience with 1974 consecutive trauma patients. *Ann Surg*. 2012;256:476–86.

41. Holcomb JB, Jenkins D, Rhee P, et al. Damage control resuscitation: directly addressing the early coagulopathy of trauma. *J Trauma Acute Care Surg*. 2007;62:307–10.

42. CRASH-2 Trial Collaborators, Shakur H, Roberts I, et al. Effects of tranexamic acid on death, vascular occlusive events, and blood transfusion in trauma patients with significant haemorrhage (CRASH-2): a randomised, placebo-controlled trial. *Lancet*. 2010;376:23–32.

43. Miller BT, Du L, Krzyzaniak MJ, Gunter OL, Nunez TC. Blood transfusion: in the air tonight? *J Trauma Acute Care Surg*. 2016;81:15–20.

44. Brown JB, Sperry JL, Fombona A, Billiar TR, Peitzman AB, Guyette FX. Pre-trauma center red blood cell transfusion is associated with improved early outcomes in air medical trauma patients. *J Am Coll Surg*. 2015;220:797–808.

45. Holcomb JB, Donathan DP, Cotton BA, et al. Prehospital transfusion of plasma and red blood cells in trauma patients. *Prehosp Emerg Care*. 2015;19:1–9.

46. O'Reilly DJ, Morrison JJ, Jansen JO, Apodaca AN, Rasmussen TE, Midwinter MJ. Prehospital blood transfusion in the en route management of severe combat trauma: a matched cohort study. *J Trauma Acute Care Surg*. 2014;77:S114–20.

47. Wilkerson RG, Stone MB. Sensitivity of bedside ultrasound and supine anteroposterior chest radiographs for the identification of pneumothorax after blunt trauma. *Acad Emerg Med*. 2010;17:11–17.

48. Heng K, Bystrzycki A, Fitzgerald M, et al. Complications of intercostal catheter insertion using EMST techniques for chest trauma. *ANZ J Surg*. 2004;74:420–3.

49. Stevens RL, Rochester AA, Busko J, et al. Needle thoracostomy for tension pneumothorax: failure predicted by chest computed tomography. *Prehosp Emerg Care*. 2009;13:14–17.

50. Rawlins R, Brown KM, Carr CS, Cameron CR. Life threatening haemorrhage after anterior needle aspiration of pneumothoraces. A role for lateral needle aspiration in emergency decompression of spontaneous pneumothorax. *Emerg Med J*. 2003;20:383–4.

51. Lockey D, O'Brien B, Wise D, Davies G. Prehospital thoracostomy. *Eur J Emerg Med*. 2008;15:283.

52. Maybauer MO, Geisser W, Wolff H, Maybauer DM. Incidence and outcome of tube thoracostomy positioning in trauma patients. *Prehosp Emerg Care*. 2012;16:237–41.

53. Sasser SM, Hunt RC, Faul M, et al. Guidelines for field triage of injured patients: recommendations of the National Expert Panel on Field Triage, 2011. *MMWR Recomm Rep*. 2012;61:1–20.

54. National Institute for Health and Care Excellence. *Major Trauma: Service Delivery*. London: National Institute for Health and Care Excellence; 2016.

55. Van PY, Schreiber MA. Contemporary thromboprophylaxis of trauma patients. *Curr Opin Crit Care*. 2016;22:607–12.

56. Guyatt GH, Akl EA, Crowther M, et al. Executive summary: Antithrombotic Therapy and Prevention of Thrombosis, 9th ed: American College of Chest Physicians Evidence-Based Clinical Practice Guidelines. *Chest*. 2012;141:7S–47S.

57. Barrera LM, Perel P, Ker K, Cirocchi R, Farinella E, Morales Uribe CH. Thromboprophylaxis for trauma patients. *Cochrane Database Syst Rev*. 2013;3:CD008303.

58. Simon B, Ebert J, Bokhari F, et al. Management of pulmonary contusion and flail chest: an Eastern Association for the Surgery of Trauma practice management guideline. *J Trauma Acute Care Surg*. 2012;73:S351–61.

59. Parry NG, Moffat B, Vogt K. Blunt thoracic trauma: recent advances and outstanding questions. *Curr Opin Crit Care*. 2015;21:544–8.

60. Andrews PL, Shiber JR, Jaruga-Killeen E, et al. Early application of airway pressure release ventilation may reduce mortality in high-risk trauma patients: a systematic review of observational trauma ARDS literature. *J Trauma Acute Care Surg*. 2013;75:635–41.

61. Gandhi RR, Overton TL, Haut ER, et al. Optimal timing of femur fracture stabilization in polytrauma patients: a practice management guideline from the Eastern Association for the Surgery of Trauma. *J Trauma Acute Care Surg*. 2014;77:787–95.

62. Patel JJ, Rosenthal MD, Miller KR, Martindale RG. The gut in trauma. *Curr Opin Crit Care*. 2016;22:339–46.

63. Cataneo AJ, Cataneo DC, de Oliveira FH, Arruda KA, El Dib R, de Oliveira Carvalho PE. Surgical versus nonsurgical interventions for flail chest. *Cochrane Database Syst Rev*. 2015;7:CD009919.

64. Slobogean GP, MacPherson CA, Sun T, Pelletier ME, Hameed SM. Surgical fixation vs nonoperative management of flail chest: a meta-analysis. *J Am Coll Surg*. 2013;216:302–11.

65. Hillman K. Critical care without walls. *Curr Opin Crit Care*. 2002;8:594–9.

Severe traumatic brain injury

Virginia Newcombe

⦿ Expert Commentary Jamie Cooper

Case history

An 18-year-old male, restrained front seat passenger was involved in a high-speed motor vehicle collision. The driver of the vehicle died at the scene. On arrival at the scene the paramedics noted that he had obstructed-sounding breathing and initial arterial blood oxygen saturation by pulse oximetry (SpO_2) of 84%. This improved with simple airway manoeuvres and administration of oxygen. His initial blood pressure was 94/63 mmHg. His initial Glasgow Coma Scale (GCS) score was 8 (E2, V1, M5), his pupils were equal and reactive at 3 mm, and he was agitated. A rapid sequence induction was performed at the scene and he was intubated without incident. He was transferred to the nearest major trauma centre by road ambulance.

On arrival, the patient was received by a trauma team. A primary survey was performed which was unremarkable except for a scalp laceration. Given the mechanism of injury, he was taken for a trauma series computed tomography (CT) scan that included head, neck, chest, abdomen, and pelvis. His initial CT head showed multiple skull fractures, bifrontal contusions, traumatic subarachnoid haemorrhage, a right-sided subdural haemorrhage, multiple intracerebral petechial haemorrhages, and signs of tentorial herniation (Figure 5.1). No other injuries were found on the rest of his imaging.

⭐ **Learning point** Imaging after traumatic brain injury

The short imaging time and ease of acquisition means that CT scanning enables early assessment of the extent of injury after traumatic brain injury (TBI) and remains the standard imaging modality used [1, 2] (Table 5.1).

Table 5.1 The National Institute for Health and Care Excellence (NICE) and Scottish Intercollegiate Guidelines Network (SIGN) guideline recommendations of indications for a head CT following TBI in adults. NICE currently advises that a provisional radiology report should be available within 1 hour of the scan

Timing of scan	NICE guidelines	SIGN guidelines
Immediate CT (within 1 hour) of risk factor being identified	GCS score <13 on initial assessment in the emergency department	Eye opening only to pain or not conversing (GCS score ≤12)
	GCS score <15 at 2 hours after the injury on assessment in the emergency department	Confusion or drowsiness (GCS score 13–14) followed by failure to improve within 1 hour of clinical observation or within 2 hours of injury (whether or not intoxication from drugs or alcohol is a possible contributory factor)
	Suspected open or depressed skull fracture	
	Any sign of basal skull fracture: panda eyes, haemotympanum, cerebrospinal fluid leakage from the ear or nose, Battle's sign	Base of skull or depressed skull fracture and/or suspected penetrating injuries
	Post-traumatic seizure	A deteriorating level of consciousness or new focal neurological signs
	Focal neurological deficit	Full consciousness (GCS score 15) with no fracture but other features, e.g. severe and persistent headache, two distinct episodes of vomiting
	More than one episode of vomiting	
		A history of coagulopathy (e.g. warfarin use) and loss of consciousness, amnesia, or any neurological feature
CT within 8 hours of injury	For adults with any of the following risk factors who have experienced some loss of consciousness or amnesia since the injury:	Age >65 (with loss of consciousness or amnesia)
	Age ≥65 years	Clinical evidence of a skull fracture (e.g. boggy scalp haematoma) but no clinical features indicative of an immediate CT scan
	Any history of bleeding or clotting disorders	Any seizure activity
	Dangerous mechanism of injury (a pedestrian or cyclist struck by a motor vehicle, an occupant ejected from a motor vehicle, or a fall from a height of >1 metre or five stairs)	Significant retrograde amnesia (>30 min)
		Dangerous mechanism of injury (pedestrian struck by motor vehicle, occupant ejected from motor vehicle, significant fall from height) or significant assault (e.g. blunt trauma with a weapon)
	More than 30 min retrograde amnesia of events immediately before the head injury	
Anticoagulation treatment	For patients (adults and children) who have sustained a head injury with no other indications for a CT head scan and who are on warfarin, perform a CT head scan within 8 hours of the injury	A history of coagulopathy (e.g. warfarin use) irrespective of clinical features (high-quality observation is an appropriate alternative to scanning in this group of patients)

NICE, National Institute for Health and Care Excellence; SIGN, Scottish Intercollegiate Guidelines Network.
Source: data from National Institute for Health and Care Excellence (NICE). *Head Injury: assessment and early management* (CG176). Copyright © 2017 NICE. Available at https://www.nice.org.uk/guidance/cg176/; and Scottish Intercollegiate Guidelines Network (SIGN). *Early management of patients with a head injury*, Guideline 110. Copyright © 2017 SIGN. Available at http://www.sign.ac.uk/pdf/sign110.pdf.

Magnetic resonance imaging (MRI) can provide more detail; however, the logistics of transporting a ventilated patient with potentially high intracranial pressure (ICP) to the MRI suite means that it can be difficult to perform early and so is performed only in select centres. Later MRIs in patients, particularly those who do not wake, may be useful.

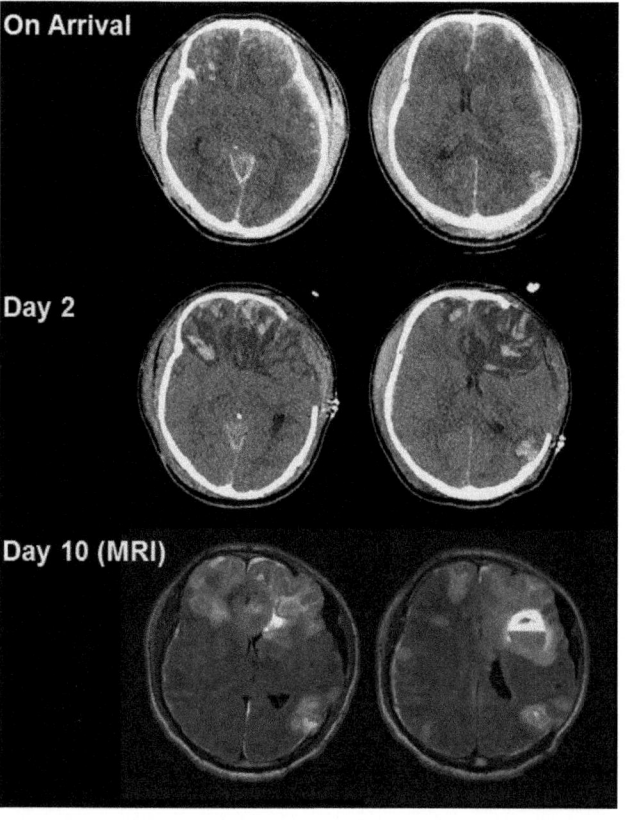

Figure 5.1 Progression of lesions after traumatic brain injury. The initial CT showed extensive bifrontal contusions, right parieto-occiptal contusion, right-sided subdural haemorrhage with midline shift, traumatic subarachnoid haemorrhage, and petechial haemorrhages. There are also signs of raised intracranial pressure with effacement of the ventricles, loss of the basal cisterns, and loss of grey/white differentiation. The CT performed on day 2 exhibits the right-sided hemicraniectomy and the progression of the contusions especially bifrontal. The MRI performed at day 10 demonstrates slices from the fluid-attenuated inversion recovery (FLAIR) sequence with the resolving haematomas still surrounded by vasogenic oedema.

> **✪ Clinical tip Spinal clearance in the unconscious patient**
>
> Cervical spine injuries occur in up to 7% of blunt trauma patients with the incidence increasing in those with coexisting TBI. Altered levels of consciousness increase the risk of missing such injuries. However, potential complications of prolonged spinal immobilization include risks of decubitus ulceration (especially cervical spine related), increased ICP, increased need for sedation and subsequent delay in extubation, delays in percutaneous tracheotomy, central venous access difficulties, deep venous thrombosis, enteral feeding intolerance due to supine positioning, increased respiratory compromise, and increased risk of cross-infection due to extra staff required for patient position changes [3]. It is therefore important to carefully exclude the possibility of a spinal injury in the TBI patient requiring intensive care unit (ICU) management as soon as is practical.
>
> Even in those not intubated, agitation and distracting injuries may render it impossible to perform an accurate clinical assessment and to safely exclude spinal injuries. Patients who require a CT head should also undergo a CT of their cervical spine to help with cervical spine clearance (Table 5.2). Spinal X-rays should be reserved for those who have no clear indication for a CT or imaging of other body areas.
>
> *(continued)*

The presence of vertebral malalignment, a fracture involving the transverse foramina or lateral processes, or a posterior circulation syndrome might indicate a vascular injury and in these cases CT or MRI angiography of the neck should be performed.

After trauma many patients undergo whole-body CT to assess for thoracoabdominal injuries. This data can be reformatted to enable review of the entire spine and enable identification of fractures, their stability, and spinal alignment.

Fractures of the spine are demonstrated more clearly with CT than with MRI. In the unconscious TBI patient, dynamic flexion–extension fluoroscopy studies of the cervical spine provide no more information than fine-cut CT and are not recommended [4, 5]. Consider cervical spine MRI if a patient has signs and symptoms of spinal cord injury, or if the CT scan in an unconscious patient is indicative or suggestive of discoligamentous injury, or they are elderly with evidence of spine degeneration.

Table 5.2 NICE and SIGN guideline recommendations of indications for cervical spine scanning following TBI in adults

	NICE guidelines	SIGN guidelines
Three-view cervical X-rays	Only if does not meet criteria for CT cervical spine If it is not considered safe to assess the range of movement in the neck Safe assessment of range of neck movement shows that the patient cannot actively rotate their neck to 45° to the left and right	
CT cervical spine scan (within 1 hour of identification of risk factor)	GCS score <13 on initial assessment The patient has been intubated Plain X-rays are technically inadequate (e.g. the desired view is unavailable) Plain X-rays are suspicious or definitely abnormal A definitive diagnosis of cervical spine injury is needed urgently (e.g. before surgery) The patient is having other body areas scanned for head injury or multi-region trauma The patient is alert and stable, there is clinical suspicion of cervical spine injury, and any of the following apply: • Age 65 years or older • Dangerous mechanism of injury (fall from a height of >1 metre or five stairs) • Axial load to the head, e.g. diving • High-speed motor vehicle collision • Rollover motor accident • Ejection from a motor vehicle • Accident involving motorized recreational vehicles • Bicycle collision • Focal peripheral neurological deficit • Paraesthesia in the upper or lower limbs	In adult patients with GCS score <15 with indications for a CT head scan, the scan should include the cervical spine Cervical spine CT scan should include the base of skull to T4 Patients who meet criteria for a CT scan should not have plain radiographs of the cervical spine taken as routine

NICE, National Institute for Health and Care Excellence; SIGN, Scottish Intercollegiate Guidelines Network.
Source: data from National Institute for Health and Care Excellence (NICE). *Head Injury: assessment and early management* (CG176). Copyright © 2017 NICE. Available at https://www.nice.org.uk/guidance/cg176/; and Scottish Intercollegiate Guidelines Network (SIGN). *Early management of patients with a head injury*, Guideline 110. Copyright © 2017 SIGN. Available at http://www.sign.ac.uk/pdf/sign110.pdf.

On return to the resuscitation bay after his CT scan, the patient's left pupil was noted to be 8 mm and unreactive and his right pupil was 3 mm and reactive. He was given a bolus of 350 mL 20% mannitol (70 g, estimated 1 mg/kg), sedation was increased, he was reparalysed, and his ventilation was increased to reduce the end-tidal carbon dioxide (CO_2) to 4.0–4.5 kPa. He was taken urgently to the operating room where an emergency right-sided decompressive hemicraniectomy was performed and an intraparenchymal pressure monitor inserted. An external ventricular drain (EVD) could not be inserted because of the small ventricular size. His initial ICP was 50 mmHg, decreasing to 23 mmHg after decompression. On arrival in the ICU, his pupils were both 2 mm and reactive.

> ✪ **Learning point** Hypocapnia/hyperventilation
>
> Hypocapnia causes cerebral vasoconstriction, reducing cerebral blood volume, which can decrease ICP rapidly and increase cerebral perfusion pressure (CPP). However, this is usually accompanied by a global decrease in cerebral blood flow that may lead to cerebral ischaemia [6]. Hyperventilation should therefore be used *only* as a temporizing measure while instituting other therapies to reduce intracranial hypertension. If it is used, brain tissue oxygen values or jugular venous oximetry should be used to monitor adequacy of oxygen delivery [7]. However, metabolic imaging with positron emission tomography scanning has shown that even moderate reductions in $PaCO_2$ may cause ischaemia in focal areas not detected with jugular venous oximetry, thus even with this monitoring, hyperventilation may be harmful [6].

> ✪ **Learning point** Osmotherapy
>
> There are multiple mechanisms by which hyperosmolar therapy, most commonly mannitol or hypertonic saline (HS), is purported to reduce raised ICP. Traditionally such therapy is thought to raise plasma osmolality and so cause an osmotic withdrawal of cerebral water though an intact blood–brain barrier. However, they may also reduce erythrocyte and endothelial cell size, improve erythrocyte deformability, and affect leucocyte adhesion. These effects are believed to contribute to improved microvascular flow. Typically they are given as boluses to reduce acute rises in ICP, and their role in long-term ICP reduction is unclear.
>
> Mannitol (0.25–2.0 g/kg, usually given as a 20% solution) is the traditionally used hyperosmolar agent. If used after the first few hours of injury, it may cause a secondary increase in ICP if the blood–brain barrier is disrupted. Hypernatraemia, intravascular depletion, and arterial hypotension may occur secondary to the osmotic diuresis. Recurrent use may cause renal impairment and so it should be discontinued if it no longer produces a significant ICP reduction, and plasma osmolality greater than 320 mOsm/L.
>
> HS solutions are available in variable concentrations (3% up to 28.4%). Usual doses are approximately 2 mL/kg of 5% saline or 10 mL of 28.4% HS. This may be repeated if serum sodium remains at less than 155 mmol/L and plasma osmolality is less than 320 mOsm/L. Targeting a specific serum sodium is unwise as total body sodium and water will progressively rise and may contribute to delayed intracranial hypertension. Treatment with HS is generally considered safe in TBI but it can cause central pontine myelinolysis if given to patients with pre-existing chronic hyponatraemia.

> ❻ **Expert comment**
>
> Equimolar doses of mannitol and HS reduce ICP equally, but HS does not cause the diuresis associated with mannitol [8] and therefore does not risk decreasing intravascular volume and cerebral blood flow. It is thought that HS may improve CPP to a greater extent than mannitol and may improve brain tissue oxygen values [9]. In a small study of 38 patients, HS provided better ICP control than mannitol with a concomitant reduction in inotropic requirements, but this physiological advantage did not translate into improved outcomes [10]
>
> HS seems to be gaining favour in most places, but a meta-analysis of randomized controlled trials (RCTs) comparing the two directly has found trials to have been underpowered and did not find statistically significant differences in outcome or mortality [11]. In practice, it is common to give mannitol or the lower-concentration HS solutions (7.5% and below) on presentation of a patient before central venous access has been established.

✪ Learning point Cerebral perfusion pressure

Current Brain Trauma Foundation guidelines focus on targeted management of ICP and CPP where:

$$CPP = mean\ arterial\ pressure\ (MAP) - ICP$$

The Neuroanaesthesia Society of Great Britain and Ireland and the Society of British Neurological Surgeons currently recommend that the arterial transducer is set at the level of the tragus (approximating the middle cranial fossa), regardless of the patient position, rather than the phlebostatic axis (heart level) to enable more accurate calculation of CPP. Individual differences in cerebral arterial and venous circulations mean that it is not possible to determine a coefficient (C) that accurately takes this into account if the transducer is left at the phlebostatic axis:

$$MAP\ brain = MAP\ heart - (water\ column\ between\ the\ heart\ and\ brain \times C)$$

A CPP target of 60–70 mmHg is commonly used as cerebral oxygenation decreases at lower pressures even with an intact cerebral autoregulation. CPP is used as a surrogate for cerebral blood flow, but cerebral vascular resistance is variable, so even with an adequate CPP there may still be areas of reduced perfusion. CPP may be increased by augmenting MAP or reducing ICP, but these interventions (including vasopressors, inotropes, or fluid resuscitation) may be harmful.

Cerebrovascular pressure reactivity is the ability of cerebral vessels to respond to changes in transmural pressure. The relationship between ICP and arterial blood pressure can be used to determine the cerebrovascular pressure reactivity index (PRx) for each patient. PRx can be interpreted as an index of cerebral autoregulation (positive implies impaired reactivity, negative intact cerebral reactivity).

To target the best blood pressure, individualized CPP thresholds or an 'optimal CPP', can be determined. This is the lowest point on a CPP versus PRx graph, that is, where cerebral autoregulation is working at its best. Use of the optimal CPP has been associated with an improved outcome and may present an avenue for more personalized care.

✪ Learning point Intracranial pressure monitoring devices

Raised ICP is associated with worse neurological outcomes. ICP monitoring is considered to be the standard of care for severe TBI worldwide [12].

Brain Trauma Foundation guidelines list the following indications for ICP monitoring:

- Patients with moderate–severe TBI who cannot be serially neurologically assessed.
- Severe head injury (GCS <8) with an abnormal CT scan.
- Severe head injury (GCS <8) with a normal CT if any two of the following are present: age over 40 years, systolic blood pressure less than 90 mmHg, or abnormal posturing [12].

The most commonly used devices to monitor ICP are intraventricular catheters (EVD or a ventriculostomy drain) and intraparenchymal fibreoptic monitors.

EVDs are the gold standard, and are placed in the lateral ventricle at the level of the foramen of Monro. Zero level is the external auditory meatus. These drains have the advantage of enabling monitoring as well as treatment of an elevated ICP via cerebrospinal fluid drainage. Risks of an EVD include parenchymal haematoma, infection (usually ventriculitis), damage to brain parenchyma, and overventing of cerebrospinal fluid.

Intraparenchymal monitors have lower complication rates including less risk of bleeding, and infection. Their smaller diameter also leads to less neuronal injury compared to an EVD. However, they are only able to be calibrated prior to insertion and are prone to drift off the zero point over time after insertion. They also do not indicate infratentorial pressure.

Extradural monitors use a catheter inserted via a burr hole but that does not penetrate the dura. They often have signal damping and so underestimate high ICP.

In general, an ICP greater than 15 mmHg is considered to be abnormally high. Most guidelines aim for either an ICP less than 20 mmHg or less than 25 mmHg, but there is little evidence for an exact cut off. Some protocols allow for a target of 20 mmHg to be relaxed to 25 mmHg if an adequate CPP is maintained.

✓ Evidence base

Benchmark Evidence from South American Trials: Treatment of Intracranial Pressure (BEST:TRIP) [13]

- 324 patients (ICP monitoring group, n = 157; imaging-clinical examination group, n = 167)
- Intervention: ICP monitoring with treatment targeted at maintaining ICP at less than 20 mmHg versus treatment based on clinical finding and CT scan results.
- Primary outcome: composite of 21 components including measures of survival, functional status, and neurocognitive status.
- No significant difference between the groups for the primary outcome measure.

❝ Expert comment

Rather than a test of ICP as a target per se this trial tested two different TBI management strategies in a resource-limited setting. It indicates that we need to refine how ICP is used in TBI management, better integrating signals from all available information and monitors.

The patient was admitted to the ICU. He was sedated with propofol and alfentanil infusions. A nasogastric tube was inserted, after a base of skull fracture was been excluded on CT, and enteral feed started. Tier one neuroprotective measures were instituted to keep his ICP at less than 20 mmHg and CPP greater than 60 mmHg (see Learning point on 'Tiered approach to management of raised ICP').

✪ Learning point Tiered approach to management of raised intracranial pressure

Protocolized management of severe TBI has been shown to improve outcomes [14]. Such protocols tend to be organized into tiers that reflect increasing intensity of therapy and increasing risk of side effects secondary to this therapy. The simplest approach is two tiers; however, some protocols break down the tiers further to encourage a step-wise progression in ICP management ensuring the simplest and safest interventions are done first. There is no clear consensus on how therapies should be split across two-, three-, or four-tier protocols and this should be considered when interpreting the results of RCTs or reading different protocols. An example of a split into tier one and tier two therapies is given in Table 5.3.

Table 5.3 Tiered treatments for management of raised ICP

Tier one	
1	Sit the patient up at 30–45°. Improve venous drainage. If this is not possible because of pelvic and other injuries, sit the patient up as much as allowed to reduce ICP without reduction in CPP, or tilt the entire bed
2	Avoid jugular compression by positioning the head facing forward
3	Remove the cervical spine collar. This may reduce ICP by approximately 4–5 mmHg. In a patient with an uncleared cervical spine, make it obvious to staff that spinal precautions are still in place, e.g. by placing sandbags on either side of the neck
4	Improve cerebral venous outflow by ensuring tracheal tube ties are not tight
5	Avoid internal jugular lines where possible, due to the increased risk of thrombus
6	Decrease PEEP if feasible while ensuring adequate oxygenation. A PEEP of 5 cmH$_2$O has no effect on ICP but in patients with raised ICP, PEEP of 10–15 cmH$_2$O may increase ICP by 1–2 mmHg
7	If there is an EVD, vent cerebrospinal fluid
8	Aim for normocarbia (PaCO$_2$ 4.5–5.0 kPa)
9	Sedation and analgesia
10	Paralysis
11	Osmotherapies (mannitol, hypertonic saline)
Tier two	
1	Barbiturate coma
2	Therapeutic hypothermia (moderate, 32–34°C)
3	Decompressive craniectomy

PEEP, positive end-expiratory pressure.

✪ Learning point Sedation

Benzodiazepines and propofol reduce cerebral metabolic rate ($CMRO_2$), cerebral blood flow, and ICP without impairing cerebral autoregulation and CO_2 reactivity. However, as the level of metabolic suppression achieved with midazolam is much less than with propofol, and it is associated with increased incidence of delirium and withdrawal symptoms, propofol is the sedative of choice.

Higher-dose, prolonged propofol infusions greater than 4 mg/kg/hour are associated with propofol infusion syndrome and the risk of propofol infusion syndrome is exacerbated by factors which may impair propofol metabolism (e.g. therapeutic hypothermia). This poorly understood syndrome is associated with progressive cardiac failure, rhabdomyolysis, metabolic acidosis, and renal failure. High propofol requirements therefore may require the addition of a benzodiazepine. Another indication includes patients with benzodiazepine dependency to avoid unrecognized withdrawal.

Opioids are not directly neuroprotective but are hypnotic sparing, provide analgesia, and have antitussive properties. This may be particularly useful to minimize ICP rises secondary to coughing, while enabling neurological assessment in suitable patients.

Barbiturates, typically thiopentone, are very effective at reducing ICP via profound cerebral metabolic suppression. They modulate the GABA chloride-ion channel, inhibiting the action potential by producing neuronal hyperpolarization. They also inhibit excitatory l-glutamate AMPA receptors, stopping calcium transport through voltage-gated calcium channels. Following a bolus of thiopentone, termination of its effects occurs mainly by redistribution of the relatively lipophilic drug into tissues, particularly fat. Prolonged infusions lead to significant accumulation in fat and continuing sedation long after infusions have been stopped. This long 'context-sensitive half-life' (thiopentone 6–46 hours) causes the kinetics to change from first order to zero order when burst suppression is achieved. Myocardial depression, central vasomotor depression, and haemodynamic instability may occur. These side effects mean that barbiturates tend to be restricted to patients with intracranial hypertension refractory to safer treatments.

✪ Learning point Nutritional support

After a severe TBI patients tend to be hypermetabolic, hypercatabolic, and hyperglycaemic. Early enteral feeding is recommended, as it helps to stimulate gut function, preserve intestinal mucosal integrity, preserve the immunological gastrointestinal tract barrier function, and reduce infection rates. A Cochrane review (284 patients) found no difference in the mortality rate of patients who were fed early compared with those fed later [17]. (See also Case 13.)

✪ Learning point Fluids

Isotonic crystalloids should be used for fluid management and 0.9% sodium chloride is the recommended solution. However, large volumes of 0.9% sodium chloride cause hyperchloraemic metabolic acidosis. Hypotonic solutions (e.g. 5% dextrose) may reduce serum osmolality and should be avoided in the acute phase of injury. In the Saline versus Albumin Fluid Evaluation (SAFE) trial, 4% albumin was associated with increased mortality in patients with TBI and therefore should be avoided [18].

✪ Learning point Venous thromboembolism prophylaxis

The hypercoagulability induced in TBI increases the risk of deep vein thrombosis, which affects approximately one in six patients [15]. However, the precise time for safe and effective chemical prophylaxis without contributing to progression of intracranial haemorrhage is uncertain. There is little evidence on which to base guidelines, which has led to considerable practice variation and clinical uncertainty. A common approach is to wait for stabilization of bleeding seen on serial CT scans, with chemical prophylaxis being started 24–48 hours after lack of progression is demonstrated [16]. In patients who are not on chemoprophylaxis, thromboembolic disease stocking and/or intermittent pneumatic compression devices should be used where possible. Other options include the use of inferior vena cava filters, these may be particularly of use in patients with a concurrent pelvic injury (see also Case 13).

Over the first few hours in ICU, his urine output increased to more than 250 mL/hour and his plasma sodium increased from an admission value of 140 mmol/L to 159 mmol/L (Figure 5.2). Matched plasma (320 mOsm/L) and urinary osmolality (< 300 mOsmol/L) were consistent with diabetes insipidus and he was administered 1-deamino-8-d-arginine vasopressin (DDAVP); this led to a rapid reduction in urine output to normal volumes.

✪ Learning point Sodium in traumatic brain injury

Disorders of sodium homeostasis are common after TBI. Repeated hyperosmolar therapy is a common cause of hypernatraemia. Mild increases in sodium may be tolerated. Approximately 1% of patients may develop central diabetes insipidus voiding large volumes of dilute urine, and are at risk of dehydration.

(continued)

The more severe hypernatraemia of diabetes insipidus will require DDAVP. Intravenous water replacement may reduce the osmolality too rapidly and enteral water is preferred. Hypernatraemia is associated with an increased risk of death even in patients without diabetes insipidus [19].

Hyponatraemia is common and may worsen cerebral oedema, decrease consciousness, and reduce the seizure threshold. It is usually considered to be secondary to either the syndrome of inappropriate antidiuretic hormone secretion or cerebral salt-wasting syndrome but the distinction is often difficult (Table 5.4). The speed at which hyponatraemia should be normalized depends on its chronicity, as rapid correction in chronic hyponatraemia may cause central pontine myelinolysis. Whether this is due to rapid sodium correction per se, or whether it is due to other factors in predisposed patients (e.g. chronic alcoholism) is unclear.

Table 5.4 Disordered sodium homeostasis after TBI

	Serum sodium	Volume status	Plasma osmolality	Urine osmolality	Management
Dehydration	Increased	Hypovolaemic	Increased	Increased	Volume replacement
Central diabetes insipidus	Increased	Hypovolaemic	Increased	Decreased	DDAVP May need 5% dextrose or 0.45% normal saline
Syndrome of inappropriate antidiuretic hormone secretion (SIADH)	Decreased	Euvolaemic or hypervolaemic	Decreased	Increased	Fluid restriction If not effective, consider hypertonic saline
Cerebral salt wasting	Decreased	Hypovolaemic	Decreased	Increased	Volume replacement with normal saline. If not effective, consider hypertonic saline and fludrocortisone

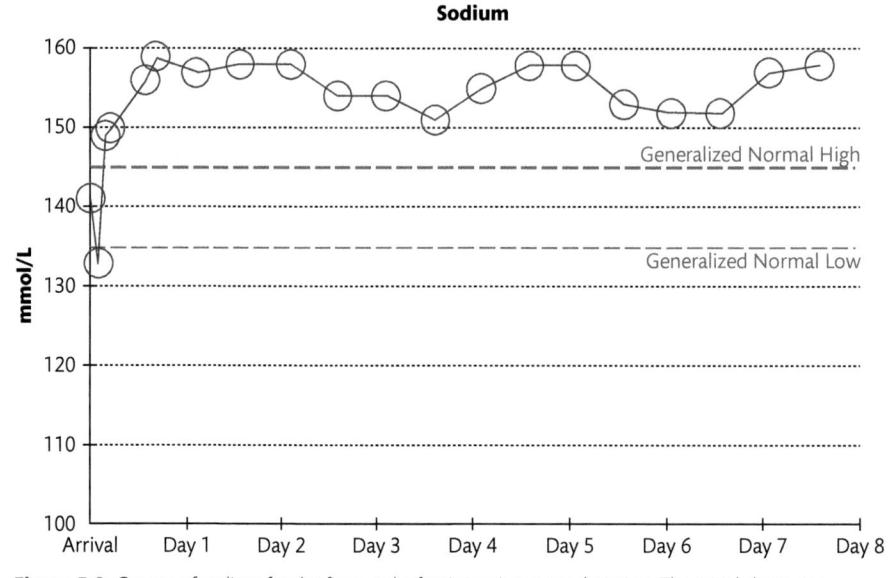

Figure 5.2 Course of sodium for the first week after intensive care admission. The initial sharp rise corresponds to the development of diabetes insipidus.

☆ Learning point
Surgical management after traumatic brain injury

Prompt evacuation of subdural and extradural haemorrhage causing mass effect is well established as appropriate therapy. However, evidence is lacking about how best to manage intraparenchymal haemorrhages and contusions, as well as raised ICP refractory to medical management. These knowledge gaps have stimulated several surgical trials over the past decade.

The patient's ICP continued to remain a problem despite the tier one interventions. While his serum sodium level remained less than 155 mmol/L and plasma osmolarity level less than 320 mOsm/L he was given HS boluses. After this, boluses of thiopentone were administered which temporarily reduced the ICP. On the second day, a CT brain scan was repeated to exclude a surgically amenable cause for the ICP rises. This scan demonstrated that the cerebral contusions had markedly increased in size.

✔ **Evidence base**

Surgical Trial in Traumatic Intracerebral Haemorrhage (STITCH(Trauma)) [20, 21]

- Halted early by the UK funding authority for failure to recruit. Results need to be interpreted in this context.
- Included 170 randomized patients (initial target 840).
- Inclusion criteria: to recruit within 48 hours of TBI. Up to two intraparenchymal haemorrhages of greater than 10 mL without an extradural or subdural haematoma that required surgery.
- Exclusion criteria: significant surface haematoma (extradural or subdural haemorrhage) needing surgery, three or more separate haematomas, cerebellar haemorrhage, or contusion.
- Intervention: early evacuation of the haematoma by a method of the surgeon's choice (within 12 hours of randomization), combined with appropriate best medical treatment versus initial conservative treatment. This was best medical treatment combined with delayed (>12 hours after randomization) evacuation if indicated by GCS score, neurology, and ICP/CPP in invasively monitored patients.
- Outcome measure: dichotomized Glasgow Outcome Scale.
- Result: no significant difference between the two groups.
- Conclusions: surgery in this group cannot currently be recommended. Study was likely under-powered.

Decompressive Craniectomy (DECRA) trial [22]

- Included 155 patients (3478 patients screened)
- Inclusion criteria: ages 15–59 years, severe non-penetrating injury (GCS score <8) or moderate diffuse injury on CT (Marshall grade III)
- Exclusion criteria: unsurvivable injury, dilated unreactive pupils, mass lesions requiring surgery, spinal cord injury, or cardiac arrest.
- Intervention: early (within 72 hours) decompressive craniectomy (n = 73) versus standard care (n = 82) of whom 15 required craniectomy.
- Trigger for intervention: spontaneous (non-stimulated) increase in ICP for longer than 15 min within 1-hour period, despite optimized first-tier interventions.
- Outcome measure: unfavourable (composite of death, vegetative state, or severe disability) on extended Glasgow Outcome Scale (eGOS) at 6 months.
- Results: patients in the craniectomy group had:
  o less time with ICP above treatment threshold (P <0.001)
  o fewer interventions for increased ICP (P <0.02)
  o fewer days in ICU (P <0.001)
  o (primary outcome) worse scores on eGOS than those who had standard care and greater risk of unfavourable outcome.
- Rates of death at 6 months were similar in the craniectomy group (19%) and the standard-care group (18%).

Randomised Evaluation of Surgery with Craniectomy for Uncontrollable Elevation of Intracranial Pressure (RESCUE-ICP) [23]

- Included 408 patients.
- Inclusion criteria: 10–65 years, abnormal CT, ICP monitoring *in situ*, raised ICP (>25 mmHg) for 1–12 hours despite tier one and tier two measures described previously. Patients could be included if they had already had surgery as long as the operation was not a craniectomy (so bone flap was replaced at the end of procedure).

(continued)

- Exclusion criteria: bilateral fixed dilated pupils, bleeding diathesis, or injury deemed to be unsurvivable.
- Primary outcome: eGOS at 6 months using a proportional odds model.
- Primary results: lower mortality and higher rates of vegetative state, lower severe disability and upper severe disability than medical care in intervention group. Rates of moderate disability and good recovery were similar.
- Secondary outcomes: at 12 months more patients with craniectomy had favourable outcomes (upper severe disability or better) than those in the medical group (45.4% vs 32.4%; P = 0.01).

Expert comment

While RESCUE-ICP showed a clear survival benefit for late decompression, more survivors in the surgical group had severe disability at 6 months. This trial supports the need for more investigation into how best to select patients for decompressive craniectomy after TBI.

On day 4, the patient became febrile to 39°C with increased respiratory secretions and a rise in his oxygen requirements. After a full septic screen, he was started on antibiotics for a ventilator-associated pneumonia. Concurrent with the rise in temperature, it became more difficult to keep his ICP and CPP within target ranges. He was cooled to normothermia with subsequent improvement in ICP and CPP control.

Learning point Temperature management

Peak temperatures below 37°C and above 39°C in the first 24 hours after ICU admission have been associated with an increased risk of death compared with normothermia [24]. There is some evidence that patients who arrive hypothermic have worse outcomes. It is likely that hypothermia is a marker of injury severity and active rewarming of such patients is generally not recommended. However, in practice many patients with TBI have multiple injuries and are often aggressively rewarmed to reduce bleeding.

In contrast, especially during the early phase of TBI, aggressive management of hyperthermia is considered beneficial because it decreases ICP and mitigates the increase in metabolic rate normally associated with fever. Fever will increase glutamate release and inflammatory activity, further compromising an already injured brain. It is important not to assume that hyperthermia has a neurogenic cause until other causes including sepsis and drugs and have been excluded.

Hypothermia reduces intracranial hypertension, may provide neuroprotection, and may prevent secondary brain injury via a variety of mechanisms including the reduction of $CMRO_2$, inflammation, and oedema. However, hypothermia also has many side effects and complications including immunosuppression, bradycardia, reduced cardiac contractility, electrolyte abnormalities (which may be secondary to cold diuresis), coagulopathy, and shivering. Whether and when therapeutic hypothermia should be used is controversial; consequently, its use is commonly limited to when elevated ICP is refractory to other therapies. Rewarming must be controlled and performed slowly (0.3–0.5°C/hour) to avoid systemic side effects including haemodynamic compromise from vasodilation, arrhythmias, and elevated ICP. Rapid rewarming has been associated with poorer neurological outcomes in small studies [25].

Evidence base

European Study of Therapeutic Hypothermia (32–35°C) for Intracranial Pressure Reduction after Traumatic Brain Injury (Eurotherm3235) [26]

- Included 387 patients (209 intervention group, 170 control group).
- ICP greater than 20 mmHg despite tier one therapy.
- Intervention: hypothermia (32–25°C) with tier two therapy only if cooling failed versus standard care with tier two therapies. Tier three therapies (barbiturates and decompressive craniectomy) were only used if tier two therapies failed to control ICP.
- Primary outcome: eGOS at 6 months.
- Results: favourable outcome (eGOS 5–8, moderate disability or good recovery) in 26% in the hypothermia group versus 37% in the control group (P = 0.03).

Expert comment

Eurotherm3235 provides evidence that using hypothermia as an early measure to control ICP is harmful [26]. However, it provides no guidance on the use of hypothermia for either refractory intracranial hypertension after the failure of tier two or other tier three interventions, or very early before intracranial hypertension and injury are established. The Prophylactic Hypothermia Trial to Lessen Traumatic Brain Injury (POLAR) is an RCT attempting to answer the second question, by using cooling within 4 hours of injury, and is currently recruiting [27].

By the second week, ICP was stable at less than 20 mmHg with no intervention required. With sedation holds the patient became hypertensive and tachycardic and he was intolerant of the tracheal tube; his neurology remained poor at E2, M4. An electroencephalogram showed no evidence of seizure activity.

> ### ✪ Learning point Post-traumatic seizures
>
> Post traumatic seizures occur 'early' (within 7 days) and/or 'late' (>7 days) with an incidence ranging between 4–25% and 9–42% respectively. The exact incidence is difficult to quantify accurately because of difficulties in clinically diagnosing seizures, as well as potentially masking signs with the use of sedatives. Risk factors for early post-traumatic seizures are a GCS score less than 10, intracranial haematoma, contusions, penetrating injuries, and depressed skull fractures.
>
> Seizures in the acute phase may increase ICP, as well as place an increased metabolic demand on damaged brain tissue and so aggravate secondary brain injury. While a recent Cochrane review found only low-quality evidence that early treatment with an antiepileptic drug compared with placebo or standard care reduced the risk of early post-traumatic seizures, the adverse sequelae of such seizures mean it is not uncommon for clinicians to prescribe 7 days of antiepileptic drugs. Phenytoin or levetiracetam are commonly used, and while there is no clear evidence favouring either, there is some literature suggesting that phenytoin may be associated with worse neurological and functional outcomes [28]. Subclinical seizures may be found using continuous electroencephalographic monitoring but the significance of these is as yet unknown. There is no evidence that using antiepileptic drugs reduces the risk of late seizures or improves neurological outcome or mortality.

> ### ✪ Expert comment
>
> This is a contentious area with a paucity of good evidence on which to base recommendations. There is no consensus on the need for prophylactic antiepileptic drugs, which drug to give, and the duration of treatment. Given the need to balance side effects of antiepileptic drugs with avoiding the detrimental effect of seizures, those at highest risk may represent a subgroup in whom to target therapy. Those wanting more detail about the pros and cons of seizure prophylaxis are directed to a pro/con debate in the literature [29].

An MRI was performed on day 10 which revealed expected progression of the contusions, and importantly that there were no brainstem lesions. A decision was made to insert a percutaneous tracheostomy. The patient continued to make slow neurological improvement and was discharged to a rehabilitation centre.

He returned 6 months later for follow-up at the neurotrauma clinic where it was found that he had made steady progress, and while he still required assistance with activities of daily living he was expected to be discharged home in the next month.

> ### ✪ Learning point Prognosis after traumatic brain injury
>
> Outcomes after TBI range from complete recovery through to severe disability, including vegetative states, and death. Being able to accurately predict outcome would help to support early clinical decision-making, improve individual management, and enable more effective clinical trials to be developed. As yet, there is no tool that is sufficiently accurate for the prediction of outcome to use on an individual basis in clinical practice. The IMPACT model (International Mission for Prognosis and Analysis of Clinical Trials; http://www.tbi-impact.org) is the most extensively validated scoring system, developed on a cohort of more than 9000 patients. There is a clear association with poor outcome with advancing age, a low GCS score (especially the motor component), bilateral fixed pupil(s), single episodes of hypotension or hypoxaemia, and certain CT abnormalities including the presence of traumatic subarachnoid haemorrhage.

(continued)

Important scoring systems

The GCS was designed for use in the acute phase of TBI [30]. It is a useful tool for the early assessment of injury severity in addition to providing some crude prognostic information (Table 5.5). Immediately after an injury, the GCS may be depressed by other factors including hypoxaemia, hypotension, and seizures. Post-resuscitation, pre-intubation GCS score is the most common score used in prognostic models but the optimal timing to assess the GCS score is unclear.

The Glasgow Outcome Scale and its extended version (eGOS) are the most common outcome scores used in clinical trials of TBI [31]. Many studies dichotomize these scores for ease of analysis. For example, the Glasgow Outcome Scale may be categorized into good outcome (score of 4–5) and poor outcome (score of 1–3). For the eGOS, a good outcome is generally judged as a score of 4–8 and poor as 1–3. The scores are relatively quick and easy to apply to large numbers of patients in the context of a clinical trial, but they do not give a true reflection of the neurocognitive status, functional status, or psychiatric issues that patients may experience after TBI.

Table 5.5 Important scoring systems

Glasgow Coma Scale		Glasgow Outcome Scale		
Eye opening		1	Dead	
Spontaneous	4	2	Vegetative	Exhibits no cortical function
To sound	3	3	Severe disability	Dependent for daily support
To pain	2			
No response	1			
Best verbal response		4	Moderate disability	Disabled but independent, no assistance with activities of daily living
Orientated	5			
Confused	4			
Inappropriate words	3	5	Good recovery	Resumption of normal life, may have minor deficits
Incomprehensible sounds	2			
None	1			
Best motor response				
Obeys commands	6	**Extended Glasgow Outcome Scale**		
Localizes pain	5	1	Dead	
Flexion (withdrawal)	4	2	Vegetative state	
Flexion (abnormal)	3	3	Lower severe disability	
Extension	2	4	Upper severe disability	
		5	Lower moderate disability	
		6	Upper moderate disability	
None	1	7	Lower good recovery	
		8	Upper good recovery	

Discussion

TBI is a major cause of death and disability, particularly in those less than 40 years of age and the elderly. In the UK alone, TBI affects 0.5–1 million people annually, resulting in nearly 150,000 hospital admissions per year (http://www.hesonline.nhs.uk). The great complexity and variability of TBI represents a significant barrier to the identification and implementation of effective treatment strategies.

Conceptually, TBI has been divided into primary and secondary injury. After the initial insult there is a complex cascade of events that occur as a result of the primary insult, as well as secondary injury that occurs because of complications of the injury including ischaemia, hypoxaemia, hypotension, and cerebral oedema. The mainstay of ICU management is supportive care aimed at minimizing secondary injury, particularly that caused by cerebral ischaemia. The pathophysiological complexity requires a coordinated approach, and there is a consensus that rigorous and continuous monitoring and management of TBI is associated with an improved outcome. Using ICP and CPP target-directed management based on the Brain Trauma Foundation guidelines remains a standard of care following TBI [7].

It is common to take a staged or tiered approach to ICP and CPP management. In general, the tiers reflect increasing intensity of therapy and increasing risk of side effects. To minimize side effects, simple measures are instituted first. In addition to neuroprotective measures, general ICU management is optimized, including optimization of cardiac and respiratory function, glycaemic control, pyrexia management, and early enteral nutrition.

The clinical neurological examination in a sedated and ventilated patient with TBI is often an insensitive tool to monitor disease progression and/or response to therapies. However, the BEST:TRIP study showed that clinical examination may still play an important role, with patients managed using clinically and CT-guided therapy having similar outcomes to ICP-guided therapy in resource-poor settings [13].

To aid clinical examination, the combination of many monitoring techniques (commonly termed 'multimodality monitoring' (MMM)) may help to guide management by providing important information about brain physiology and metabolism, to assist titration of medical and surgical therapies. The European Society of Intensive Care Medicine in collaboration with the Neurocritical Care Society has released a consensus summary statement on the use of MMM [32].

ICP measurement is the most commonly used neurointensive care-specific monitor but it simply reflects the severity of disease. In patients at particular risk of cerebral ischaemia, hypoxaemia, energy failure, and glucose deprivation, it may be useful to use more specialized techniques such as cerebral microdialysis and brain parenchymal oxygen tension in addition to ICP monitoring. Some specialist monitors (e.g. brain tissue oxygen) are becoming increasingly used outside of the academic environment, and the concepts of MMM are more commonly being applied across all neurointensive care units. The invasive and labour intensive nature of these more specialized monitors, along with difficulties in integrating and interpreting large amounts of temporal data, is challenging. Tools are being developed which enable such integration to be done in a clinically meaningful way (Figures 5.3 and 5.4).

There are many benefits to using MMM in TBI and these include the following:

- Monitoring the temporal changes in a patient's pathophysiology and their response to treatment.
- Better and earlier detection of secondary events that may be amenable to intervention.
- Potential to enable more targeted and individualized therapy.
- Enables cross-validation between the different monitors to enable artefact rejection and improved confidence in treatment decisions.

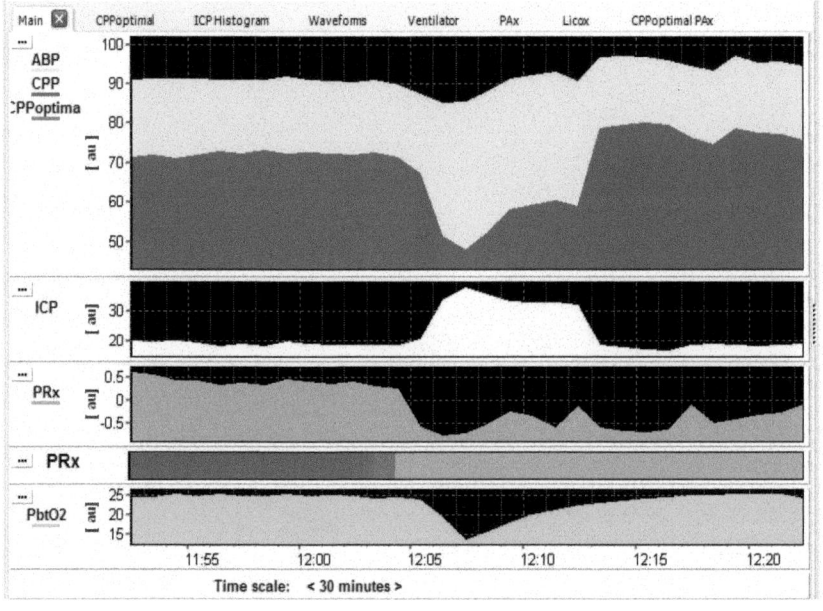

Figure 5.3 Example of the ICM+ software which enables continuous measurement and visualization of variables. In this example, about midway along the graph, the CPP suddenly drops despite a constant arterial blood pressure. This corresponds to a rise in ICP above 30 mmHg and may represent a plateau wave. Lagging slightly behind, the brain tissue oxygen tension (PbtO$_2$) decreases, indicating ischaemic stress. The rise in PbtO$_2$ is secondary to a rise in the fraction of inspired oxygen (FiO$_2$) as part of the therapeutic intervention.

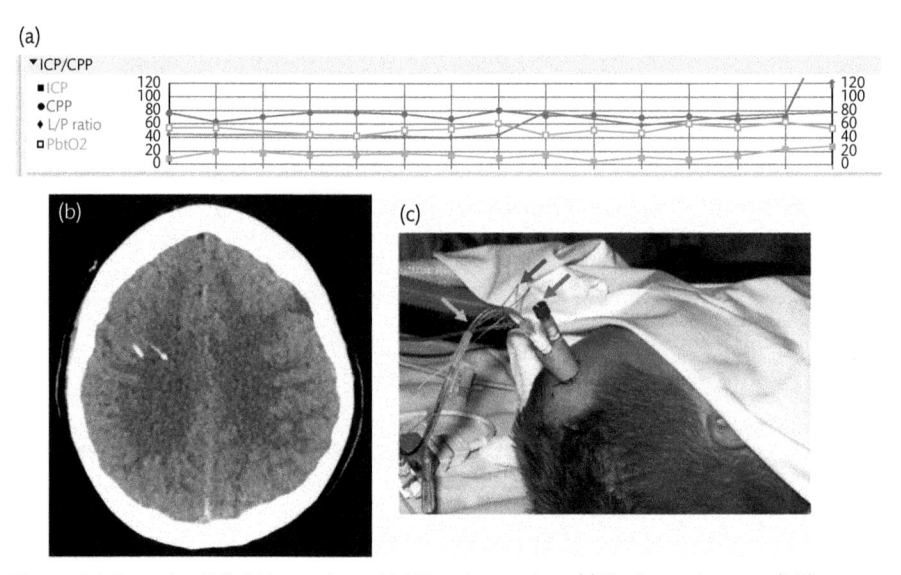

Figure 5.4 Example of MMM in a patient with bifrontal contusions. (a) The lactate/pyruvate (L/P) ratio was high in this patient (up to 78) despite an ICP less than 20 mmHg and adequate brain tissue oxygenation. The L/P ratio was reflected by a low cerebral glucose (not shown) and resolved with a higher blood glucose level. Panel (b) shows the location of the monitors on CT which were in normal-appearing white matter. Panel (c) gives an example of a triple bolt through which an intraparenchymal pressure transducer (red arrow), brain tissue oxygen monitor (green arrow), and a cerebral microdialysis catheter (blue arrow) have been inserted.

> ## ✪ Learning point Intracranial pressure waveforms
>
> There are three distinct peaks to an ICP waveform, synchronous with the arterial pulse (Figure 5.5). Each peak is only 10–30% of mean ICP (so usually <4 mmHg in amplitude):
>
>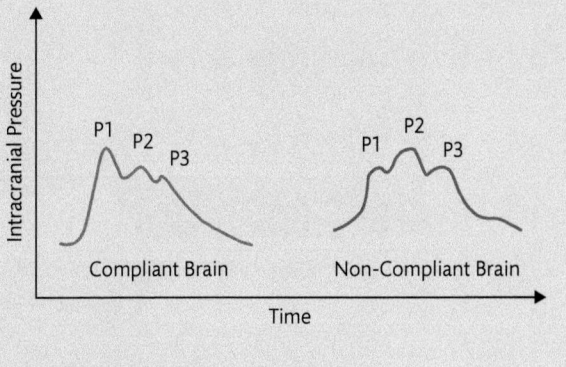
>
> **Figure 5.5** ICP waveforms.
>
> - Percussion wave (P1): correlates with the arterial pulse being transmitted.
> - Tidal wave (P2): represents cerebral compliance.
> - Dicrotic wave (P3): correlates with the closure of the aortic valve.

> ## ✪ Learning point Examples of specialized monitoring
>
> ### Oxygenation
>
> *Global: jugular bulb oxygen saturation ($SjvO_2$)*
>
> A venous catheter is sited in the jugular bulb to detect ischaemia (oxygen saturation <55%) and hyperaemia (oxygen saturation >75%). However, it is a global measurement and even normal values cannot rule out clinically important ischaemia; for this reason it is not commonly used.
>
> *Focal: brain parenchymal oxygen tension ($PbtO_2$)*
>
> Typically sited in the right frontal white matter or on the side of a focal lesion, it enables a continuous focal measurement of cerebral oxygenation. Normal values are 23–35 mmHg and values below 20 mmHg represent compromised brain oxygen and intervention should be considered. It is not yet clear if targeting parenchymal oxygen tension improves outcome.
>
> ### Focal metabolism
>
> *Cerebral microdialysis*
>
> A fine coaxial catheter is inserted into frontal white matter. It has a dialysis membrane on its outer surface and low flow rates of dialysis fluid are passed through the catheter using a pump mechanism. Vials of fluid are removed every 10–60 min which enables the measurement of concentrations of substances in the cerebral extracellular fluid which commonly include lactate, pyruvate, and glucose, but neurotransmitters and cytokines may also be measured. Being a focal monitor, the values obtained must be interpreted in the context of catheter location, for example, is it located in normal-appearing brain or is it peri-contusional? Persistently low glucose or an elevated lactate/pyruvate ratio, or both, is a strong predictor of mortality and poor outcome. These abnormalities in the microdialysis measurements are also associated with long-term atrophy.

> ## ✪ Learning point
> ### Systemic complications of traumatic brain injury
>
> The presence of extracranial injuries has a significant impact on outcome after TBI, both in the acute phase and through rehabilitation and beyond. However, even in the absence of direct extracranial organ injury, more than 80% of patients exhibit dysfunction of at least one non-neurological organ system after severe TBI. Multiorgan dysfunction occurs in 60% and is independently associated with poorer outcomes. Iatrogenic injuries may also occur, for example, cardiorespiratory complications may be associated with interventions to optimize CPP.

> ## ✪ Learning point Neuroprotective agents
>
> As yet, while many agents have shown promise as neuroprotective agents in animal models, there have been no phase III trials that support the use of any agent. The lack of translation from animals to humans is thought to be, at least in part, because animal models do not reflect accurately the complex
>
> *(continued)*

pathophysiological processes that occur in humans after TBI, as well as the great heterogeneity of disease patterns. Examples of therapies studied include the following:

- Steroids: the Medical Research Council (MRC) Corticosteroid Randomization After Significant Head injury (CRASH) trial investigated 10,000 patients of all severities of TBI [33]. Intervention was 48 hours of intravenous steroids versus placebo. The trial was stopped early as mortality was increased within 14 days and at 6 months, and there was an increased risk of severe disability in the intervention group. As a result, steroids are not recommended in the management of TBI. A low dose of steroids to replace endogenous deficiency was not studied in CRASH and in selected patients such therapy may be appropriate.
- Erythropoietin: experimentally it has neuroprotective, anti-inflammatory properties but two recent studies showed no improvement in neurological status in patients who received the drug.
- Progesterone: in animal models, progesterone had multifactorial effects including inhibition of inflammatory cytokines, reduction of apoptosis, and reduction of vasogenic oedema. However, two phase III trials found no treatment effect.

> ⊗ **Learning point**
> **Tranexamic acid**
>
> CRASH-2 showed that tranexamic acid reduced mortality in trauma patients with significant extracranial bleeding when given within 8 hours of injury. The CRASH-3 trial is being conducted to assess the effect of tranexamic acid on risk of death or disability in patients with TBI.

A final word from the expert

The intensive care management of TBI is centred on a comprehensive, multimodal, and often protocolized approach that is aimed at the prevention of secondary cerebral insults, maintenance of adequate CPP, and prevention of cerebral ischaemia. Improved understanding of the pathophysiology after TBI, as well as the effects of different management strategies, may provide an opportunity for more personalized care in the future.

References

1. National Institute for Health and Care Excellence. *Head Injury: Assessment and Early Management*. Clinical guideline [CG176]. London: National Institute for Health and Care Excellence; 2014. Available from: https://www.nice.org.uk/guidance/cg176/.
2. Scottish Intercollegiate Guidelines Network. *Early Management of Patients with a Head Injury*. Guideline 110. Edinburgh: Scottish Intercollegiate Guidelines Network; 2009. Available from: http://www.sign.ac.uk/assets/sign110.pdf.
3. Ackland H, Cooper D, Malham G, Kossmann T. Factors predicting cervical collar-related decubitus ulceration in major trauma patients. *Spine*. 2007;32:423–8.
4. Padayachee L, Cooper D, Irons S, et al. Cervical spine clearance in unconscious traumatic brain injury patients: dynamic flexion-extension fluoroscopy versus computed tomography with three-dimensional reconstruction. *J Trauma*. 2006;60:341–5.
5. Oh J, Asha S, Curtis K. Diagnostic accuracy of flexion-extension radiography for the detection of ligamentous cervical spine injury following a normal cervical spine computed tomography. *Emerg Med Australas*. 2016;28:450–5.
6. Coles J, Minhas P, Fryer T, et al. Effect of hyperventilation on cerebral blood flow in traumatic head injury: clinical relevance and monitoring correlates. *Crit Care Med*. 2002;30:1950–9.
7. Brain Trauma Foundation, American Association of Neurological Surgeons, Congress of Neurological Surgeons, et al. Guidelines for the management of severe traumatic brain injury. VIII. Intracranial pressure thresholds. *J Neurotrauma*. 2007;24:S55–8.

8. Francony G, Fauvage B, Falcon D, et al. Equimolar doses of mannitol and hypertonic saline in the treatment of increased intracranial pressure. *Crit Care Med.* 2008;36:795–800.

9. Oddo M, Levine J, Frangos S, et al. Effect of mannitol and hypertonic saline on cerebral oxygenation in patients with severe traumatic brain injury and refractory intracranial hypertension. *J Neurol Neurosurg Psychiatry.* 2009;80:916–20.

10. Jagannatha A, Sriganesh K, Devi B, Rao G. An equiosmolar study on early intracranial physiology and long term outcome in severe traumatic brain injury comparing mannitol and hypertonic saline. *J Clin Neurosci.* 2016;27:68–73.

11. Burgess S, Abu-Laban R, Slavik R, Vu EN, Zed P. A systematic review of randomized controlled trials comparing hypertonic sodium solutions and mannitol for traumatic brain injury: implications for emergency department management. *Ann Pharmacother.* 2016;50:291–300.

12. Carney N, Totten A, O'Reilly BS, et al. Guidelines for the management of severe traumatic brain injury, 4th edition. *Neurosurgery.* 2017;80:6–15.

13. Chesnut R, Temkin N, Carney N, et al. A trial of intracranial-pressure monitoring in traumatic brain injury. *N Engl J Med.* 2012;367:2471–81.

14. Patel H, Menon D, Tebbs S, Hawker R, Hutchinson P, Kirkpatrick P. Specialist neurocritical care and outcome from head injury. *Intensive Care Med.* 2002;28:547–53.

15. Nichol A, French C, Little L, et al. Erythropoietin in traumatic brain injury (EPO-TBI): a double-blind randomised controlled trial. *Lancet.* 2015;386:2499–506.

16. Paydar S, Sabetian G, Khalili H, et al. Management of deep vein thrombosis (DVT) prophylaxis in trauma patients. *Bull Emerg Trauma.* 2016;4:1–7.

17. Perel P, Yanagawa T, Bunn F, Roberts I, Wentz R, Pierro A. Nutritional support for head-injured patients. *Cochrane Database Syst Rev.* 2006;4:CD001530.

18. Finfer S, Bellomo R, Boyce N, et al. A comparison of albumin and saline for fluid resuscitation in the intensive care unit. *N Engl J Med.* 2004;350:2247–56.

19. Maggiore U, Picetti E, Antonucci E, et al. The relation between the incidence of hypernatremia and mortality in patients with severe traumatic brain injury. *Critical care* 2009;13:R110.

20. Gregson B, Rowan EN, Francis R, et al. Surgical Trial In Traumatic intraCerebral Haemorrhage (STITCH): a randomised controlled trial of early surgery compared with initial conservative treatment. *Health Technol Assess.* 2015;19:1–138.

21. Mendelow A, Gregson B, Rowan E, et al. Early Surgery versus Initial Conservative Treatment in Patients with Traumatic Intracerebral Hemorrhage (STITCH[Trauma]): the first randomized trial. *J Neurotrauma.* 2015;32:1312–23.

22. Cooper D, Rosenfeld J, Murray L, et al. Decompressive craniectomy in diffuse traumatic brain injury. *N Engl J Med.* 2011;364:1493–502.

23. Hutchinson P, Kolias A, Timofeev I, et al. Trial of decompressive craniectomy for traumatic intracranial hypertension. *N Engl J Med.* 2016;375:1119–30.

24. Saxena M, Young P, Pilcher D, et al. Early temperature and mortality in critically ill patients with acute neurological diseases: trauma and stroke differ from infection. *Intensive Care Med.* 2015;41:823–32.

25. Thompson H, Kirkness C, Mitchell P. Hypothermia and rapid rewarming is associated with worse outcome following traumatic brain injury. *J Trauma Nurs.* 2010;17:173–7.

26. Andrews PJ, Sinclair HL, Rodriguez A, et al. Hypothermia for intracranial hypertension after traumatic brain injury. *N Engl J Med.* 2015;373:2403–12.

27. Nichol A, Gantner D, Presneill J, et al. Protocol for a multicentre randomised controlled trial of early and sustained prophylactic hypothermia in the management of traumatic brain injury. *Crit Care Resusc.* 2015;17:92–100.

28. Szaflarski J. Is there equipoise between phenytoin and levetiracetam for seizure prevention in traumatic brain injury? *Epilepsy Curr.* 2015;15:94–7.

29. Verduzco-Gutierrez M, Reddy C, O'Dell MW. Is there a need for early seizure prophylaxis after traumatic brain injury? *PM R.* 2016;8:169–75.

30. Teasdale G, Jennett B. Assessment of coma and impaired consciousness. A practical scale. *Lancet*. 1974;2:81–4.

31. Jennett B, Snoek J, Bond MR, Brooks N. Disability after severe head injury: observations on the use of the Glasgow Outcome Scale. *J Neurol Neurosurg Psychiatry*. 1981;44:285–93.

32. Le Roux P, Menon D, Citerio G, et al. Consensus summary statement of the International Multidisciplinary Consensus Conference on Multimodality Monitoring in Neurocritical Care: a statement for healthcare professionals from the Neurocritical Care Society and the European Society of Intensive Care Medicine. *Intensive Care Med*. 2014;40:1189–209.

33. Roberts I, Yates D, Sandercock P, et al. Effect of intravenous corticosteroids on death within 14 days in 10008 adults with clinically significant head injury (MRC CRASH trial): randomised placebo-controlled trial. *Lancet*. 2004;364:1321–8.

6 Post-cardiac arrest care and prognostication

Justine Barnett

Ⓓ **Expert Commentary** Jerry Nolan

Case history

A 73-year-old man sustained a witnessed out-of-hospital cardiac arrest (OHCA) at home. Cardiopulmonary resuscitation was started by a family member immediately and the emergency services were called. Paramedics arrived 7 min later. The electrocardiogram (ECG) showed the initial heart rhythm was ventricular fibrillation (VF). A standard resuscitation protocol was followed and after four shocks and a single dose of adrenaline return of spontaneous circulation (ROSC) was achieved. The time from collapse to ROSC was approximately 15 min. During resuscitation, the patient's airway was managed with an i-gel supraglottic airway device and after ROSC he remained unconscious. He was transferred to hospital with his lungs ventilated via the i-gel.

> Ⓓ **Expert comment**
>
> Paramedics are increasingly using supraglottic airways instead of tracheal intubation when treating patients with OHCA. This is because it has been difficult to get sufficient training in tracheal intubation and to maintain these skills. A supraglottic airway is easier to insert, is associated with shorter interruptions in chest compressions, and, unlike tracheal intubation, is not associated with a risk of unrecognized oesophageal intubation. A recent cluster randomized trial (AIRWAYS-2) reported no overall difference in neurological outcome, improved outcome in the i-gel group as this enabled advanced airway management in a larger number of patients.

On hospital arrival, he remained in sinus rhythm with a heart rate of 88 beats/min (bpm) and arterial blood pressure of 115/55 mmHg. The patient's Glasgow Coma Scale (GCS) score was 5 (E1, V1, M3). Invasive arterial monitoring was established and intravenous anaesthesia commenced, the i-gel was then exchanged for a tracheal tube and mechanical ventilation continued. During laryngoscopy, there was no evidence of aspiration and his chest X-ray confirmed clear lung fields.

> ✪ **Learning point** Post-cardiac arrest syndrome
>
> Of the 60,000 people who have an OHCA in England each year, the emergency medical services attempt resuscitation in approximately 29,000 (roughly 50%) and about 25% of these survive to be admitted to an intensive care unit (ICU). Of those admitted, 30–40% (approximately 7–9% of the original 29,000) survive to hospital discharge, the majority with good neurological function [1].
>
> Resuscitation care does not stop at the return of circulation and the immediate and longer-term care, usually undertaken in an ICU, is vital to ensure the best possible outcomes for these patients.
>
> *(continued)*

> Post-cardiac arrest syndrome is the term given to the pathophysiological changes that occur after a period of whole-body ischaemia. These changes are exacerbated by the primary cause of the arrest and any pre-existing comorbidities of the patient [2].
>
> It includes:
>
> - post-cardiac arrest brain injury
> - post-cardiac arrest myocardial dysfunction
> - systemic ischaemia/reperfusion
> - precipitating pathology.

In the emergency department, oxygen was titrated to maintain arterial blood oxygen saturation at 94–96%. His lungs were ventilated with a tidal volume of 6 mL/kg ideal body weight and positive end-expiratory pressure of 5 cmH$_2$O. The ventilation rate was adjusted to achieve a partial pressure of carbon dioxide of 5.3–6.0 kPa (40–45 mmHg).

The patient did not have a history of hypertension so an initial mean arterial pressure (MAP) of at least 65 mmHg was targeted. His temperature was 35.9°C. With sedation established, he was administered boluses of a neuromuscular blocking drug to prevent shivering.

> ✪ **Learning point** **Best practice guidelines**
>
> The optimal management of those in cardiac arrest and after ROSC is reviewed regularly by the International Liaison Committee on Resuscitation (ILCOR). Guidance is updated every 5 years after evidence reviewers use the most recent literature to answer specific resuscitation questions. The 'Consensus on Cardiopulmonary Resuscitation Science and Treatment Recommendations' are graded on the quality of the evidence and are then used as the basis for national resuscitation guidelines. The latest ILCOR guidelines were published in 2015 [3].
>
> Best practice guidelines do not cite a specific GCS score at which a post-cardiac arrest patient should be intubated and sedated; instead, tracheal intubation is considered for any such patient who is obtunded.
>
> Hyper- and hypoxaemia is harmful to vulnerable neurons; for this reason, when it can be measured reliably, arterial blood oxygen saturation should be maintained in the range of 94–98%. A randomized clinical trial (RCT) of air versus supplemental oxygen in ST-elevation myocardial infarction documented increased myocardial injury, recurrent myocardial infarction, major cardiac arrhythmia, and larger infarct size at 6 months in the group given supplemental oxygen therapy [4].
>
> Normocapnia is targeted because hypocapnia causes cerebral ischaemia in the post-cardiac arrest population [5]. Although two observational studies have documented an association between mild hypercapnia and better neurological outcome among post-cardiac arrest patients, a recent systematic review documented better outcomes among those with normocapnia in comparison with those with hypercapnia [6]. A recent phase II RCT documented an attenuated increase in neuron-specific enolase (NSE) values in post-arrest patients treated with targeted mild hypercapnia compared with targeted normocapnia [7]. A larger RCT comparing mild hypercapnia with normocapnia is planned and will include long-term survival as the primary outcome.
>
> The optimal MAP in the post-cardiac arrest patient is unknown but likely needs to be individualized. Although some guidelines advocate a target MAP of 65–70 mmHg, there is increasing evidence that higher blood pressures are preferable (e.g. MAP of 85–105 mmHg), particularly in the first few hours after ROSC, when cerebrovascular resistance tends to be high [8]. The degree of myocardial dysfunction after cardiac arrest varies and can be evaluated by serial echocardiography. Fluid, dobutamine, and noradrenaline are the most commonly used agents to support the circulation. Try to achieve a systolic pressure sufficient to achieve a urine output of 1 mL/kg/hour and a normal or decreasing lactate [9].

A 12-lead ECG showed marked ST depression in the inferior leads and an acute coronary event was thought the likely cause of his cardiac arrest; 300 mg aspirin per rectum was administered.

After a discussion with the interventional cardiologist on call, the patient was transferred directly to the coronary catheterization laboratory where he underwent coronary angiography. This demonstrated a culprit lesion in the right coronary artery; he was treated with primary percutaneous coronary intervention (PCI) involving placement of a single stent which re-established good distal flow.

The current recommendations on the management of patients undergoing PCI were followed. These included giving aspirin and ticagrelor as antiplatelet drugs, starting a statin, and introducing a beta blocker and angiotensin-converting enzyme (ACE) inhibitor when his cardiac and renal function allowed.

An echocardiogram after PCI demonstrated moderate left ventricular systolic dysfunction and hypokinetic segments in the basal and mid-inferior region consistent with a recent right coronary artery occlusion. The right ventricle had good function and there were no valve abnormalities identified.

> ### ✪ Learning point Timing of coronary angiography
>
> If the ECG shows ST elevation, immediate coronary angiography and PCI is indicated because over 80% of patients will have an acute coronary lesion [10]. Consider immediate angiography in patients with ROSC in whom acute coronary syndrome (ACS) is suspected, for example, left bundle branch block or minor ST or T-wave changes, particularly in those resuscitated from a shockable rhythm [11]. There is currently no consensus on the timing of angiography among post-arrest patients without ST elevation on their 12-lead ECG but they should be discussed with the nearest centre that provides emergency PCI.
>
> The use of troponins at 0 and 2 hours as a stand-alone measure for excluding the diagnosis of ACS is strongly discouraged [12]. Follow standard guidelines for the use of antiplatelet and anticoagulant therapy in the management of ACS [13]. The management of ACS is a subject under frequent review as stent technology and drug therapy progresses. In general, it will include antiplatelet drugs, statins, beta blockade, and ACE inhibitors. The timing of starting these drugs in post-cardiac arrest patients will be determined by the amount of organ dysfunction they develop after ROSC.
>
> Identifying patients who have a non-cardiac cause for their arrest is important, especially those with intracranial haemorrhage for whom anticoagulation would be harmful. However, delaying PCI by computed tomography (CT) scanning all arrest patients is also unhelpful. If there is evidence of a prodrome of neurological or respiratory symptoms (e.g. headache, seizure, focal deficits, shortness of breath, or hypoxia) before the cardiac arrest, then a CT head and chest is obtained before coronary angiography [14].

> ### ⓬ Expert comment
>
> Immediately after resuscitation from cardiac arrest, the 12-lead ECG is unreliable for detecting acute coronary occlusion [15]. Although there is general agreement that post-cardiac arrest patients with ST elevation on the 12-lead ECG should undergo urgent coronary angiography with PCI as required, there is no consensus on the management of post-cardiac arrest patients with other ECG changes. Many experts now advocate urgent coronary angiography for all post-cardiac arrest patients without a clear non-cardiac cause of their cardiac arrest [11]; others restrict this intervention to those patients with an initial rhythm of VF/pulseless ventricular tachycardia. Following a pilot trial [16], a randomized trial of expedited transfer to a cardiac arrest centre for non-ST elevation VF OHCA is about to start in London, UK.
>
> *(continued)*

There is no consensus on whether a CT brain scan should be undertaken routinely before coronary angiography is performed in the comatose survivor of OHCA. A group from Paris with considerable experience in the treatment of such patients recommends direct transfer to the cardiac catheterization laboratory without an initial brain CT scan in those patients that have no prodrome before their sudden cardiac arrest—these are highly likely to be primary cardiac arrests [14]. Patients with neurological or respiratory prodromes undergo immediate CT brain and, if this is normal, chest CT with pulmonary angiography to rule out pulmonary embolism and other potential respiratory causes of cardiac arrest.

After tracheal intubation, the patient was sedated with infusions of propofol and alfentanil. With his MAP consistently above 65 mmHg his urine output was greater than 1 mL/kg/hour. His temperature was monitored closely and, with sedation and exposure during the PCI, it remained between 35°C and 36°C without intervention.

After PCI, the patient had a CT of his brain to exclude intracranial pathology. He was then admitted to the ICU for ongoing care including targeted temperature management (TTM).

In ICU, mechanical ventilation with a routine lung protective strategy was continued. An intravascular temperature control catheter was inserted into the femoral vein and a temperature-sensing urinary catheter sited. With this, his temperature was maintained at 36°C. Neuromuscular blocking drugs were used intermittently to prevent shivering and during their use sedation was titrated to a Richmond Agitation–Sedation Scale (RASS) of −4 (deep sedation) to avoid potential awareness.

⭐ **Learning point**
Sedation

Sedatives are given to reduce cerebral and cardiac oxygen consumption by reducing the metabolic rate and hence oxygen demand. Short-acting drugs such as propofol, alfentanil, and remifentanil are advocated so that residual sedation does not interfere with clinical examination findings when assessing neurological function. Metabolism of even short-acting drugs is reduced by 30% in mild hypothermia. The optimal duration of sedation is not clear but is generally continued for at least 24 hours and while TTM is occurring.

⭐ **Learning point Therapeutic hypothermia and targeted temperature management**

Cooling injured brains has long been hypothesized as a form of neuroprotection. The cerebral metabolic rate for oxygen drops by 6% for every 1°C reduction in core temperature although this is probably not the main mechanism for potential benefit in cardiac arrest patients. It is also thought to modify or abort apoptosis.

Two RCTs showing improved neurological outcome following therapeutic hypothermia for those with VF/pulseless ventricular tachycardia OHCA were published in 2002 [17, 18]. Observational studies suggested benefit for comatose survivors (usually defined as unresponsive to voice or GCS score ≤8) for all arrest rhythms and 12–24 hours of therapeutic hypothermia was recommended in international guidelines from 2003. The TTM randomized trial, published in 2013, compared outcomes of 950 all-rhythm OHCA patients treated with a target temperature of either 33°C or 36°C. There was no difference in survival or neurological outcome between the two groups: good neurological outcome occurred in 46% in the 33°C group compared with 48% in the 36°C group (risk ratio 1.01; 95% confidence interval 0.89–1.14) [19]. The current European Resuscitation Council and European Society of Intensive Care Medicine (ERC/ESICM) guidelines recommend maintaining a constant, target temperature between 32°C and 36°C for at least 24 hours [9]. More high-quality trials are needed to determine the optimal temperature and duration of temperature control.

⑥ Expert comment

All patients enrolled in the TTM trial had their temperature controlled. That the outcomes were the same in the 36°C and 33°C groups is not a reason to abandon active temperature control, because hyperthermia is associated with worse neurological outcome. Animal data indicate improved outcomes with mild hypothermia after a global hypoxic–ischaemic cerebral injury but the results of the TTM trial makes it difficult to make a firm recommendation about a specific target temperature. There will be fewer physiological changes (e.g. bradycardia, electrolyte shifts, and shivering) at 36°C compared with 33°C but some post-cardiac arrest patients (e.g. those with more severe neurological injury) might get better neuroprotection from the lower temperature. The forthcoming TTM2 study will compare comatose all-rhythm post-cardiac arrest patients treated with either TTM at 33°C or temperature control only when the temperature exceeds 37.5°C.

⊕ Clinical tip Inducing and maintaining hypothermia

Options to induce hypothermia or TTM include the following:

- Ice packs, these work rapidly and are easily available but do not stop temperature fluctuations or enable controlled rewarming.
- Air cooling blankets or water-filled pads.
- Intravascular cooling catheters, which circulate cold fluid in a counter-current manner. Usually placed in the femoral or internal jugular vein and maintain the intended temperature by using feedback from a centrally placed thermometer (usually bladder or oesophagus).
- Transnasal evaporative cooling.
- Extracorporeal circulation. Available in only a few centres in the UK but in many other developed countries is used increasingly commonly to treat refractory cardiogenic shock after cardiac arrest [20]. Accurate temperature control is a benefit as a heater is included in the extra corporal circuit.

It would seem logical to start TTM as soon as possible after ROSC. However, trials comparing pre-hospital cooling with cooling delayed until hospital arrival have not shown benefit. This may have been because of the cooling method used [21]. The target temperature is maintained for at least 24 hours.

Monitor core temperature continuously during cooling. Options include oesophageal, bladder, or intravascular probes. Other sites may not reflect core temperature during cooling; consider a second site when using a closed feedback cooling system [22].

Shivering can occur at both 36°C and 33°C and should be avoided because it increases oxygen consumption and core body temperature. Muscle relaxation, with adequate sedation, is the most effective treatment. Magnesium sulphate may also decrease the shivering threshold [23].

After hypothermia, rewarming is undertaken slowly at no more than 0.25–0.5°C/hour. Avoid hyperthermia at 37.5°C or higher which is harmful to vulnerable neurons. Rebound hyperthermia is associated with poorer neurological outcomes.

⑥ Expert comment

Until recently, the use of 2 L of 4°C 0.9% saline or Hartmann's solution was considered to be a safe and effect method for initiating cooling—it reduces core temperature by 1.0–1.5°C. An RCT of prehospital cooling with up to 2 L of 4°C 0.9% saline versus no prehospital cooling following ROSC after all-rhythm OHCA showed no difference in survival to hospital discharge or neurological recovery [21]. Among those treated with prehospital cooling, there were significantly more rearrests during transport to hospital and a higher incidence of pulmonary oedema seen on the first chest X-ray. In a further study, infusion of up to 2 L of cold fluid during prehospital cardiac arrest was associated with a decrease in the rate of ROSC in patients with shockable rhythm [24]. Based on these results, cold intravenous fluid should not be used prehospital or pre-ROSC, but its use to initiate cooling after ROSC in a closely monitored environment, such as the emergency department, may still be reasonable.

> ⊗ **Learning point** Side effects of hypothermia
>
> Side effects of hypothermia include:
>
> - shivering
> - an increase in systemic vascular resistance
> - arrhythmias—most commonly bradycardia which may have a beneficial effect in reducing diastolic dysfunction and frequently does not need treating
> - diuresis
> - hypokalaemia via intracellular redistribution
> - hypomagnesaemia and hypophosphataemia
> - hyperglycaemia from decreased insulin secretion and sensitivity
> - elevated serum amylase
> - decreased clearance of drugs including sedatives and neuromuscular blockade
> - mild coagulopathy
> - mild immunosuppression—the incidence of pneumonia in this population is high and should be actively sought and treated.

Frequent assessments of volume status and end-organ perfusion were made. The MAP did drop below target intermittently. This was clinically thought to be due to the sedatives reducing the systemic vascular resistance rather than worsening left or ventricular or right ventricular function. This was consistent with readings from a pulse index contour cardiac output catheter that had been inserted into a femoral artery. Small boluses of fluid were given to restore intravascular volume and then noradrenaline was started to maintain blood pressure. He developed a bradycardia of 45 bpm; a 12-lead ECG confirmed it was a sinus bradycardia and it was not treated. Serum potassium values were maintained above 4.0 mmol/L and serum magnesium values above 0.8 mmol/L.

A nasogastric tube was inserted and enteral feed started. Blood glucose values were controlled between 4 and 10 mmol/L with an intravenous insulin infusion. A statin was started on the evening of admission. Prophylactic low-molecular-weight heparin was used along with compression stockings and an intermittent pneumatic compression device to reduce the risk of venous thromboembolism.

After 24 hours at 36°C the patient was allowed to rewarm slowly. The intravascular cooling catheter remained in place until 72 hours post ROSC for further cooling in case his temperature went above 37°C and to ensure it did not exceed 37.5°C. Sedation was stopped but would have been restarted if he was shivering or displayed ventilator dyssynchrony.

Without sedation the noradrenaline was weaned off. He was commenced on a small dose of cardioselective beta blocker (bisoprolol) and an ACE inhibitor; both were titrated up over the next 2 weeks.

At 72 hours after ROSC his best GCS score was 5T (E2, VT, M3). It was noted he had some abnormal movements of his facial muscles that could have been a focal seizure. These were intermittent, not associated with stimulation, and resolved spontaneously in less than 1 min. An electroencephalogram (EEG) did not show epileptiform activity.

> ⊗ **Learning point** Treatment of seizures
>
> Seizures are common in patients with ROSC: myoclonus occurs in up to 25% and post-anoxic status epilepticus in up to 31% depending on the diagnostic criteria used [25]. Not all clinical seizures will be epileptic in origin. Seizures are treated because they increase the cerebral metabolic rate and will mask clinical examination findings. Sodium valproate, levetiracetam, phenytoin, benzodiazepines, propofol, or barbiturates have all been used for this indication. There is no strong evidence for the first choice of drug in this population; however, experts now recommend the use of sodium valproate and/or levetiracetam for myoclonic status epilepticus [26]. Seizure control may be challenging and
>
> *(continued)*

may require several drugs used at maximal doses. EEGs to confirm seizure control and exclude non-convulsive status epilepticus may be indicated and assistance from a neurologist may be helpful in these cases. There is no role for prophylactic anticonvulsants.

Myoclonic status epilepticus is defined as spontaneous, repetitive, unrelenting, generalized multifocal myoclonus in a comatose patient and is usually, but not always, associated with severe cortical damage and poor outcome. Other forms of myoclonus (e.g. intention myoclonus) may not represent irreversible brain injury and the sedative effects of treatment instigated for myoclonus should be considered when assessing neurological recovery [25, 27].

Over the next 48 hours, the patient's motor score continued to improve. When he was localizing consistently, breathing spontaneously with minimal pressure support, and a strong cough, his trachea was extubated. He was delirious but not agitated, for the next 2 days, which resolved without needing pharmacological intervention. He was discharged to the neurology ward for rehabilitation 8 days after his cardiac arrest.

After a further 2 weeks of inpatient care the patient was discharged home with support from his wife and rehabilitation within the community. He reported mild problems with memory and severe fatigue but otherwise made an uneventful recovery.

> ✪ **Learning point** Predicting outcome
>
> Time to ROSC or initial rhythm is not a reliable predictor of outcome. Similarly, no examination finding or clinical test has demonstrated 100% sensitivity at predicting poor neurological outcome after hypoxic brain injury while avoiding false positives. Prognostication studies can be separated into to those before and after TTM became a standard of care. The quality of evidence in most studies is limited by the lack of blinding and the fact that the outcome predictor under investigation is subsequently used in treatment decisions including the withdrawal of life-sustaining therapies; thus, becoming a self-fulfilling prophecy of poor prognosis. First, it is important to define what is meant by good outcome.
>
> **Classifying outcomes**
>
> The American Heart Association published a consensus statement on the best outcome measures for clinical trials in resuscitation medicine [28]. Neurological outcome is frequently graded into several categories and then dichotomized into 'good' or 'poor' outcomes.
>
> The time point at which these assessments are made is relevant, as neurological function may improve for several months after a cardiac arrest. The dependence described in a 'good' outcome in research terms may not correspond to the hopes or expectations of individual patients and relatives.
>
> Cerebral performance category (CPC) is used in many studies to describe good (CPC 1 and 2) and poor (CPC 4 and 5) neurological outcomes. Authors of earlier studies often included CPC 3 as a good outcome but in the vast majority of studies in recent years, CPC 3 is defined as a poor outcome.
>
> CPCs are defined as follows:
>
> 1. Conscious and alert with normal function or only slight disability
> 2. Conscious and alert with only moderate disability. Sufficient cerebral function for independent activities of daily living and able to work in a sheltered environment. May have hemiplegia, seizures, ataxia, dysarthria, dysphasia, or permanent memory or mental changes.
> 3. Conscious with severe disability. Dependent on others for daily support because of limited brain function. Ranges from ambulatory state to severe dementia or paralysis.
> 4. Comatose or persistent vegetative state.
> 5. Brain dead or death from other causes.
>
> CPC at hospital discharge is often used as a surrogate measure of long-term survival because these data are easy to collect; however, several recent studies have shown marked improvement in CPC scores between hospital discharge and 6–12 months later. A study of 980 patients documented a 5-year survival in each CPC domain as follows: CPC 1, 74%; CPC 2, 55%; CPC 3, 44%; and CPC 4, 22% [29].
>
> The modified Rankin score (mRS) and the extended Glasgow Outcome Scale are alternative neurological outcome descriptors used in cardiac arrest research [30, 31].

> ### ✪ Learning point Prognostication
>
> #### Clinical assessment
>
> Most deaths in ICU patients who are admitted after ROSC are from withdrawal of life-sustaining treatment, based on the expectation of poor neurological outcome [32].
>
> As no prognostication tool fully predicts outcome, neurological examination remains the most important tool for assessing progress after cardiac arrest. It may be confounded by hypotension, seizures, sedatives, or neuromuscular blocking drugs. Clearance of sedatives is reduced during even mild hypothermia, which necessitates waiting longer after stopping sedation before reliable neurological assessment can be undertaken.
>
> A markedly reduced motor component of the GCS is a poor prognostic sign but even an absent or extensor motor response (GCS M1 or M2) 72 hours after ROSC does not reliably predict a poor prognosis—there is a false-positive rate of 5% (95% confidence interval 2–9%). Bilateral absence of pupillary light and corneal reflexes at 72 hours after ROSC has a very low false-positive rate but also low sensitivity in identifying patients with a poor prognosis [33–35].
>
> #### Electroencephalogram
>
> The EEG is non-invasive, mobile, and more readily available than other outcome predictors. It can detect non-convulsive status epilepticus that occurs in up to 25% of comatose post-cardiac arrest patients. Specific EEG abnormalities that persist beyond rewarming can be associated with a poor outcome. They include:
>
> - absence of reactivity
> - burst suppression pattern
> - status epilepticus.
>
> However, interpretation can be hindered by a lack of universal classification systems, observer variability, and drug and metabolic effects. No single EEG abnormality has a 0% false-positive rate when predicting poor outcome. Normal and abnormal EEGs are shown in Figures 6.1–6.3.

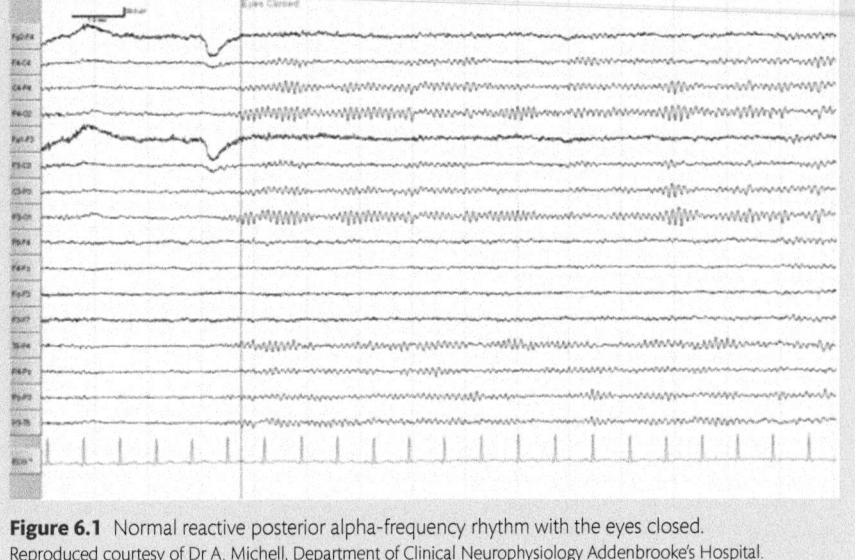

Figure 6.1 Normal reactive posterior alpha-frequency rhythm with the eyes closed.
Reproduced courtesy of Dr A. Michell, Department of Clinical Neurophysiology Addenbrooke's Hospital.

(continued)

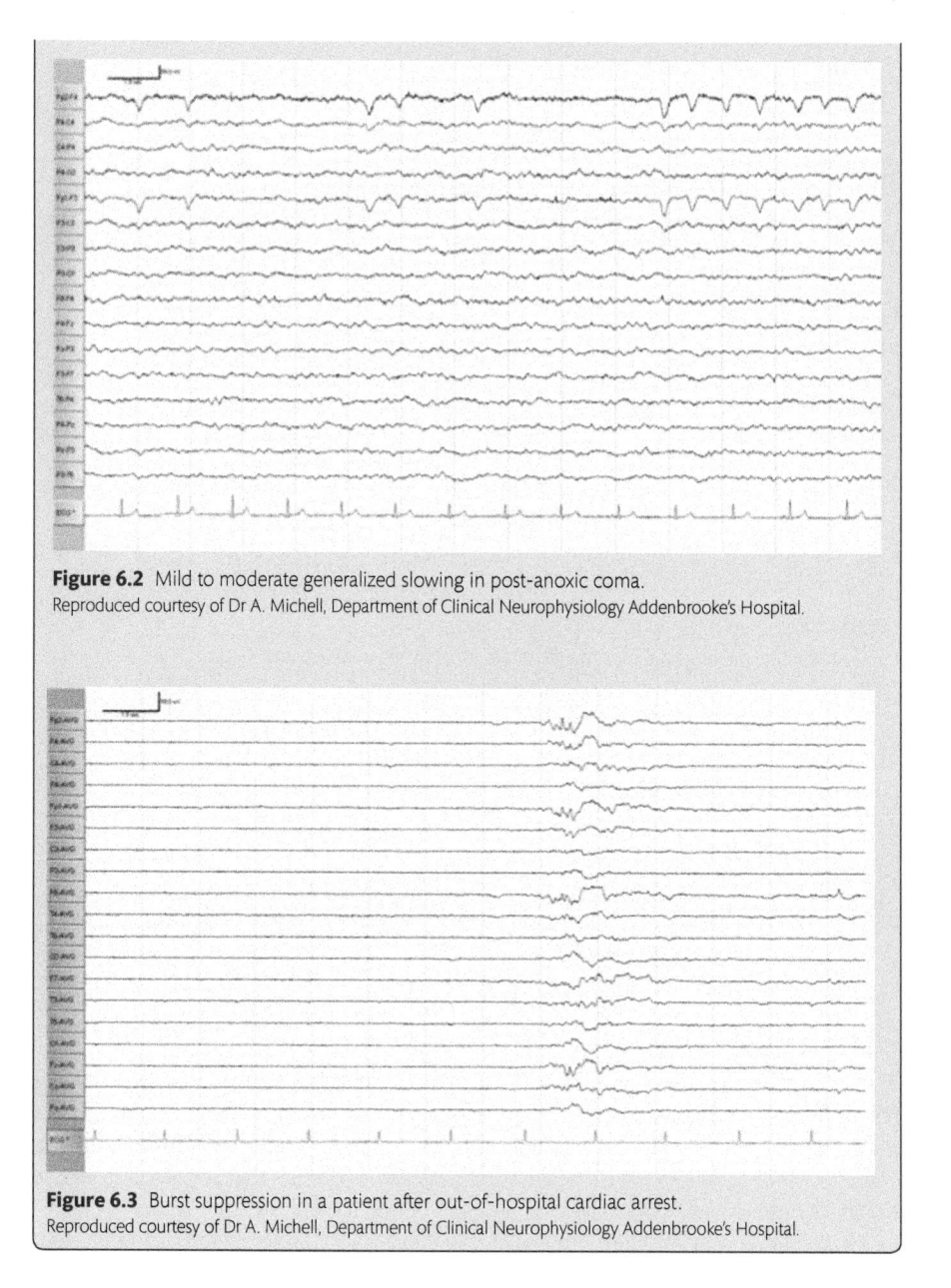

Figure 6.2 Mild to moderate generalized slowing in post-anoxic coma.
Reproduced courtesy of Dr A. Michell, Department of Clinical Neurophysiology Addenbrooke's Hospital.

Figure 6.3 Burst suppression in a patient after out-of-hospital cardiac arrest.
Reproduced courtesy of Dr A. Michell, Department of Clinical Neurophysiology Addenbrooke's Hospital.

> ⊛ **Learning point** Prognostication
>
> **Evoked potentials**
>
> Somatosensory evoked potentials (SSEPs) test the integrity of neuronal pathways between the peripheral and central nervous system [37]. They are less affected than other tests by drugs and metabolic abnormalities. Bilateral absence of the N20 cortical response to median nerve SSEPs during hypothermia or after rewarming does predict a poor outcome with a false-positive rate less than 1% [38]. However, presence of the N20 response does not reliably predict a good outcome and the test is not yet widely available.
>
> **Neuroimaging**
>
> Multiple modalities of neuroimaging have been studied for prognostication after a cardiac arrest but most have a small sample size and have inherent selection bias. The level of evidence is not high and therefore no single imaging test can be recommended for prognostication at present.
>
> CT changes that reflect brain swelling after anoxic coma include loss of grey–white matter differentiation and sulcal effacement. These are visible within 24 hours of ROSC.
>
> Magnetic resonance imaging (MRI) has been used to demonstrate abnormalities in the cortical or deep grey matter in several sequences around 3–5 days after ROSC. Diffusion-weighted imaging is the most extensively studied and the apparent diffusion coefficient is a quantitative measure of these ischaemic changes [39].
>
> **Biomarkers**
>
> Serum NSE is the most studied biomarker of neuronal damage after cardiac arrest. It is a cytoplasmic glycolytic enzyme found in neurons and neuroendocrine tumours. NSE values are consistently raised in neuronal injury and with more severe injury tend to increase in the first 72 hours but, despite early promise, like other tests, this biomarker is not completely reliable in predicting a poor outcome. NSE values may also be elevated in haemolysis and in the presence of neuroendocrine tumours. S100 beta is a calcium binding protein from astroglial and Schwann cells and is another potential biomarker.
>
> Variability in the assay used, cut-off values, and clinical availability currently limit biomarker use in predicting outcome. Increasing values of NSE between 48 and 72 hours after ROSC is associated with a poor outcome [40, 41].

Discussion

A multimodal prognostication strategy is advocated rather than relying on a single test to predict outcome. Clinical examination is the first step once confounding factors including sedation, metabolic derangement, and hypothermia are excluded. Figure 6.4 summarizes the 2015 ERC/ESICM algorithm for those patients that remain GCS M1 or M2 at 72 hours after ROSC [35].

Bilaterally absent pupillary and corneal reflexes at 72 hours or later or bilaterally absent N20 SSEP at 24 hours or later are the most robust predictors of poor outcome (i.e. with very low false-positive rates). If these reflexes are present, observe for a further 24 hours and consider other tests including EEG, CT, or MRI or serial biomarkers to aid treatment decisions. A combination of a least two of these predictors is suggested. All these test neurological function only and do not take into account the outcome from coexisting organ failure, premorbid conditions, and frailty. Most survivors will recover consciousness within 10 days [42]. In a series of 194 comatose post-cardiac arrest patients who awoke, 30% did not awake until more than 48 hours after sedation was stopped [43]. Age over 59 years (odds ratio (OR) 2.1), post-arrest shock (OR 2.6), and renal failure on admission (OR 3.1) were all associated with delayed awakening.

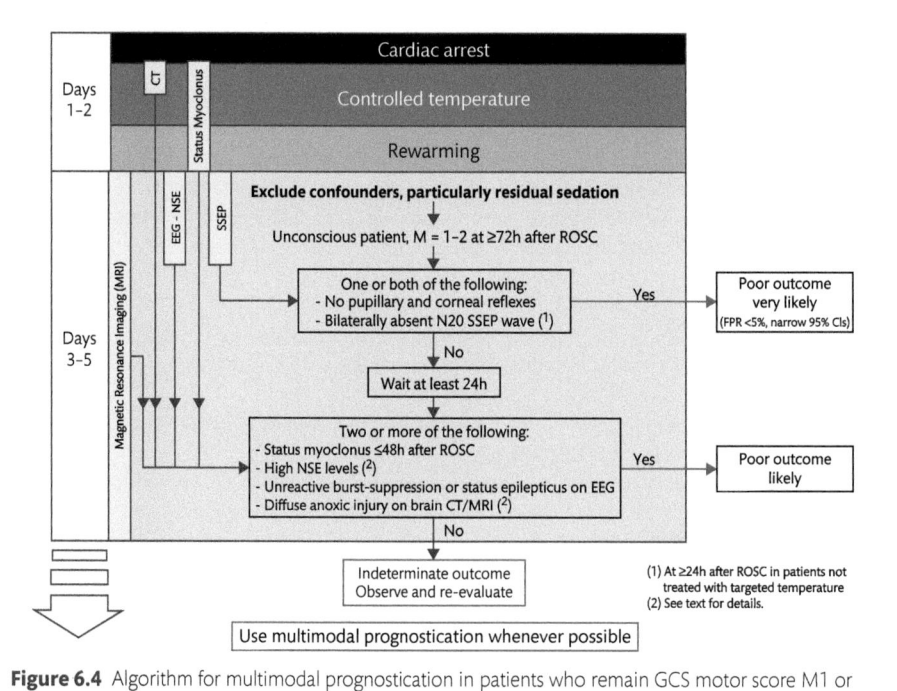

Figure 6.4 Algorithm for multimodal prognostication in patients who remain GCS motor score M1 or M2 72 hours after ROSC.

Reproduced from Sandroni, C., et al. Prognostication in comatose survivors of cardiac arrest: An advisory statement from the European Resuscitation Council and the European Society of Intensive Care Medicine. *Resuscitation*. 2014;85:1779–1789. Copyright © Elsevier Inc. All rights reserved. Open Access.

There has been a considerable increase in the volume of data relating to the prediction of outcome in the comatose post-cardiac arrest patient. Inevitably, these are all observational studies. Recent international guidelines recommend a multimodal approach to prognostication (clinical examination plus at least one other modality, typically an electrophysiological investigation such as EEG or SSEP, or imaging) [19, 33]. Generally, prognostication should not be attempted until at least 72 hours after ROSC. There is evidence that withdrawal of life-sustaining treatment decisions are being increasingly delayed but many are still made prematurely [1]. The increasing tendency to regionalize post-resuscitation care, which is generally predicated on the need for 24/7 access to a cardiac catheterization laboratory, may enable more of these patients to access the full range of prognostic investigations [44].

A final word from the expert

Patients with ROSC after cardiac arrest now account for more than 12% of mechanically ventilated ICU admissions [1]. Optimal treatment of post-cardiac arrest syndrome may be prolonged and accurate early prognostic factors have not been identified. Avoiding premature prognostication of futility without creating unreasonable hopes of recovery or survivors with severe neurological impairment is the goal of post-cardiac arrest care. Allowing sufficient time for the patient to recover is important. Combining clinical assessment, ancillary tests, multidisciplinary opinion, premorbid status, and the likely wishes of the patient is currently the best way of approaching this difficult scenario.

References

1. Hawkes C, Booth S, Ji C, et al. Epidemiology and outcome from out-of-hospital cardiac arrests in England. *Resuscitation*. 2017;110:133–40.
2. Nolan J, Neumar R, Adrie C, et al. Post-cardiac arrest syndrome: epidemiology, pathophysiology, treatment, and prognostication. A Scientific Statement from the International Liaison Committee on Resuscitation; the American Heart Association Emergency Cardiovascular Care Committee; the Council on Cardiovascular Surgery and Anesthesia; the Council on Cardiopulmonary, Peri-operative, and Critical Care; the Council on Clinical Cardiology; the Council on Stroke. *Resuscitation*. 2008;79:350–79.
3. Nolan J, Hazinski M, Aickin R. 2015 International Consensus on Cardiopulmonary Resuscitation and Emergency Cardiovascular Care Science with Treatment Recommendations. *Resuscitation*. 2015;92:e1–31.
4. Stub D, Smith K, Bernard S, et al. Air versus oxygen in ST-segment elevation myocardial infarction. *Circulation*. 2015;131:2143–50.
5. Bouzat P, Suys T, Sala N, Oddo M. Effect of moderate hyperventilation and induced hypertension on cerebral tissue oxygenation after cardiac arrest and therapeutic hypothermia. *Resuscitation*. 2013;84:1540–5.
6. McKenzie N, Williams T, Tohira H, Ho K, Finn J. A systematic review and meta-analysis of the association between arterial carbon dioxide tension and outcomes after cardiac arrest. *Resuscitation*. 2017;111:116–26.
7. Eastwood G, Schneider A, Suzuki S, et al. Targeted therapeutic mild hypercapnia after cardiac arrest: a phase II multi-centre randomised controlled trial (the CCC trial). *Resuscitation*. 2016;104:83–90.
8. Van den Brule J, Vinke E, van Loon L, van der Hoeven J, Hodemaekers C. Middle cerebral artery flow, the critical closing pressure, and the optimal mean arterial pressure in comatose cardiac arrest survivors—an observational study. *Resuscitation*. 2017;110:85–9.
9. Nolan J, Soar J, Cariou A. European Resuscitation Council and European Society of Intensive Care Medicine Guidelines for Post-resuscitation Care 2015 Section 5 of the European Resuscitation Council Guidelines for Resuscitation 2015. *Resuscitation*. 2015:95;202–22.
10. Garcia-Tejada J, Jurado-Roman A, Rodriguez J, et al. Post-resuscitation electro-cardiograms, acute coronary findings and in-hospital prognosis of survivors of out-of-hospital cardiac arrest. *Resuscitation*. 2014;85:1245–50.
11. Dumas F, Bougouin W, Geri G, et al. Emergency percutaneous coronary intervention in post-cardiac arrest patients without ST-segment elevation pattern: insights from the PROCAT II Registry. *JACC Cardiovasc Interv*. 2016;9:1011–18.
12. Soar J, Callaway C, Aibiki B, et al. Part 4: Advanced Life Support 2015 International Consensus on Cardiopulmonary Resuscitation and Emergency Cardiovascular Care Science with Treatment Recommendations. *Resuscitation*. 2015;95:e71–120.
13. Roffi M, Patrono C, Collet J, et al. 2015 ESC Guidelines for the management of acute coronary syndromes in patients presenting without persistent ST-segment elevation: Task Force for the Management of Acute Coronary Syndromes in Patients Presenting without Persistent ST-Segment Elevation of the European Society of Cardiology (ESC). *Eur Heart J*. 2016;37:267–315.
14. Chilly J, Mongardon N, Dumas F, et al. Benefit of an early and systematic imaging procedure after cardiac arrest: insights from the PROCAT (Parisian Region Out of Hospital Cardiac Arrest) registry. *Resuscitation*. 2012;83:1444–50.
15. Sideris G, Voicu S, Dillinger JG, et al. Value of post-resuscitation electrocardiogram in the diagnosis of acute myocardial infarction in out-of-hospital cardiac arrest patients. *Resuscitation*. 2011;82:1148–53.
16. Patterson T, Perkins G, Joseph J, et al. A randomised trial of expedited transfer to a cardiac arrest centre for non-ST elevation ventricular fibrillation out-of-hospital cardiac arrest: the ARREST pilot randomised trial. *Resuscitation*. 2017;115:185–91.

17. Hypothermia after Cardiac Arrest Study Group. Mild therapeutic hypothermia to improve the neurologic outcome after cardiac arrest. *N Engl J Med*. 2002;346:549–56.

18. Bernard S, Gray T, Buist M, et al. Treatment of comatose survivors of out-of-hospital cardiac arrest with induced hypothermia. *N Engl J Med*. 2002;346:557–63.

19. Nielsen N, Wetterslev J, Cronberg T, et al. Targeted temperature management at 33 degrees C versus 36 degrees C after cardiac arrest. *N Engl J Med*. 2013;369:2197–206.

20. Pineton de Chambrun M, Bréchot N, Lebreton G, et al. Venoarterial extracorporeal membrane oxygenation for refractory cardiogenic shock post-cardiac arrest. *Intensive Care Med*. 2016;42:1999–2007.

21. Kim F, Nichol G, Maynard C, et al. Effect of pre-hospital induction of mild hypothermia on survival and neurological status among adults with cardiac arrest: a randomized clinical trial. *JAMA*. 2014;311:45–52.

22. Knapik P, Rychlik W, Duda D, Golyszny R, Borowik D, Ciesla D. Relationship between blood, nasopharyngeal and urinary bladder temperature during intravascular cooling for therapeutic hypothermia after cardiac arrest. *Resuscitation*. 2012;83:208–12.

23. Wadhwa A, Sengupta P, Durrani J, et al. Magnesium sulphate only slightly reduces the shivering threshold in humans. *Br J Anaesth*. 2005;94:756–62.

24. Bernard S, Smith K, Finn J, et al. Induction of therapeutic hypothermia during out-of-hospital cardiac arrest using a rapid infusion of cold saline: the RINSE Trial (Rapid Infusion of Cold Normal Saline). *Circulation*. 2016;134:797–805.

25. Seder D, Sunde K, Rubertsson S, et al. Neurologic outcomes and postresuscitation care of patients with myoclonus following cardiac arrest. *Crit Care Med*. 2015;43:965–72.

26. Reynolds AS, Claassen J. Treatment of seizures and postanoxic status epilepticus. *Semin Neurol*. 2017;37:33–9.

27. English W, Giffin N, Nolan J. Myoclonus after cardiac arrest: pitfalls in diagnosis and prognosis. *Anaesthesia*. 2009;64:908–11.

28. Becker L, Aufderheide T, Geocadin G, et al. Primary outcomes for resuscitation science studies. A Consensus Statement from the American Heart Association. *Circulation*. 2011;124:2158–77.

29. Phelps R, Dumas F, Maynard C, Silver J, Rea T. Cerebral performance category and long-term prognosis following out-of-hospital cardiac arrest. *Crit Care Med*. 2013;41:1252–7.

30. Bonita R, Beaglehole R. Modification of Rankin Scale: recovery of motor function after stroke. *Stroke*. 1988;19:1497–500.

31. Wilson J, Pettigrew L, Teasdale G. Structured interviews for the Glasgow Outcome Scale and the Extended Glasgow Outcome Scale: Guidelines for Their Use. *J Neurotrauma*. 1997;15:573–85.

32. Cronberg T, Kuiper M. Withdrawal of life-sustaining therapy after cardiac arrest. *Semin Neurol*. 2017;37:81–7.

33. Dragancea I, Horn J, Kuiper M, et al. Neurological prognostication after cardiac arrest and targeted temperature management 33°C versus 36°C: results from a randomised controlled clinical trial. *Resuscitation*. 2015;93:164–70.

34. Sandroni C, Cavallaro F, Callaway CW, et al. Predictors of poor neurological out-come in adult comatose survivors of cardiac arrest: a systematic review and meta-analysis. Part 2: patients treated with therapeutic hypothermia. *Resuscitation*. 2013;84:1324–38.

35. Sandroni C, Cariou A, Cavallaro F, et al. Prognostication in comatose survivors of cardiac arrest: an advisory statement from the European Resuscitation Council and the European Society of Intensive Care Medicine. *Resuscitation*. 2014;85:1779–89.

36. Rossetti A, Rabinstein A, Oddo M. Neurological prognostication of outcome in patients in coma after cardiac arrest. *Lancet Neurol*. 2016;15:597–609.

37. Horn J, Tjepkema-Cloostermans MC. Somatoensory evoked potentials in patients with hypoxic-ischaemic brain injury. *Semin Neurol*. 2017;37:60–5.

38. Young G, Doig G, Ragazzoni A. Anoxic–ischemic encephalopathy: clinical and electro-physiological associations with outcome. *Neurocrit Care*. 2005;2:159–64.

39. Hahn D, Geocadin R, Green D. Quality of evidence in studies evaluating neuroimaging for neurologic prognostication in adult patients resuscitated from cardiac arrest. *Resuscitation*. 2014;85:165–72.
40. Stammet P, Collignon O, Hassager C, et al. Neuron-specific enolase as a predictor of death or poor neurological outcome after out-of-hospital cardiac arrest and targeted temperature management at 33°C and 36°C. *J Am Coll Cardiol*. 2015;65:2104–14.
41. Stammet P. Blood biomarkers of hypoxic-ischemic brain injury after cardiac arrest. *Semin Neurol*. 2017;37:75–80.
42. Gold B, Puertas L, Davis S, et al. Awakening after cardiac arrest and post resuscitation hypothermia: are we pulling the plug too early? *Resuscitation*. 2014;85:211–14.
43. Paul M, Bougouin W, Geri G, et al. Delayed awakening after cardiac arrest: prevalence and risk factors in the Parisian registry. *Intensive Care Med*. 2016;42:1128–36.
44. Elmer J, Rittenberger J, Coppler P, et al. Long-term survival benefit from treatment at a specialty center after cardiac arrest. *Resuscitation*. 2016;108:48–53.

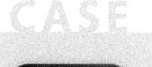

Subarachnoid haemorrhage

Matthew A. Kirkman

Expert Commentary Martin Smith

Case history

A 66-year-old female presented to her local emergency department via ambulance having developed a sudden-onset, severe headache while at work. She described it as the 'worst headache' of her life, reaching maximal intensity within minutes of onset. Associated symptoms included nausea, vomiting, neck stiffness, and photophobia. Except for treated hypertension she had no past medical history of note, although she was a smoker with a 40 pack-year history and drank 20 units of alcohol per week.

On examination, the patient was eye opening to speech, disorientated but obeying commands; her Glasgow Coma Scale (GCS) score was 13 out of 15 (E3, V4, M6). Her pupils were 3 mm and reactive to light bilaterally, and she had no other cranial nerve or limb focal neurological deficits. She had nuchal rigidity and a positive Kernig's sign. Based on the history and examination, a subarachnoid haemorrhage (SAH) was suspected, and this was confirmed by an urgent non-enhanced computed tomography (CT) scan of the head. The clinical grade of the SAH, according to the World Federation of Neurosurgical Societies (WFNS) classification, was 2.

Expert comment

Headache alone is non-discriminatory for SAH; only around 1% of patients presenting to emergency departments with headache have a confirmed SAH. Associated clinical features such as neck stiffness, vomiting, altered consciousness, and seizures make the diagnosis of SAH more likely and should prompt further investigation. Standard non-contrast CT is diagnostic in around 95% of cases, although a normal scan, particularly early after symptom onset, does not exclude SAH. In the presence of a good history for SAH and normal CT scan, a lumbar puncture should be performed. Demonstration of red blood cells or their metabolites in the cerebrospinal fluid (CSF) identifies an additional 3% of patients who subsequently have positive cerebral angiography. The diagnostic sensitivity of lumbar puncture is increased when performed at least 6 to 12 hours after SAH onset, although waiting leads to a delay in diagnosis and definitive treatment.

Learning point Clinical grading of subarachnoid haemorrhage

There are several grading systems used in SAH, based on clinical and/or radiological criteria, which can be used to communicate disease severity and for prognostication. The most frequently used clinical grading scale is the WFNS scale, which incorporates the GCS and the presence or absence of a focal neurological deficit (Table 7.1) [1]. The higher the WFNS score, the worse the patient's likely outcome.

(continued)

Table 7.1 World Federation of Neurosurgical Societies subarachnoid haemorrhage grading system

Grade	Glasgow Coma Scale score	Focal neurological deficit
1	15	Absent
2	13–14	Absent
3	13–14	Present
4	7–12	Present or absent
5	<7	Present or absent

Note: if a patient has hydrocephalus which is likely to affect the conscious level, WFNS grading should be applied after treatment of the hydrocephalus to ensure optimal prognostic value. A patient who is alert and orientated (GCS score of 15) but has a neurological deficit, such as a hemiparesis, is classified as grade 3.
Source: data from Drake, CG., et al. Report of World Federation of Neurological Surgeons Committee on a Universal Subarachnoid Hemorrhage Grading Scale. *Journal of Neurosurgery.* 1988; 68: 985–6. Copyright © 1988 American Association of Neurological Surgeons.

🔾 Expert comment

Approximately 85% of cases of SAH are caused by spontaneous rupture of an intracranial aneurysm. Non-aneurysmal peri-mesencephalic bleeds, with haemorrhage centred anterior to the midbrain or pons, account for 10% of cases. The remaining 5% are divided between multiple rarer pathologies, including traumatic SAH.

🔾 Expert comment

Patients should be transferred to a neuroscience centre as soon as the diagnosis of SAH has been confirmed and the patient stabilized. Definitive treatment of the ruptured aneurysm should be undertaken within 24–48 hours of SAH onset. Treatment in high-volume centres with timely access to multidisciplinary teams is associated with improved outcomes after SAH.

The CT scan demonstrated blood within the basal cisterns, particularly around the region of the right internal carotid artery but also in the posterior horns of both lateral ventricles and over the right cerebral convexity, and early signs of hydrocephalus (Figure 7.1a, b). A computed tomography angiogram (CTA) was subsequently performed and demonstrated a 6 × 4 mm bilobed aneurysm of the right terminal internal carotid artery (Figure 7.1c).

The patient was transferred urgently to the local neuroscience centre where she was placed on bed rest and commenced on nimodipine, laxatives, analgesia, and intravenous fluid therapy. An admission electrocardiogram (ECG) was normal.

Shortly after admission to the neurosciences centre, the patient's GCS deteriorated to 8/15 (E2, V2, M4) and a repeat cranial CT scan showed worsening hydrocephalus. An external ventricular drain was inserted to treat the hydrocephalus. After discussion between the neurosurgical and interventional neuroradiology teams, the patient underwent endovascular coiling of the right internal carotid artery aneurysm (Figure 7.1d), during the same anaesthetic.

🔾 Expert comment

Early (within 24 hours) neurological deterioration after SAH is most likely to be related to rebleeding or the development of hydrocephalus.

Rebleeding was previously the primary cause of death following poor-grade SAH but rates have dramatically reduced since the shift towards early securing of the ruptured aneurysm. Antifibrinolytic therapy may reduce the risk of rebleeding by up to 40% but does not improve outcome, possibly because of treatment-related microthrombosis and cerebral ischaemia. The short-term use of antifibrinolytics can be considered in selected cases at high risk of rebleeding in whom definitive treatment of the aneurysm is delayed.

Hydrocephalus develops in around 50% of patients after SAH, and deterioration due to worsening of hydrocephalus requires immediate insertion of an external ventricular drain. Up to 30% of patients with poor-grade SAH improve neurologically with CSF drainage even in the absence of overt hydrocephalus.

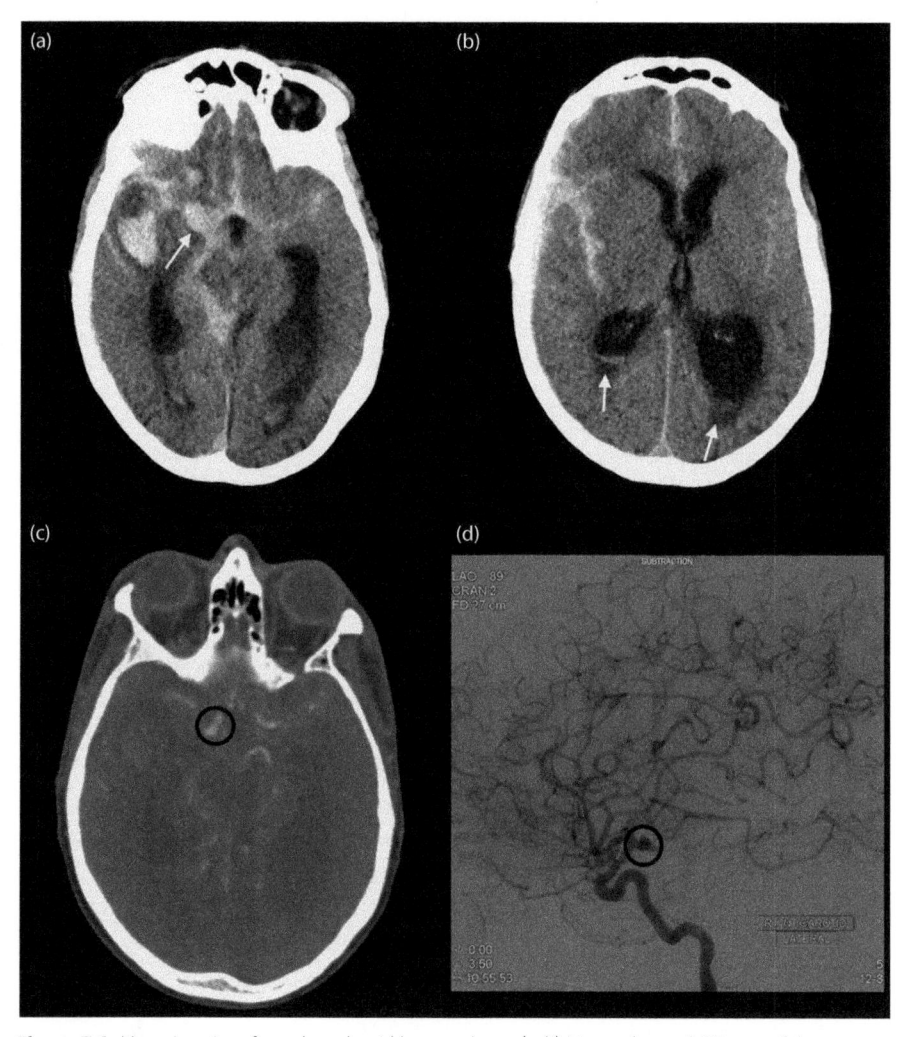

Figure 7.1 Neuroimaging after subarachnoid haemorrhage. (a, b) Non-enhanced CT scan of the head demonstrating a large amount of subarachnoid blood, largely on the right side in the region of the terminal internal carotid artery and middle cerebral artery (arrow in (a)). The blood has tracked into the ventricular system (arrows in (b)) and is associated with hydrocephalus. The ventricles are dilated asymmetrically, the left side being more dilated than the right. (c) CT angiogram and (d) subsequent digital subtraction angiography demonstrate a terminal right internal carotid artery aneurysm (circled).

⊘ Learning point Treatment of aneurysms: coiling or clipping?

Prior to the introduction of coil embolization technology in the early 1990s, aneurysms were treated through craniotomy and placement of a clip around the aneurysm neck. Since then, the role of endovascular treatment of intracranial aneurysms has expanded, allowing minimally invasive and effective treatment even in the sickest patients. This is important because early aneurysm control reduces the risk of rebleeding and allows higher arterial blood pressure to prevent or treat cerebral hypoperfusion.

The most important trial to date investigating the treatment of ruptured intracranial aneurysms is the International Subarachnoid Aneurysm Trial (ISAT) [2]. Between 1994 and 2002, this study randomized 2143 patients from 42 centres (largely within the UK and Europe) with ruptured intracranial aneurysms

(continued)

to receive either neurosurgical clipping or endovascular coiling. The primary outcome measure was death or dependency (defined as a modified Rankin scale of 3–6) at 1 year, and secondary outcomes included rebleeding and seizure rate. ISAT found a significantly reduced risk of death or dependency at 1 year in the endovascular coiling group compared to the neurosurgical clipping group. The risk of rebleeding was low overall, but late rebleeding was more common following coiling. The risk of seizures following coiling was substantially lower than following neurosurgical clipping. Many concerns were raised following the publication of ISAT, particularly with regards to the durability of coil technology and the risk of rebleeding. Subsequent follow-up of the ISAT cohort has shown that, although rebleeding was more likely in the endovascular coiling group at 10 years following treatment, the overall risk of rebleeding remains small [3]. Of the 1003 patients followed up at 10 years, rebleeding from the treated aneurysm occurred in only 13 of 531 in the endovascular coiling group and in 4 of 472 in the neurosurgical clipping group. Although rates of dependency alone were similar in the two groups at 10-year follow-up, the probability of death or dependency was significantly greater in the neurosurgical clipping group. Thus endovascular coiling appears to be effective and durable.

ISAT has been criticized for many reasons [4]. Sixty-nine per cent of the 9559 patients eligible for recruitment into the study were excluded because of lack of equipoise and, since almost all intracranial aneurysms can be treated by surgery, it follows that a large proportion of patients were excluded because of a local assessment that their aneurysm was not suitable for coiling. There was also underrepresentation of middle cerebral artery and posterior circulation aneurysms in the study and, because these are preferentially treated by clipping and coiling respectively, this also raises the possibility of sample bias. Larger aneurysms were also underrepresented in the study. There have been significant developments in endovascular technology in recent years, including the development of stents and flow diverters, and this may significantly influence the outcomes following endovascular coiling. Such developments may also enable aneurysms that were unsuitable for coiling at the time of ISAT (such as larger aneurysms) to be treated by this method today. The authors of ISAT have therefore established another randomized controlled trial (RCT) (ISAT 2) that aims to include a wider range of aneurysm types, including many of those that were excluded from the original study [5]. This study will need to take account of any effects on rebleeding rates and outcome of dual antiplatelet therapy which is often required following the deployment of stents and flow diverters.

Decisions about the optimal treatment for an intracranial aneurysm require multidisciplinary consensus between neurosurgeons and neuroradiologists. This must account for the healthcare resources available (including surgical and endovascular expertise), the age and clinical status of the patient, and the anatomy and location of the aneurysm. At present, factors favouring surgical clipping include the presence of intraparenchymal haematomas requiring surgical evacuation, wide-necked aneurysms, and those causing acute brainstem compression. In contrast, endovascular coiling is often preferred in elderly and comorbid patients, posterior circulation aneurysms, and in poor-grade patients.

Following the procedure, which was uneventful, the patient was transferred sedated and ventilated to the intensive care unit (ICU) for neurological and cardiovascular monitoring, and systemic physiological optimization. Treatment targets included euvolaemia, systolic blood pressure at 20% above baseline level, normoglycaemia, and normothermia.

⊕ Clinical tip   Principles of ICU management

Optimization of systemic physiological variables, particularly arterial blood gases, arterial blood pressure, blood glucose, and temperature, is the cornerstone of the ICU management of SAH. Abnormalities of fluid balance are common, with hypovolaemia occurring in 17–30% of patients. Isotonic crystalloids are the replacement fluid of choice. Mineralocorticoids, such as fludrocortisone or hydrocortisone, have been shown to limit natriuresis and associated water loss, and the amount of fluid required to maintain euvolaemia. However, they are not used routinely since no outcome benefits have been demonstrated. Hyperglycaemia occurs in around 30% of patients after SAH and is associated with poor outcome. A blood glucose target of 6–10 mmol/L is recommended; very tight

(continued)

glycaemic control is avoided to minimize the risk of hypoglycaemia which is harmful to the injured brain. Fever occurs in up to 70% of patients, is more common in poor-grade SAH, and is associated with worse outcome. An infective cause should be excluded or treated, but fever is often related to the hypothalamic or inflammatory effects of subarachnoid blood. Temperature should be monitored frequently and standard measures used to maintain normothermia, particularly during the period of risk of delayed cerebral ischaemia (DCI). Anaemia is also very common after SAH and is associated with a poor outcome, although blood transfusion is similarly associated with an adverse outcome. Current guidance recommends transfusion to maintain the haemoglobin concentration between 80–100 g/L [6], although higher thresholds might be appropriate in patients at high risk of DCI. SAH patients are at risk of venous thromboembolism, and intermittent compression devices should be applied in all patients on admission to the ICU. Pharmacological thromboprophylaxis can be started 24 hours after aneurysm treatment.

The sedation was stopped and the patient awoke and was extubated later that day. Her GCS at this stage was 12/15 (E3, V4, M5). Daily testing of full blood count and serum electrolytes was performed, with particularly close monitoring of serum sodium levels. Daily serial transcranial Doppler (TCD) examinations and ECG were obtained.

> ✪ **Learning point** Aneurysmal subarachnoid haemorrhage management protocol
>
> The general principles of managing SAH are shown in Figure 7.2. Close and frequent neurological and cardiorespiratory monitoring is important in SAH. Although SAH patients are often managed in high dependency unit or ICU settings that facilitate such monitoring, some, including many that are WFNS grade 1, can be safely managed in a neurosurgical ward. However, irrespective of care location, close clinical observation with regular neurological assessment is crucial with a low threshold for escalation of care. Strict bed rest minimizes fluctuations in blood pressure that may adversely affect outcome, and the use of laxatives minimizes straining and hence intracranial hypertension. All patients should be commenced on nimodipine immediately after symptom onset where clinical suspicion is high, and those in whom SAH is subsequently confirmed should complete a 21-day course as a standard of care. Nimodipine is typically administered at a dose of 60 mg orally or via nasogastric tube every 4 hours. Intravenous nimodipine, at a dose of 1 mg/hour (or 500 mcg/hour if body weight <70 kg or blood pressure unstable) increased to 2 mg/hour after 2 hours if blood pressure remains stable, can be used in the presence of poor enteral absorption. Maintenance of adequate hydration is important since many patients with SAH have intravascular fluid depletion. Maintenance of euvolaemia minimizes the risk of cerebral ischaemia. ECG and chest X-ray are essential for the assessment of cardiopulmonary complications.
>
> Urgent identification of an aneurysm as the cause of the SAH is imperative. Early treatment of an unsecured aneurysm, ideally as soon as possible but within 48 hours of symptom onset, is recommended to prevent rebleeding. Early transfer to a neuroscience centre with appropriate facilities and continuous availability of all members of the multidisciplinary team are crucial to facilitate early intervention. Early treatment may not always be possible or appropriate, for example in a poor-grade, elderly patient with multiple comorbidities or patients with highly complex aneurysm anatomy.
>
> Hypertension is a normal response to SAH, although high blood pressure increases the risk of rebleeding. On the other hand, excessive reductions in blood pressure risk the development of cerebral ischaemia. Extreme hypertension should be treated cautiously with a short-acting agent. Current guidelines recommend that before the aneurysm is treated, systolic and mean blood pressure should be no higher than 160 mmHg and 110 mmHg, respectively [6]. Hypotension is meticulously avoided, and chronic antihypertensive medications are withheld initially. Once the aneurysm is secured, systolic blood pressure is often managed at 20% above baseline. In the presence of hydrocephalus, CSF diversion is required. External ventricular drainage through a transfrontal catheter is the most common method. Use of antibiotic- or silver-impregnated catheters can reduce the infection risk associated with this intervention [7]. Insertion of an external ventricular drain, in addition to permitting therapeutic drainage of CSF, also enables measurement of intracranial pressure. Lumbar puncture or insertion of a lumbar drain can also be used for therapeutic CSF drainage, although it is relatively contraindicated in the presence of obstructive hydrocephalus that may result from the
>
> *(continued)*

presence of intraventricular blood. Lumbar drainage of CSF can also be used to clear blood from the CSF and prevent stasis of clots, but there is currently no conclusive evidence of benefit. Overall, what evidence there is does not support a concern about the safety of lumbar drains [8].

Anticonvulsants are generally not recommended unless there are documented seizures, as their use has been associated with unfavourable outcomes [6]. However, these data are based primarily on the use of phenytoin and it is unclear whether the same holds true for newer anticonvulsants. Levetiracetam is being increasingly used in this context, because of its superior pharmacodynamic and kinetic profiles compared to phenytoin: levetiracetam has minimal protein binding and no hepatic metabolism, resulting in a lower risk of drug interactions and better tolerability. At present, there are no outcome data demonstrating benefits of levetiracetam over phenytoin after SAH.

The monitoring and management of DCI is covered later in this chapter.

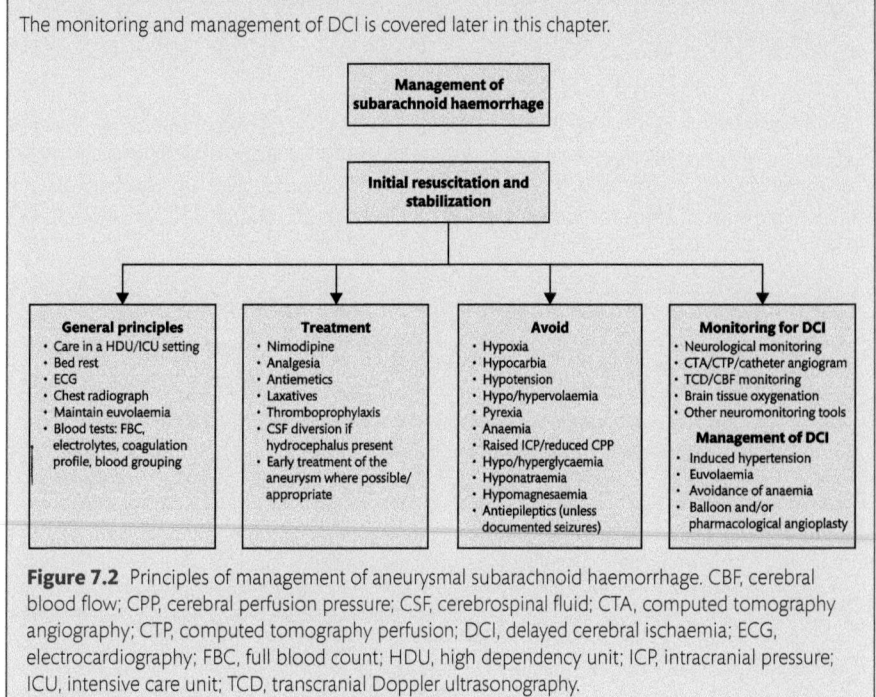

Figure 7.2 Principles of management of aneurysmal subarachnoid haemorrhage. CBF, cerebral blood flow; CPP, cerebral perfusion pressure; CSF, cerebrospinal fluid; CTA, computed tomography angiography; CTP, computed tomography perfusion; DCI, delayed cerebral ischaemia; ECG, electrocardiography; FBC, full blood count; HDU, high dependency unit; ICP, intracranial pressure; ICU, intensive care unit; TCD, transcranial Doppler ultrasonography.

On the first postoperative day, the ECG showed T-wave inversion in the lateral leads and a prolonged QTc interval. There was a modest rise in serum troponin, but an echocardiogram was normal. A 'watch and review' approach was taken.

⑥ Expert comment

Cardiac complications are common after SAH and related to sympathetic hyperactivity and catecholamine-induced myocyte dysfunction. They may result in minimal clinical effects but, in severe cases, can lead to cardiogenic shock and pulmonary oedema. Cardiovascular dysfunction often resolves spontaneously after a variable period, emphasizing the importance of general supportive critical care during periods of instability. There is no specific curative therapy. Although modification of the sympathetic response might limit cardiac dysfunction after SAH, there is no strong evidence to recommend this line of therapy which may risk hypotension and the development of cerebral ischaemia. Vasopressors and inotropes may be used for haemodynamic augmentation, but there is no definitive evidence to recommend one agent over another.

> ✪ **Learning point** Management of cardiac abnormalities after subarachnoid haemorrhage
>
> Cardiac complications are common after SAH and associated with DCI and poor outcome [9]. These manifest as ECG abnormalities, elevated cardiac troponin I (cTnI), and a spectrum of ventricular dysfunction collectively referred to as the neurogenic stunned myocardium (NSM) syndrome. ECG abnormalities are extremely common after SAH. ST-segment changes have been reported in up to 50% of patients, inverted or isoelectric T waves in up to 90%, QTc prolongation in almost two-thirds, and cardiac arrhythmias in more than one-third [10]. Elevation of cTnI occurs in approximately one-third of patients, and left ventricular dysfunction in around 18% [11]. The underlying mechanism of NSM is believed to relate to sympathetic nervous system activation and excessive noradrenaline release from myocardial sympathetic nerve terminals [12]. This causes a physiological denervation in the presence of normal coronary perfusion and a characteristic pattern of left ventricular regional wall motion abnormalities involving the basal and middle portions of the anteroseptal and anterior ventricular walls with relative apical sparing, reflecting the distribution of sympathetic nerves rather than specific vascular territories [13].
>
> Left ventricular dysfunction is usually temporary, although some patients require cardiovascular support [14]. Risk factors for the development of NSM include worse SAH clinical grade at presentation, smoking, and increasing age [15]. A known history of hypertension before SAH has been associated with a lower risk of NSM [15]. Nuclear imaging in a cohort of 30 patients with aneurysmal SAH has shown that the majority had altered cardiac glucose metabolism (83%) and sympathetic innervation (90%) but preserved cardiac perfusion (100%) [16], suggesting that many SAH patients may have subclinical alterations in cardiac metabolism.
>
> Although cardiopulmonary and haemodynamic status should be optimized, no class I data (i.e. from RCTs) exists to guide the management of cardiac abnormalities after SAH. Characterizing cardiac performance using echocardiography and continuous cardiac output monitoring may be useful in guiding therapy in patients with symptomatic NSM. Dobutamine has been used to increase cardiac output, but the influence on outcomes is unclear [17]. Potassium and magnesium values should be checked and corrected if necessary. Crucially important is the avoidance of delays in securing the aneurysm in patients with ECG and other cardiac abnormalities in the presence of clinical stability.

On the third day after admission the patient developed acute hyponatraemia. Her serum sodium decreased to 121 mmol/L from 135 mmol/L on the previous day. She was treated with infusion of hypertonic saline (1.8%), and this corrected her sodium values slowly over 48 hours.

> ⓘ **Expert comment**
>
> Aneurysmal SAH is commonly associated with abnormalities of fluid balance and electrolyte derangements, which can negatively affect outcome. Hyponatraemia (serum sodium <135 mmol/L) may be related to iatrogenic haemodilution, the cerebral salt-wasting syndrome, or the syndrome of inappropriate antidiuretic hormone secretion. The major risk of acute hyponatraemia is the development of cerebral oedema secondary to fluid shifts as plasma tonicity reduces. Fluid restriction to treat hyponatraemia from whatever cause is no longer recommended after SAH because of the risk of cerebral infarction caused by hypovolaemic hypoperfusion. Hypertonic (1.8%) saline can be used to maintain euvolaemia in hyponatraemic patients, particularly those at high risk of DCI. Prophylactic use of mineralocorticoids may limit natriuresis and hyponatraemia, but careful electrolyte monitoring is essential as hypokalaemia and hyperglycaemia may ensue. The correction of hyponatraemia can itself lead to neurological sequelae, particularly osmotic demyelination syndrome. This risk is minimized by gradual correction of sodium deficits. Hypertonic saline infusion should be discontinued when serum sodium reaches 125–130 mmol/L.

> **✪ Learning point** Management of hyponatraemia in subarachnoid haemorrhage
>
> Hyponatraemia is the most common electrolyte abnormality in hospital inpatients [18]. It is particularly common in patients with SAH [19], with some studies suggesting an incidence greater than 50% [20]. Correct and timely management of hyponatraemia is important as it is associated with an increased risk of cerebral oedema, vasospasm, and cerebral infarction following SAH.
>
> The underlying pathophysiology of hyponatraemia following SAH is unclear, but it is associated with elevated values of atrial [21, 22] and brain natriuretic peptides [23, 24]. Cerebral salt wasting (CSW) is thought to be the predominant mechanism of hyponatraemia in patients with SAH, although the syndrome of inappropriate antidiuretic hormone (SIADH) is also common. SIADH occurs because of excess antidiuretic hormone secretion causing water retention and volume overload, and leads to a dilutional hyponatraemia. CSW on the other hand is associated with raised atrial and brain natriuretic peptide and excessive renal sodium and water loss, leading to circulating volume contraction. The administration of large volumes of isotonic saline can increase extracellular fluid volume, activate atrial natriuretic peptides (ANPs), and suppress aldosterone. Significant fluid administration can also result in a 'normal' physiological pressure natriuresis [25].
>
> A detailed management protocol for hyponatraemia in patients with SAH is beyond the scope of this chapter, and for this the reader is referred elsewhere [25]. Accurately establishing the underlying cause of hyponatraemia in SAH is vital for appropriate management. Several therapies used in the management of SAH can complicate the assessment of the underlying cause of hyponatraemia. For example, the calcium channel antagonist nimodipine can lead to hyponatraemia through activation of atrial natriuretic peptides [26] and inhibition of aldosterone activity [27]. Noradrenaline, often used to augment blood pressure, may lead to a pressure diuresis and hypovolaemic hyponatraemia [28]. Whether a clinically significant difference between CSW and SIADH exists is unclear [29]—most laboratory criteria cannot distinguish between the two. However, the consensus is that the clinical and laboratory assessment of extracellular fluid status is important for differentiation (Table 7.2).
>
> **Table 7.2** Features of the syndrome of inappropriate antidiuretic hormone secretion and cerebral salt wasting
>
> | | SIADH | CSW |
> |---|---|---|
> | Serum sodium (mmol/L) | <135 | <135 |
> | Serum osmolality (mOsm/kg) | <285 | <285 |
> | Urine osmolality (mOsm/kg) | >200 | >200 |
> | Urinary sodium (mmol/L) | >25 | >25 |
> | Extracellular fluid volume | Increased or no change | Reduced |
> | Central venous pressure (cmH$_2$O) | ≥6 | <6 |
> | Fluid balance | Positive | Negative |
>
> CSW, cerebral salt-wasting syndrome; SIADH, syndrome of inappropriate antidiuretic hormone secretion.
>
> The management of hyponatraemia depends on the underlying cause, and whether it is acute and symptomatic (e.g. seizures, coma, dilated pupils, and neurogenic pulmonary oedema) or chronic. The volume of hypertonic saline administered should be individualized, guided by frequent serum sodium level monitoring to minimize the risk of overcorrecting, or correcting hyponatraemia too rapidly. Acute symptomatic hyponatraemia can be corrected with hypertonic saline (1.8%) to raise plasma sodium by 1–2 mmol/hour to a total of 4–6 mmol [30], after which guidelines for correction of chronic hyponatraemia are followed by correcting sodium values by no more than 0.5 mmol/hour, to a maximum of 8–10 mmol/24 hours, to avoid the risk of osmotic demyelination syndrome. For SIADH, lithium and demeclocycline can also be used. Fludrocortisone [31] and hydrocortisone [32] may also have a role in reducing natriuresis, but further evidence is required before these can be considered routine options. Vasopressin-2 receptor antagonists are currently licensed in the UK for the treatment of SIADH (and in the US for treatment of chronic hyponatraemia), but there is little evidence for their use specifically in patients with SAH and extreme caution is advised because of the risk of hypovolaemia.

Five days after admission, the patient developed a left-sided hemiparesis that correlated with TCD-derived indices of vasospasm (middle cerebral artery velocity 180 cm/s; Lindegaard ratio 5.2—see later). Induced hypertension to a target systolic blood pressure of 160–180 mmHg using a noradrenaline infusion improved her neurological deficit.

> **⚑ Expert comment**
>
> Euvolaemia is the target for both prophylaxis and treatment of DCI, and induced hypertension can be effective in reversing established DCI. Systemic blood pressure is increased slowly while monitoring for evidence of neurological or perfusion improvement, and after 2–3 days can be gradually weaned while continuing monitoring for deterioration. There is preliminary evidence that early goal-directed haemodynamic therapy might reduce the risk of DCI and improve outcome after SAH, but large, randomized controlled outcome studies are required before its widespread adoption into clinical practice.

---

❸ Learning point   Diagnosis and management of vasospasm and delayed cerebral ischaemia

There are many causes of delayed (>24 hours) neurological deterioration after SAH, which can be related to systemic and intracranial causes (Figure 7.3). DCI is a term applied to any neurological deterioration, including focal neurological deficits and altered consciousness, which persists for more than 1 hour and is not attributable to other causes including a complication of aneurysm occlusion, hyponatraemia, or fever. Although death caused by DCI is infrequent in patients with SAH [33], the associated morbidity is high and it doubles the risk of a poor outcome.

Factors associated with delayed cerebral ischaemia include:

- severe early brain injury (from the acute effects of subarachnoid blood and the transient global ischaemia that may accompany aneurysm rupture)
- volume, density, and persistence of the subarachnoid blood
- extent and severity of angiographic vasospasm
- increased cerebral metabolic demand/factors reducing the supply of oxygen and glucose
- low cardiac output
- raised intracranial pressure
- hypotension
- existing collateral and anastomotic blood flow (protective)
- genetics (e.g. apolipoprotein E ε4 allele)
- choice of treatment used for the aneurysm (rates of DCI are higher following neurosurgical clipping compared to endovascular coiling) [56]
- smoking
- pre-existing hypertension
- diabetes and hyperglycaemia
- systemic inflammatory response syndrome
- hydrocephalus.

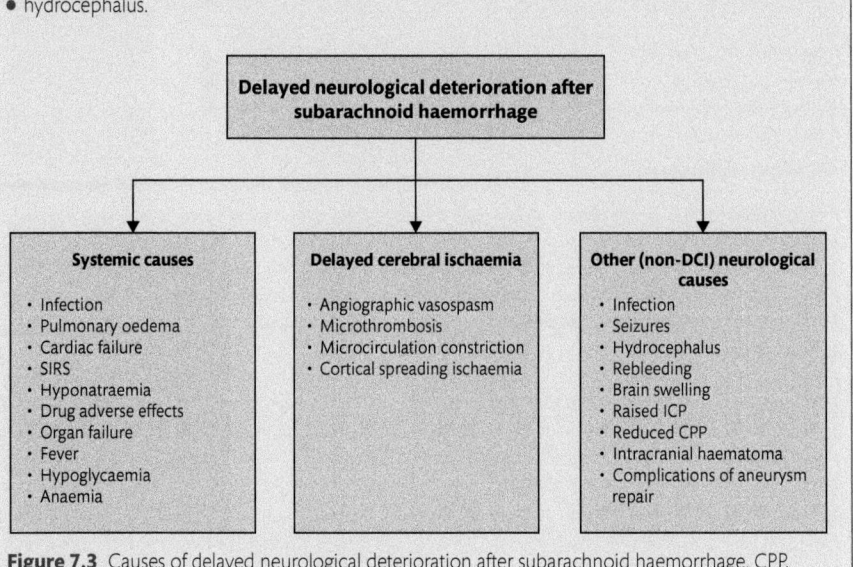

Figure 7.3 Causes of delayed neurological deterioration after subarachnoid haemorrhage. CPP, cerebral perfusion pressure; DCI, delayed cerebral ischaemia; ICP, intracranial pressure; SIRS, systemic inflammatory response syndrome.

(continued)

Pathophysiology

The pathophysiology of DCI is complex and incompletely understood. Angiographic vasospasm is associated with DCI, but vasospasm and DCI are not synonymous. While approximately two-thirds of patients with SAH develop angiographic vasospasm approximately 3–14 days after the initial injury [34], symptoms develop in only 20–30% [35]. Ischaemia often involves more than one vascular territory, suggesting that mechanisms other than simple vessel constriction contribute to the development of DCI. These mechanisms include cortical spreading ischaemia, microthrombosis, and microcirculation constriction and have been comprehensively reviewed elsewhere (Figure 7.3) [36].

Diagnosis

The diagnosis of DCI can be made on clinical and radiological grounds (Figure 7.2), after exclusion of other neurological and systemic causes for the neurological deterioration. Clinically, patients may present with a spectrum of impaired consciousness, focal neurological deficits, or pupillary abnormalities. The clinical diagnosis is often difficult or impossible in poor-grade and sedated and ventilated patients, in whom it is necessary to rely on other diagnostic criteria. Of the potential contributors to DCI, angiographic vasospasm is the most readily detectable and cerebrovascular imaging therefore plays a key role in the investigation of DCI. Although catheter angiography is the gold standard test for diagnosing vasospasm, CTA is increasingly being used. The main limitations of CTA include the possibility of overestimating the degree of vessel narrowing, and the presence of artefacts from the treated aneurysm (clips and coils), although this can be overcome with adjustment of the image reconstruction plane and appropriate windowing and levelling of the CT. CT perfusion permits calculation of the mean transit time taken for blood to perfuse a tissue region of interest, and is also used as a marker of cerebral vasospasm. A meta-analysis has confirmed a high diagnostic accuracy for both CTA and CT perfusion in the diagnosis of cerebral vasospasm in SAH [37].

TCD is widely used as a bedside tool for diagnosing and monitoring vasospasm, and can also be used to detect impaired cerebral autoregulation [38]. Increased middle cerebral artery flow velocity to greater than 120 cm/s is consistent with vasospasm, but increases in flow velocity can also be related to hyperaemia. The Lindegaard ratio, which compares the mean flow velocity in the middle cerebral artery and that in the ipsilateral extracranial internal carotid artery, overcomes this issue and is often preferred. A ratio greater than 3 is considered diagnostic of vasospasm [39]. Although a sensitivity of 97% for the TCD detection of severe vasospasm has been reported [40], TCD is a user-dependent tool that requires skilled personnel for interpretation and only assesses a small number of large arteries. Treatment decisions should not be based on TCD values alone [41].

Prevention and treatment

The only drug with class I evidence of improving outcomes following SAH is the L-type calcium channel antagonist nimodipine, which reduces the risk of both DCI and poor outcome [42]. Interestingly, in most clinical trials, nimodipine does not reduce the incidence of angiographic vasospasm, suggesting that its action is at least in part through the inhibition of cortical spreading ischaemia and antifibrinolytic activity that reduces microthrombus formation [43, 44]. The prevention of DCI focuses on the avoidance of factors that adversely affect the delivery of oxygen and glucose to the brain. These include optimization of fluid status and blood pressure. Traditionally, hypervolaemia, hypertension, and haemodilution (triple-H therapy) were central to the prevention and management of DCI, without evidence of outcome benefits from RCTs. In recent years, evidence has accumulated to suggest that not all aspects of triple-H therapy are beneficial, and that some are detrimental. A multimodality neuromonitoring study found that induced hypertension improved cerebral blood flow and brain tissue oxygenation (measured using brain tissue oxygen tension ($PbtO_2$) monitoring) after SAH, whereas hypervolaemia had an adverse effect on $PbtO_2$ [45]. Hypervolaemic haemodilution is also associated with increased systemic complications, including acute lung injury, and reduction of haemoglobin to dangerously low values [46]. In the latest guidelines on the management of SAH from the Neurocritical Care Society, euvolaemia and induced hypertension are recommended, with firm advice to avoid haemodilution [6].

Significant efforts have been directed into RCTs of drug treatment for SAH. While many have been shown to minimize the development of vasospasm and/or DCI, most have not resulted in improved

(continued)

clinical outcomes [47]. In particular, high-profile trials of magnesium [48] and statins [49] have been disappointing. Endothelin-A antagonists have been studied extensively after SAH because of the key role that endothelin plays in maintaining vascular tone. The endothelin-A antagonist clazosentan reduces angiographic vasospasm but has no significant effect on outcome [50]. There are also no robust data to support approaches targeting pathophysiological aspects of DCI other than vasospasm, including microthromboembolism and platelet aggregation. A meta-analysis of RCTs of antiplatelet therapies to target microthromboembolism reported a reduction in poor outcomes and increased risk of intracranial complications, neither of which was statistically significant [51].

Data on other drugs for SAH are promising, but methodological limitations of the studies necessitate caution in their interpretation. The rho-kinase inhibitor fasudil has been shown in several studies to reduce the incidence of angiographic vasospasm and cerebral infarction, and improve the odds ratio for good recovery compared to placebo or nimodipine and other drugs (odds ratio 1.58; 95% confidence interval 1.12–2.23) [52]. However, these studies had several limitations and the drug is not used in Europe or North America. The delivery of localized intrathecal thrombolytic agents to remove the clot have been found in RCTs to significantly reduce the incidence of vasospasm, delayed neurological deficits, hydrocephalus, and poor outcomes [53], although these studies also had several limitations. A small RCT of erythropoietin showed fewer cerebral infarcts, less protracted cerebral autoregulatory dysfunction, and improved clinical outcomes [54], although further data are required to confirm these preliminary findings.

Several study limitations might have accounted for the multiple 'negative' results, including inappropriate or insensitive outcome measures, lack of selection of high-risk patients, and higher reliance on rescue therapy in the placebo arm of trials which may have offset any benefit of the intervention arm. Although future studies should aim to address these and other methodological limitations, it also seems clear that targeting a single pathway in a disease with a complex pathophysiology is unlikely to lead to dramatic improvements in outcome.

'Rescue' therapies are often used when a patient with SAH develops DCI. This can include haemodynamic therapy or endovascular angioplasty. Attention should be paid to the fluid status and blood pressure. Euvolaemia and induced hypertension is recommended. Systemic blood pressure should be increased in a stepwise fashion guided by assessment of neurological function, neuromonitoring, or radiological evidence of improved perfusion. The higher blood pressure is maintained for 2–3 days and gradually weaned while monitoring for deterioration in clinical and neuromonitoring variables. Although balloon angioplasty and intra-arterial injections of vasodilating drugs are commonly used in clinical practice, particularly if a patient does not respond to induced hypertension or is intolerant of it, these interventions have not yet been subjected to the rigours of a clinical trial [55]. Examples of vasodilating drugs used in this setting include papaverine, nicardipine, nimodipine, verapamil, and milrinone. All are short acting, can cause hypotension in high doses, and should be considered only when medical treatment has failed or is considered too risky because of cardiac or other comorbidities.

The patient made a good recovery, and the noradrenaline infusion was slowly weaned after 2 days. Ten days following the endovascular procedure, the patient was transferred to a neurosurgical ward for ongoing care and rehabilitation.

Discussion

SAH comprises less than 5% of all strokes, but its societal impact is profound because the mean age of affected patients is lower than that of other stroke subtypes [57]. There has been a marked (up to 50%) reduction in SAH-related mortality in recent decades [58, 59], but morbidity remains high in the approximately 60% of patients who survive. Survivors often have profound cognitive, neurological, or functional deficits that impair their quality of life and ability to work [60].

Several factors are associated with poor outcome after SAH (see the following list) [61]. The recent improvements in outcome are likely to be multifactorial and related to earlier and improved diagnosis, greater understanding of both the early and late patho-physiology of SAH and their effects on outcome, and more aggressive management approaches including early aneurysm repair, treatment of DCI, and improved medical management of complications [62].

Factors associated with poor outcome following SAH include [61]:

- increased age
- worse neurological grade
- large blood load on admission CT scan
- symptomatic vasospasm
- cerebral infarction
- presence of intracerebral or intraventricular haemorrhage
- larger aneurysm size
- ruptured posterior circulation aneurysm
- elevated systolic blood pressure on admission
- previous diagnosis of hypertension, myocardial infarction, liver disease, or SAH
- temperature greater than 38°C 8 days after SAH
- anticonvulsant use.

Early brain injury

Delayed neurological deterioration due to DCI and other causes (Figure 7.3) was de-scribed in detail earlier in this chapter. Early brain injury is also an important patho-physiological process in patients with SAH. Aneurysm rupture is associated with extravasation of blood into the subarachnoid space and often into the ventricles and brain tissue. This is associated with an acute increase in ICP that may result in impaired cerebral perfusion, transient global ischaemia, and temporary loss of consciousness. Early brain injury after SAH results from this chain of events in combination with the direct effects of the blood itself [36]. The underlying pathophysiological changes asso-ciated with early brain injury include impaired cerebral blood flow and autoregulation, disruption of the blood–brain barrier, activation of cell death pathways, cerebral oe-dema, impaired calcium homeostasis, oxidative stress, and inflammation. These pathophysiological pathways have recently been comprehensively reviewed [63]. It is anticipated that, in the future, pharmacological treatments will be able to target this early damage associated with SAH and improve outcomes.

Pending the development of treatments that target the early and delayed brain injury associated with SAH, clinical management should focus on early securing of the ruptured aneurysm and optimization of systemic physiology and modifiable risk factors for DCI that are known to influence outcome.

A final word from the expert

Aneurysmal SAH is a devastating disease associated with high mortality and poor outcome in many survivors. Aggressive treatment by a comprehensive multidisciplinary team in a high-volume centre is associated with improved outcome. The critical care management of SAH presents significant challenges and should focus on the following key points:

1. Rapid intervention to secure the ruptured aneurysm to minimize the risk of rebleeding, followed by implementation of measures to minimize secondary brain injury.
2. Identification and treatment of acute intracranial complications such as hydrocephalus.
3. Optimization of fluid balance to target euvolaemia, and careful control of blood pressure.
4. Avoidance of hyperglycaemia, hyperthermia, and liberal blood transfusions which are all associated with longer ICU and hospital length of stay, higher mortality, and worse neurological outcome in survivors.
5. Identification and management of non-neurological complications including SAH-related cardiac dysfunction and hyponatraemia.
6. Prevention and treatment of DCI through meticulous fluid management, and induced hypertension in established DCI.
7. Early, aggressive treatment should be offered to all but the most hopeless cases since substantial numbers of even poor-grade patients may do well.

References

1. Drake CG, Hunt WE, Kassell N, et al. Report of World Federation of Neurological Surgeons Committee on a Universal Subarachnoid Hemorrhage Grading Scale. *J Neurosurg.* 1988;68:985–6.
2. Molyneux AJ, Kerr RSC, Yu L-M, et al. International subarachnoid aneurysm trial (ISAT) of neurosurgical clipping versus endovascular coiling in 2143 patients with ruptured intracranial aneurysms: a randomised comparison of effects on survival, dependency, seizures, rebleeding, subgroups, and aneurysm occlusion. *Lancet.* 2005;366:809–17.
3. Molyneux AJ, Birks J, Clarke A, et al. The durability of endovascular coiling versus neurosurgical clipping of ruptured cerebral aneurysms: 18 year follow-up of the UK cohort of the International Subarachnoid Aneurysm Trial (ISAT). *Lancet.* 2015;385:691–7.
4. Britz GW. ISAT trial: coiling or clipping for intracranial aneurysms? *Lancet.* 2005;366:783–5.
5. Darsaut TE, Jack AS, Kerr RS, Raymond J. International Subarachnoid Aneurysm Trial—ISAT part II: study protocol for a randomized controlled trial. *Trials.* 2013;14:156.
6. Diringer MN, Bleck TP, Hemphill C, et al. Critical care management of patients following aneurysmal subarachnoid hemorrhage: recommendations from the Neurocritical Care Society's Multidisciplinary Consensus Conference. *Neurocrit Care.* 2011;15:211–40.
7. Keong NC, Bulters DO, Richards HK, et al. The SILVER (Silver Impregnated Line Versus EVD Randomized trial): a double-blind, prospective, randomized, controlled trial of an intervention to reduce the rate of external ventricular drain infection. *Neurosurgery.* 2012;71:394–403.
8. Wolf S. Rationale for lumbar drains in aneurysmal subarachnoid hemorrhage. *Curr Opin Crit Care.* 2015;21:120–6.
9. van der Bilt IAC, Hasan D, Vandertop WP, et al. Impact of cardiac complications on outcome after aneurysmal subarachnoid hemorrhage: a meta-analysis. *Neurology.* 2009;72:635–42.
10. Wartenberg KE, Schmidt JM, Claassen J, et al. Impact of medical complications on outcome after subarachnoid hemorrhage. *Crit Care Med.* 2006;34:617–23.
11. Bruder N, Rabinstein A, Participants in the International Multi-Disciplinary Consensus Conference on the Critical Care Management of Subarachnoid Hemorrhage. Cardiovascular and pulmonary complications of aneurysmal subarachnoid hemorrhage. *Neurocrit Care.* 2011;15:257–69.
12. Hinson HE, Sheth KN. Manifestations of the hyperadrenergic state after acute brain injury. *Curr Opin Crit Care.* 2012;18:139–45.

13. Nguyen H, Zaroff JG. Neurogenic stunned myocardium. *Curr Neurol Neurosci Rep*. 2009;9:486–91.

14. Mazzeo AT, Micalizzi A, Mascia L, et al. Brain-heart crosstalk: the many faces of stress-related cardiomyopathy syndromes in anaesthesia and intensive care. *Brit J Anaesth*. 2014;112:803–15.

15. Malik AN, Gross BA, Rosalind Lai PM, et al. Neurogenic stress cardiomyopathy after aneurysmal subarachnoid hemorrhage. *World Neurosurg*. 2015;83:880–5.

16. Prunet B, Basely M, D'Aranda E, et al. Impairment of cardiac metabolism and sympathetic innervation after aneurysmal subarachnoid hemorrhage: a nuclear medicine imaging study. *Crit Care*. 2014;18:R131.

17. Joseph M, Ziadi S, Nates J, et al. Increases in cardiac output can reverse flow deficits from vasospasm independent of blood pressure: a study using xenon computed tomographic measurement of cerebral blood flow. *Neurosurgery*. 2003;53:1044–51.

18. Boscoe A, Paramore C, Verbalis JG. Cost of illness of hyponatremia in the United States. *Cost Eff Resour Alloc*. 2006;4:10.

19. Qureshi AI, Suri MF, Sung GY, et al. Prognostic significance of hypernatremia and hyponatremia among patients with aneurysmal subarachnoid hemorrhage. *Neurosurgery*. 2002;50:749–55.

20. Sherlock M, O'Sullivan E, Agha A, et al. The incidence and pathophysiology of hyponatraemia after subarachnoid haemorrhage. *Clin Endocrinol (Oxf)*. 2006;64:250–4.

21. Nakagawa I, Kurokawa S, Nakase H. Hyponatremia is predictable in patients with aneurysmal subarachnoid haemorrhage – clinical significance of serum atrial natriuretic peptide. *Acta Neurochir (Wien)*. 2010;152:2147–52.

22. Espiner EA, Leikis R, Ferch RD, et al. The neuro-cardio-endocrine response to acute subarachnoid haemorrhage. *Clin Endocrinol (Oxf)*. 2002;56:629–35.

23. Berendes E, Walter M, Cullen P, et al. Secretion of brain natriuretic peptide in patients with aneurysmal subarachnoid haemorrhage. *Lancet*. 1997;349:245–9.

24. Sviri GE, Feinsod M, Soustiel JF. Brain natriuretic peptide and cerebral vasospasm in subarachnoid hemorrhage. Clinical and TCD correlations. *Stroke*. 2000;31:118–22.

25. Kirkman MA, Albert AF, Ibrahim A, Doberenz D. Hyponatremia and brain injury: historical and contemporary perspectives. *Neurocrit Care*. 2013;18:406–16.

26. Shamiss A, Peleg E, Rosenthal T, Ezra D. The role of atrial natriuretic peptide in the diuretic effect of Ca2 + entry blockers. *Eur J Pharmacol*. 1993;233:113–17.

27. Kosaka H, Hirayama K, Yoda N, et al. The L-, N-, and T-type triple calcium channel blocker benidipine acts as an antagonist of mineralocorticoid receptor, a member of nuclear receptor family. *Eur J Pharmacol*. 2010;635:49.

28. Singh S, Bohn D, Carlotti AP, et al. Cerebral salt wasting: truths, fallacies, theories, and challenges. *Crit Care Med*. 2002;30:2575–9.

29. Sterns RH, Silver SM. Cerebral salt wasting versus SIADH: what difference? *J Am Soc Nephrol*. 2008;19:194–6.

30. Mount DB. Fluid and electrolyte disturbances. In: Longo DL, Kasper DL, Jameson JL, et al. (eds) *Harrison's Principles of Internal Medicine*, 18th edn. Boston, MA: McGraw-Hill Medical; 2001, pp. 341–59.

31. Mori T, Katayama Y, Kawamata T, Hirayama T. Improved efficiency of hypervolemic therapy with inhibition of natriuresis by fludrocortisone in patients with aneurysmal subarachnoid hemorrhage. *J Neurosurg*. 1999;91:947–52.

32. Katayama Y, Haraoka J, Hirabayashi H, et al. A randomized controlled trial of hydrocortisone against hyponatremia in patients with aneurysmal subarachnoid hemorrhage. *Stroke*. 2007;38:2373–5.

33. Macdonald RL, Rosengart A, Huo D, Karrison T. Factors associated with the development of vasospasm after planned surgical treatment of aneurysmal subarachnoid hemorrhage. *J Neurosurg*. 2003;99:644–52.

34. Dorsch N. A clinical review of cerebral vasospasm and delayed ischaemia following aneurysm rupture. *Acta Neurochir Suppl*. 2011;110:5–6.

35. Dehdashti AR, Mermillod B, Rufenacht DA, et al. Does treatment modality of intracranial ruptured aneurysms influence the incidence of cerebral vasospasm and clinical outcome? *Cerebrovasc Dis*. 2004;17:53–60.

36. Macdonald RL. Delayed neurological deterioration after subarachnoid haemorrhage. *Nat Rev Neurol*. 2014;10:44–58.

37. Greenberg ED, Gold R, Reichman M, et al. Diagnostic accuracy of CT angiography and CT perfusion for cerebral vasospasm: a meta-analysis. *AJNR Am J Neuroradiol*. 2010;31:1853–60.

38. Aries MJH, Elting JW, De Keyser J, et al. Cerebral autoregulation in stroke: a review of transcranial Doppler studies. *Stroke*. 2010;41:2697–704.

39. Lindegaard KF, Nornes H, Bakke SJ, et al. Cerebral vasospasm diagnosis by means of angiography and blood velocity measurements. *Acta Neurochir (Wien)*. 1989;100:12–24.

40. Fontanella M, Valfrè W, Benech F, et al. Vasospasm after SAH due to aneurysm rupture of the anterior circle of Willis: value of TCD monitoring. *Neurol Res*. 2008;30:256–61.

41. Carrera E, Schmidt JM, Oddo M, et al. Transcranial Doppler for predicting delayed cerebral ischemia after subarachnoid hemorrhage. *Neurosurgery*. 2009;65:316–23.

42. Dorhout Mees SM, Rinkel GJE, Feigin VL, et al. Calcium antagonists for aneurysmal subarachnoid haemorrhage. *Cochrane Database Syst Rev*. 2007;3:CD000277.

43. Vergouwen MDI, Vermeulen M, Coert BA, et al. Microthrombosis after aneurysmal subarachnoid hemorrhage: an additional explanation for delayed cerebral ischemia. *J Cereb Blood Flow Metab*. 2008;28:1761–70.

44. Dreier JP. The role of spreading depression, spreading depolarization and spreading ischemia in neurological disease. *Nat Med*. 2011;17:439–47.

45. Muench E, Horn P, Bauhuf C, et al. Effects of hypervolemia and hypertension on regional cerebral blood flow, intracranial pressure, and brain tissue oxygenation after subarachnoid hemorrhage. *Crit Care Med*. 2007;35:1844–51.

46. Treggiari MM, Deem S. Which H is the most important in triple-H therapy for cerebral vasospasm? *Curr Opin Crit Care*. 2009;15:83–6.

47. Etminan N, Vergouwen MDI, Ilodigwe D, Macdonald RL. Effect of pharmaceutical treatment on vasospasm, delayed cerebral ischemia, and clinical outcome in patients with aneurysmal subarachnoid hemorrhage: a systematic review and meta-analysis. *J Cereb Blood Flow Metab*. 2011;31:1443–51.

48. Dorhout Mees SM, Algra A, Vandertop WP, et al. Magnesium for aneurysmal subarachnoid haemorrhage (MASH-2): a randomised placebo-controlled trial. *Lancet*. 2012;380:44–9.

49. Kirkpatrick PJ, Turner CL, Smith C, et al. Simvastatin in aneurysmal subarachnoid haemorrhage (STASH): a multicentre randomised phase 3 trial. *Lancet Neurol*. 2014;13:666–75.

50. Vergouwen MDI, Algra A, Rinkel GJE. Endothelin receptor antagonists for aneurysmal subarachnoid hemorrhage: a systematic review and meta-analysis update. *Stroke*. 2012;43:2671–6.

51. Dorhout Mees SM, van den Bergh WM, Algra A, Rinkel GJE. Antiplatelet therapy for aneurysmal subarachnoid haemorrhage. *Cochrane Database Syst Rev*. 2007;4:CD006184.

52. Liu GJ, Wang ZJ, Wang YF, et al. Systematic assessment and meta-analysis of the efficacy and safety of fasudil in the treatment of cerebral vasospasm in patients with subarachnoid hemorrhage. *Eur J Clin Pharmacol*. 2012;68:131–9.

53. Kramer AH, Fletcher JJ. Locally-administered intrathecal thrombolytics following aneurysmal subarachnoid hemorrhage: a systematic review and meta-analysis. *Neurocrit Care*. 2011;14:489–99.

54. Tseng M-Y, Hutchinson PJ, Richards HK, et al. Acute systemic erythropoietin therapy to reduce delayed ischemic deficits following aneurysmal subarachnoid hemorrhage: a phase II randomized, double-blind, placebo-controlled trial. *J Neurosurg*. 2009;111:171–80.

55. Kimball MM, Velat GJ, Hoh BL, Participants in the International Multi-Disciplinary Consensus Conference on the Critical Care Management of Subarachnoid Hemorrhage. Critical care guidelines on the endovascular management of cerebral vasospasm. *Neurocrit Care*. 2011;15;336–41.

56. Dorhout Mees SM, Kerr RS, Rinkel GJE, et al. Occurrence and impact of delayed cerebral ischemia after coiling and after clipping in the International Subarachnoid Aneurysm Trial (ISAT). *J Neurol*. 2012;259:679–83.

57. Macdonald RL, Schweizer TA. Spontaneous subarachnoid haemorrhage. *Lancet*. 2016;389:655–66.

58. Lovelock CE, Rinkel GJE, Rothwell PM. Time trends in outcome of subarachnoid hemorrhage: population-based study and systematic review. *Neurology*. 2010;74:1494–501.

59. Nieuwkamp DJ, Setz LE, Algra A, et al. Changes in case fatality of aneurysmal subarachnoid haemorrhage over time, according to age, sex, and region: a meta-analysis. *Lancet Neurol*. 2009;8:635–42.

60. Al-Khindi T, Macdonald RL, Schweizer TA. Cognitive and functional outcome after aneurysmal subarachnoid hemorrhage. *Stroke*. 2010;41:e519–36.

61. Rosengart AJ, Schultheiss KE, Tolentino J, Macdonald RL. Prognostic factors for outcome in patients with aneurysmal subarachnoid hemorrhage. *Stroke*. 2007;38:2315–21.

62. Smith M, Citerio G. What's new in subarachnoid hemorrhage. *Intensive Care Med*. 2015;41:123–6.

63. Sehba FA, Hou J, Pluta RM, Zhang JH. The importance of early brain injury after subarachnoid hemorrhage. *Prog Neurobiol*. 2012;97:14–37.

8 Acute-on-chronic respiratory failure

Richard Hunt

⊕ Expert Commentary Peter MacNaughton

Case history

A 61-year-old male with acute respiratory distress was referred for consideration for admission to the intensive care unit (ICU). He had presented to the emergency department the day before with a 4-day history of worsening dyspnoea. He had a 40 pack-year smoking history with a past medical history of chronic obstructive pulmonary disease (COPD). He had been seen by his general practitioner 3 days earlier who had prescribed 40 mg prednisolone once daily. His regular medications were an inhaled, combined long-acting beta$_2$ agonist with a steroid and an inhaled short-acting beta$_2$ agonist. He was fully independent with activities of daily living and could manage a flight of stairs, but would struggle to walk around a supermarket without stopping to catch his breath. He had never been admitted to hospital before and was not on oxygen therapy at home.

In the emergency department, examination showed a lean man in significant respiratory distress using his accessory muscles. He was fully conscious and orientated with a respiratory rate of 24 breaths/min, hyperinflated chest with poor expansion, quiet breath sounds with occasional wheeze and no focal signs. Circulation was unremarkable with warm peripheries, no peripheral oedema, and jugular venous pressure did not appear to be raised. His initial arterial blood gas (ABG) analysis, taken breathing air, showed a moderate respiratory acidosis: pH 7.28, partial pressure of oxygen (PaO$_2$) 7.92 kPa, partial pressure of carbon dioxide (PaCO$_2$) 7.37 kPa, bicarbonate 27.2 mmol/L (alveolar–arterial oxygen gradient 2.8 kPa and PaO$_2$/fraction of inspired oxygen (FiO$_2$) 37.7 kPa). He was treated with oxygen at 2 L/min via a Hudson mask, salbutamol nebulizers 6-hourly, ipratropium nebulizers 8-hourly, and oral prednisolone was continued. Admission bloods were unremarkable with a white blood count of 7.4 × 10^9/L and C-reactive protein of 11 mg/L. An initial chest X-ray (CXR) showed chronic changes associated with COPD but no focal changes (Figure 8.1). His respiratory distress improved and he was transferred to the medical admissions unit with a diagnosis of an acute exacerbation of COPD (AECOPD).

Following admission to the medical admissions unit, he developed worsening respiratory distress and arterial blood oxygen saturation by pulse oximetry (SpO$_2$) decreased to 80%. The oxygen mask was changed to a Venturi mask with an FiO$_2$ of 0.4 and urgent medical review requested. A repeat ABG showed pH 7.26, PaO$_2$ 17.8 kPa, PaCO$_2$ 8.37 kPa, and bicarbonate 27.1 mmol/L. He was reviewed by the medical registrar who decreased his FiO$_2$ to 0.28, started an intravenous aminophylline infusion, and transferred him to the respiratory high dependency unit for non-invasive ventilation (NIV).

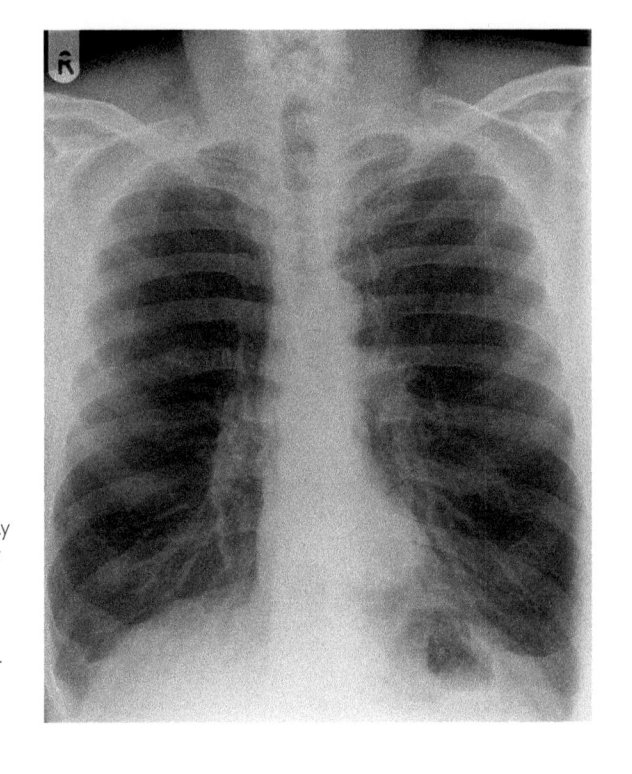

Figure 8.1 Admission chest X-ray shows chronic changes classically seen in COPD (increased lung markings, hyperexpansion, small cardiac shadow, bullae, and old rib fractures secondary to steroid-induced osteoporosis) with no focal signs.

Bi-level NIV was commenced using a full facemask and inspiratory and expiratory airway pressures (IPAP/EPAP) of 15 cmH$_2$O and 5 cmH$_2$O respectively with an FiO$_2$ of 0.30. His respiratory distress improved and a repeat ABG showed pH 7.30, PaO$_2$ 8.5 kPa, PaCO$_2$ 7.21 kPa, and bicarbonate 27.2 mmol/L.

> ✪ **Learning point** Controlled oxygen therapy
>
> Significant worsening of hypercapnia in response to supplemental oxygen exposure occurs in approximately 25% of patients with an exacerbation of COPD. The cause of this clinically important phenomenon is often incorrectly stated by clinicians.
>
> **Loss of hypoxic drive**
>
> This mechanism was first proposed in 1949 [1]. Despite several subsequent clinical studies that could not confirm this theory, this mechanism of oxygen-induced hypercapnia continues to be perpetuated in clinical texts. This has resulted in an inappropriate reluctance to administer oxygen to patients with COPD and severe hypoxaemia. Clinical studies have revealed that minute ventilation is not significantly reduced and that respiratory drive remains high in patients with COPD who develop hypercapnia following oxygen exposure [2]. Hypercapnia occurs because of an inability to increase minute ventilation to compensate for an increased pulmonary arterial carbon dioxide (CO$_2$) load from two main mechanisms:
>
> - *Hyperoxia-induced ventilation/perfusion (V/Q) mismatch*: hypoxic pulmonary vasoconstriction ensures that blood flow to poorly ventilated alveolar capillary units is minimized, maintaining optimal V/Q matching. If a high inspired oxygen concentration is administered, hypoxic vasoconstriction will be supressed in poorly ventilated lung units. This results in V/Q mismatch
>
> *(continued)*

and impaired CO_2 clearance. If the patient has ventilatory failure and is unable to increase minute ventilation significantly in order to increase CO_2 clearance from other lung units, then arterial CO_2 tension will inevitably rise.

- *The Haldane effect*: this describes the process by which CO_2 is bound more readily to deoxygenated haemoglobin than oxygenated haemoglobin. Administration of high inspired oxygen concentrations will result in less CO_2 bound to haemoglobin thereby increasing $PaCO_2$.

Oxygen-induced hypercapnia is not restricted to patients with severe COPD but may occur in any patient with chronic respiratory failure who is unable to increase minute ventilation to compensate for the mechanisms described. This includes COPD, morbid obesity hypoventilation syndrome, and neuromuscular disorders. The British Thoracic Society oxygen administration guidelines highlight the priority in all patients of preventing severe hypoxaemia and that therapy should be titrated to a target arterial blood oxygen saturation of 88–92% in patients with chronic respiratory disease at risk of hypercapnia [3].

> **Learning point Chronic obstructive pulmonary disease**
>
> COPD is characterized by long-standing airflow obstruction with limited reversibility. Smoking is the major cause, although occupational exposures and genetic factors may contribute. Smoking induces chronic inflammation resulting in both airway and parenchymal damage. In England, it is the fifth most common cause of mortality with more than 30,000 deaths per year and is a major cost burden on the National Health Service [4].

> **Learning point Management of AECOPD**
>
> The British Thoracic Society and National Institute for Health and Care Excellence (NICE) recommend the following on admission for any patient with AECOPD [5]:
>
> **Baseline investigations**
> - ABG with documented FiO_2.
> - Full blood count, urea and electrolytes, blood cultures if pyrexial.
> - CXR.
> - Electrocardiogram (ECG).
> - Theophylline concentration.
> - Sputum microscopy and culture (if purulent).
>
> **Medical therapy**
> - Oxygen to maintain SpO_2 88–92%.
> - Inhaled bronchodilators; the driving gas should be prescribed for nebulizers.
> - Prednisolone 30 mg (7 to no longer than 14 days).
> - Antibiotics (see next section).
> - Methylxanthines: only if there is an inadequate response to nebulized bronchodilators. Check levels after 24 hours.
> - Doxapram: is rarely used and should be considered only in obtunded patients with hypercapnia when NIV is unavailable or inappropriate.
>
> **Antibiotics**
> - Prescribe in patients with a history of more purulent sputum and/or evidence of consolidation on CXR or clinical signs of pneumonia.
> - Adhere to local microbiology guidelines.
> - Change from broad-spectrum cover to targeted antibiotics when sensitivities are available.

The following morning, when reviewed by the ICU team, the patient had developed worsening respiratory distress, despite full medical therapy. The patient was receiving NIV via a full face mask at pressures of 20/5 cmH_2O. He was agitated, was not tolerating the NIV, and was struggling to speak single words because of respiratory distress. His vital signs were respiratory rate 34 breaths/min, blood pressure 134/78 mmHg, and pulse 114 beats/min. His SpO_2 was 85% with FiO_2 0.30, and ABG showed worsening hypoxaemia with hypercapnia: pH 7.28, PaO_2 6.70 kPa, $PaCO_2$ 7.68 kPa, and bicarbonate 26.3 mmol/L.

> ### ✪ Learning point Causes of AECOPD
>
> Although the cause for acute deterioration is unknown in around 30% of cases [5], it is important to consider and, where appropriate, to investigate/exclude the likely cause to ensure optimal treatment. The most common causes are as follows:
>
> **Infective exacerbation**
> - Viral in up to 60%. Most commonly rhinovirus [6].
> - Bacterial. Most commonly *Haemophilus influenza*, *Streptococcus pneumoniae*, and *Moraxella catarrhalis* [7].
>
> **Environmental pollution**
> - Epidemiological studies suggest this can be a significant factor in urban areas. Exposure to nitrogen dioxide and sulphur dioxide are implicated.
>
> **Pulmonary embolus**
> - This is present in 16% of patients with AECOPD who have no evidence of infection [8].
> - Consider when there is no evidence of infection and the CXR is clear.
> - Hypercapnia may be caused by increased alveolar dead space.
> - The ECG and echocardiogram may show right heart strain/right ventricular dilation as a result of chronic respiratory failure, which reduces sensitivity in this patient group.
> - A CT pulmonary angiogram is required for diagnosis.
>
> **Heart failure**
> - Acute left heart failure is present in up to 30% of patients with AECOPD [9].
> - Right heart failure may be precipitated by hypoxia-induced pulmonary hypertension, pneumonia, or pulmonary embolus.
> - Useful investigations include B-type natriuretic peptide, CXR, and echocardiography.
> - Pulmonary oedema in emphysematous lungs is associated with predominately basal airspace shadowing on CXR and can be misinterpreted as 'bilateral pneumonia'.
>
> **Pneumothorax**
> - Exclude using CXR or thoracic ultrasonography.
> - Do not confuse emphysematous bullae with pneumothorax

> ### ⓘ Expert comment
>
> The classic ABG pattern associated with a pulmonary embolus of hypoxaemia and hypocapnia may be surprising when you consider the underlying pathophysiology of reduced perfusion to lung units (increased alveolar dead space). However, diversion of lung perfusion to other less well ventilated lung units results in hypoxaemia (V/Q mismatch) and the severe tachypnoea associated with pulmonary embolus results in a marked increase in minute ventilation overcompensating for the increase in alveolar dead space producing a low $PaCO_2$. Patients with chronic lung disease such as COPD are unable to increase minute ventilation significantly to compensate for the increase in alveolar dead space with the result that a pulmonary embolus will be associated with an increase in $PaCO_2$.

In view of the failure of NIV, a decision was made to transfer the patient to ICU for intubation and ventilatory support.

> ### ✪ Learning point Non-invasive ventilation
>
> NIV refers to the provision of ventilatory support without the use of an artificial airway (tracheal tube or tracheostomy). It is typically applied via a mask or hood to deliver either continuous positive airway pressure (CPAP) or bi-level positive airway pressure. In bi-level support, the airway pressure delivered during inspiration is termed IPAP and the expiratory pressure, EPAP. The difference represents
>
> *(continued)*

the pressure support level. Bi-level NIV is considered a standard of care for patients with severe exacerbations of COPD who do not improve with standard medical care.

A Cochrane review assessed NIV in the management of AECOPD and reported the following benefits [10]:

- Decreased need for intubation and ventilation (relative risk 0.42 (0.31–0.59)).
- Fewer treatment complications (relative risk 0.32 (0.18–0.56)).
- Shorter length of stay (mean 3.24 days).
- Decreased mortality (relative risk 0.41 (0.26–0.64)).

British Thoracic Society guidelines for the initiation of NIV [11] advise the following:

- Begin NIV if the patient has decompensated hypercapnic respiratory failure (pH <7.35) despite optimal medical therapy.
- NIV should be administered by appropriately trained staff in a setting optimized for the management of such patients (e.g. respiratory wards, medical high dependency unit (HDU), or ICU).
- Patients with pH less than 7.26 should be considered for admission to an HDU or ICU if appropriate.
- Start at EPAP 5 cmH$_2$O and IPAP 15 cmH$_2$O and titrate IPAP upwards at increments of 2–5 cm at a rate of approximately 5 cmH$_2$O every 10 min until a therapeutic response is achieved or the patient is unable to tolerate higher pressures.
- Take ABGs at 1 hour and every hour after settings are changed. Otherwise after 4 hours.
- Success in NIV is considered to be correction of acidaemia to pH greater than 7.35.
- Plan what to do in the event of deterioration and agree ceilings of therapy.

✪ Learning point Indications of non-invasive ventilation in other conditions

Other causes of acute-on-chronic respiratory failure, which are likely to benefit from NIV, are outlined as follows:

Heart failure

Evidence suggests that bi-level and CPAP have a similar efficacy in the treatment of patients with cardiogenic pulmonary oedema. A Cochrane review [12] concluded that bi-level or CPAP were both effective in reducing need for intubation, ICU length of stay, and mortality.

NICE guidance for the management of patients with acute cardiogenic pulmonary oedema recommends that NIV is not used routinely but is started without delay in those with severe dyspnoea and acidaemia at acute presentation and also in patients who do not improve with initial medical management [13].

Obesity hypoventilation syndrome

Acute-on-chronic respiratory failure caused by obesity-associated diseases is becoming more prevalent. The cost of treating these diseases is projected to reach £2 billion/year in the UK by 2030 [14]. Obesity hypoventilation syndrome is defined as [15]:

- obesity (body mass index (BMI) >30 kg/m^2)
- daytime hypoventilation (PaCO$_2$ >6 kPa or bicarbonate >27 mmol/L)
- sleep-disordered breathing (e.g. obstructive sleep apnoea)
- absence of an alternative explanation (it is a diagnosis of exclusion).

NIV is indicated in patients with obesity hypoventilation syndrome with acute respiratory failure; indeed, outcomes appear to be as good as, if not better, than for COPD patients [16].

Postoperative surgical patients

Postoperative NIV may improve outcome in patients at high risk of respiratory complications although strong evidence is lacking [17]. A Cochrane review found weak evidence to support the use of CPAP in patients after major abdominal surgery [18].

Post extubation in high-risk patients

See Case 16.

(continued)

Contraindications to NIV

An inability to maintain an airway is an absolute contraindication to NIV.

Other contraindications include:

- very poor gas exchange (e.g. need for high levels of positive end-expiratory pressure (PEEP))
- emergency indication for intubation (e.g. cardiorespiratory arrest)
- excessive secretion load
- mucous plugging
- agitation/intolerance
- severely impaired consciousness unless due to hypercapnia
- vomiting
- upper gastrointestinal haemorrhage
- recent surgery to the upper gastrointestinal tract
- recent surgery or trauma to the face or upper respiratory tract
- base of skull fracture
- cardiovascular instability.

✚ Clinical tip Do patients on non-invasive ventilation need a nasogastric tube?

Placement of a nasogastric tube during NIV to prevent gastric distension is unnecessary in the majority of patients. Nasogastric tubes can impair patient ventilator synchrony because they can cause significant mask leak and may paradoxically increase gastric distension by splinting open the gastro-oesophageal junction. Most patients will not require enteral feeding and will tolerate oral feeding as their condition improves. Enteral feeding is undertaken cautiously and not early in the treatment of patients during NIV because of the risk of aspiration if the patient vomits. Where a nasogastric tube is required, use of a fine-bore tube will limit mask leak.

❝ Expert comment

The keys to successful initiation of NIV are:

- patient selection
- effective communication with the patient
- selecting an appropriate interface
- taking time to ensure an optimal fit to minimize any leaks
- adjusting ventilator settings to optimize synchrony
- gradual increase of pressures to ensure patient tolerance.

Once NIV has been established, ensure there is an escalation plan in case NIV fails. This details whether admission to ICU for intubation and ventilation is appropriate and whether the patient is for resuscitation. Alternatively, document a plan for palliation [19].

✚ Clinical tip Interfaces for non-invasive ventilation

There is a range of devices that can be used to apply NIV. Nasal masks are commonly used for patients receiving home ventilation but are generally unsuitable in the acute setting when patients are breathing through their mouth, hence a facemask will be required. Facemasks need to be correctly sized to the patient to ensure any leak is minimized. If correctly positioned, the mask should provide an effective seal without the need for excessive tension in the mask straps. Total face masks which seal around the perimeter of the face above the eyes appear to be better tolerated and avoid the complication of pressure damage to the nasal bridge. The helmet also appears to be well tolerated. It was initially used to apply only CPAP because the dead space is large; however, subsequent reports have described successful use in hypercapnic respiratory failure.

> **✪ Learning point   High-flow nasal oxygenation**
>
> High-flow nasal oxygenation (HFNO) is increasingly used as an alternative to NIV in patients with acute hypoxaemic respiratory failure. HFNO provides humidified oxygen at flow rates of up to 60 L/min and has a number of beneficial effects including:
>
> - effective delivery of high FiO_2
> - augments CO_2 clearance by flushing out upper airway dead space
> - small PEEP-like effect
> - improved secretion clearance.
>
> HFNO is well tolerated and easy to implement. In the Clinical Effect of the Association of Noninvasive Ventilation and High Flow Nasal Oxygen Therapy in Resuscitation of Patients with Acute Lung Injury (FLORALI) study, which involved predominately patients with pneumonia, and excluded patients with COPD and heart failure [20], mortality was lower in patients who received HFNO compared to NIV or conventional oxygen therapy. HFNO also appears to be effective in the management of respiratory failure following cardiac surgery [21] and when used prophylactically following planned extubation it reduces the need for reintubation [22].

> **✪ Learning point   Indications for invasive mechanical ventilation**
>
> Intubation and mechanical ventilation is indicated in appropriate patients who are not improving despite optimal NIV support, if they are unable to tolerate NIV, or if there are contraindications to NIV. Early recognition of the need for intubation is vital as delayed intubation and ventilation results in much poorer outcomes. In patients with severe acidaemia (e.g. pH <7.26), receiving NIV outcome is improved if they are managed in an ICU setting so that intubation can be undertaken without delay if needed [23].
>
> There is some evidence that clinicians have been overly pessimistic about the outcome of patients with AECOPD resulting in a failure to refer or admit to ICU for invasive ventilation. A large, international, multicentre study reported that the outcome of patients ventilated in ICU with a diagnosis of AECOPD is significantly better than other ventilated patients (mortality 22% in COPD, 52% in ARDS) [24, 25].
>
> The largest study undertaken to date assessing the outcome of patients with AECOPD admitted to an ICU in England and Wales is the COPD and Asthma Outcome (CAOS) study. This prospective cohort study assessed 180-day survival and quality of life in 832 patients admitted to 92 ICUs. Overall survival was 62% at 180 days and of the 80% who responded to a questionnaire assessing quality of life, 96% would choose to have a similar treatment again [26]. This study assessed outcome only in those patients admitted to ICU, thus representing those who had been assessed as having a realistic chance of survival.
>
> The challenge for the clinician is to assess which patients are likely to benefit from ICU admission and invasive ventilation. Factors which have been associated with a high hospital mortality rate include increasing age, poor nutritional status, acute comorbidity, and previous admissions for acute exacerbations [27]. Additional factors, associated with a high mortality after hospital discharge, include poor functional status, cor pulmonale, and inability to perform activities of daily living [28]. All these factors need to be considered when assessing suitability for ICU admission.

> **✪ Learning point   Scoring systems in chronic respiratory failure**
>
> **DECAF score for AECOPD**
>
> The DECAF score uses five variables to classify patients with an AECOPD into low-, intermediate-, or high-risk groups [29]. Its use was recommended by the 2014 UK national COPD audit. The five variables are:
>
> *(continued)*

• Dyspnoea (eMRCD)	5a	1
	5b	2
• Eosinopenia	(<0.05 × 10^9/L)	1
• Consolidation	(On CXR)	1
• Acidaemia	(pH <7.3)	1
• Fibrillation	(Atrial fibrillation, including paroxysmal atrial fibrillation)	1

eMRCD = extended MRC dyspnoea scale: patients should only score 5a (independent in washing or dressing) or 5b (dependant for both washing and dressing) if they cannot leave the house without assistance. Patients with a DECAF score greater than 3 are considered high risk and may be suitable for escalation planning or early palliation.

BODE Index

The BODE index is a composite score which can be used to predict long-term prognosis in COPD. It is based on BMI, severity of airflow obstruction (forced expiratory volume in 1 second), dyspnoea (Modified Medical Research Council Dyspnoea Scale), and exercise capacity as assessed by the 6 min walk distance. NICE recommends that it is calculated when the component values are available.

Body mass index

Low BMI is an indicator of poor prognosis in chronic respiratory failure [30] and it becomes a more important prognosticator as disease severity progresses. Reasons for a low BMI predicting a poor outcome include:

- increased work of breathing
- decreased nutritional intake because of shortness of breath
- mitochondrial dysfunction because of chronic hypoxaemia [31]
- apoptosis and skeletal muscle wasting [32].

Shortly after arriving on the ICU the patient was intubated and invasive ventilation initiated using synchronized intermittent mandatory ventilation using a target tidal volume of 7 mL/kg based on predicted body weight.

> **✪ Learning point Mechanical ventilation in chronic obstructive pulmonary disease**
>
> Increased airway resistance in patients with COPD may significantly impair expiration during mechanical ventilation. The characteristic slow and incomplete exhalation may mean that expiration is not complete before the ventilator cycles to inspiration. This leads to gas trapping or 'dynamic hyperinflation' also termed 'breath stacking'. Intrinsic PEEP is a measure of the degree of dynamic hyperinflation. Suggested initial ventilator settings include:
>
> - volume controlled mode
> - tidal volume of 6–8 mL/kg predicted body weight
> - low respiratory rate (10–12 breaths/min)
> - shorter inspiratory time to ensure adequate expiration.
>
> Monitor hyperinflation from the end inspiratory pressure (i.e. plateau pressure) and measurement of the intrinsic PEEP level following an end-expiratory pause. Pressure control modes are not recommended as the plateau pressure will not be apparent and as the pressure delivered in the ventilator will not reflect the pressure within the lungs at end inspiration it is difficult to set an acceptable and effective inspiratory pressure. With volume control, the peak and plateau pressures are readily appreciated with the goal of ensuring a plateau pressure of less than 30 cmH_2O and not being concerned about a high peak airway pressure. These patients are at increased risk of barotrauma and this is associated with increased plateau pressures, not peak pressures.
>
> Adjust the minute volume to target pH rather than $PaCO_2$ to ensure that patients with chronic CO_2 retention are not made alkalaemic. If attempts to control pH cause significant dynamic hyperinflation, reduce the respiratory rate and allow the $PaCO_2$ to rise (permissive hypercapnia).
>
> Minimizing equipment dead space by using an active humidifier rather than a heat and moisture exchanger is a simple and safe method to help reduce $PaCO_2$.

> ⓘ **Expert comment**
>
> The use of external PEEP to offset intrinsic PEEP during mechanical ventilation in patients with severe obstructive airways disease is controversial. Intrinsic PEEP results in a significant load to the inspiratory muscles during spontaneous breathing that needs to be offset before inspiration is initiated. This may lead to either failure to trigger if inspiratory efforts are weak or a high work of breathing if the patient is able to generate strong inspiratory efforts.
>
> Applying external PEEP towards but not exceeding the value of the intrinsic PEEP does not add to the total PEEP but will offset the inspiratory load reducing failure to trigger and work of breathing. External PEEP may also prevent dynamic collapse of the airways during expiration in patients with severe emphysema.
>
> It is recommended that external PEEP is applied during spontaneous modes of ventilatory support if high levels of intrinsic PEEP were recorded during controlled ventilation
>
> Controlled modes of ventilation are appropriate when initiating invasive ventilatory support in patients with an acute exacerbation of COPD. They ensure full respiratory muscle rest in order to correct fatigue, reduce CO_2 production as metabolic rate is lowered, and enable respiratory rate to be adjusted to ensure that intrinsic PEEP is minimized.

The patient was established on volume-controlled ventilation and kept sedated for 48 hours. Intrinsic PEEP was measured at 10 cmH_2O. An echocardiogram revealed good left ventricular function with a moderately dilated right ventricle with reasonable function and a dilated inferior vena cava. In view of the lack of evidence for acute infection precipitating the acute deterioration, and the echocardiogram findings, a CT pulmonary angiogram was performed which excluded pulmonary embolus but revealed severe pan-lobar emphysema throughout both upper lobes and moderate emphysematous changes to the middle and lower lobes (Figure 8.2).

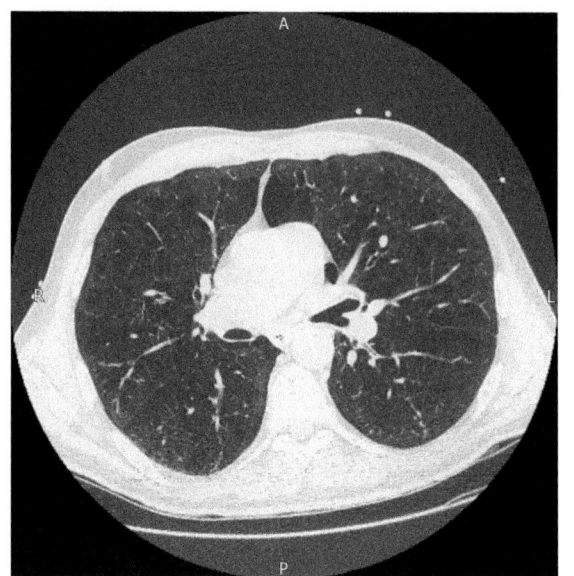

Figure 8.2 CT scan showing multiple bullae leading to loss of alveoli and hyperexpansion.

On day 3 of ICU admission, sedation was discontinued and the patient commenced on pressure support ventilation set at 15 cmH_2O with a PEEP level of 10 cm in order to offset the measured intrinsic PEEP.

An attempt to extubate from this level of pressure support ventilation directly to NIV failed because of worsening respiratory acidosis and fatigue. A further attempt at extubation 3 days later also failed. At this point the patient had limited capacity, so following discussion with his family and in view of the failure to wean, a percutaneous tracheostomy was performed 10 days after ICU admission. Initial attempts to wean using pressure support ventilation failed.

Subsequently, respiratory support was slowly weaned by gradually increasing twice-daily short periods of unsupported spontaneous breathing on a tracheostomy mask with respiratory rest and pressure support ventilation in between. After 21 days of weaning, the patient was fully liberated from mechanical ventilation. Two days later, the tracheostomy was removed and he was discharged to the respiratory ward the following day having been in ICU for 30 days. He was discharged to his home 38 days after admission.

Discussion

> ✪ **Learning point** Weaning from ventilator support
>
> Patients with chronic respiratory diseases are challenging to liberate from mechanical ventilator support. Weaning is usually undertaken by first establishing the patient on a spontaneous mode of ventilatory support such as pressure support. Patient ventilator dyssynchrony is common in patients with COPD and may be a significant factor contributing to respiratory distress during spontaneous ventilator modes and preventing successful weaning.
>
> Weaning can be undertaken by daily unsupported spontaneous breathing periods using a tracheostomy mask or by a gradual reduction in pressure support. The use of a protocol or guideline to support weaning is associated with a reduction in the time taken, independent of the mode used, though there is little evidence to support one mode of weaning over another [33, 34].
>
> **Weaning and nutrition**
>
> A low BMI is common in severe COPD and associated with a poor prognosis. Critical illness and ICU admission leads to further weight loss. Delayed initiation of nutritional support will increase loss of muscle mass and impair ability to wean from ventilatory support. Provision of adequate nutritional support is therefore an important aspect of the management of patients with chronic respiratory failure. Enteral nutrition should be commenced as soon as possible, aiming for a calorie intake of 25–30 kcal/kg/day. Excessive feeding should be avoided as it will increase CO_2 production and impair weaning. The use of pulmonary feeds with a high fat content (reduced respiratory quotient to reduce CO_2 production) are not recommended as they have only been shown to be effective with overfeeding and may have a proinflammatory effect [35].

> ✚ **Clinical tip** Ventilator dyssynchrony during pressure support ventilation
>
> Patient ventilator dyssynchrony is a common but often unrecognized problem during spontaneous modes of ventilatory support in patients with COPD. Failure to trigger (missed breaths) due to the effect of intrinsic PEEP (see earlier discussion) and delayed inspiratory to expiratory cycling are common manifestations. These can be significant factors contributing to an apparent failure to wean.
>
> In pressure support ventilation, the inspiratory phase is typically terminated when inspiratory flow falls to 25% of the measured peak value. In many patients with COPD, the peak inspiratory flow is low because of the increased airway resistance and therefore does not fall to 25% before the patient starts to breathe out. The result is that the patient has to actively exhale against the pressure support level before the ventilator cycles to expiration. This can be noted by observing an increase in end inspiratory pressure immediately before the onset of the expiratory phase. Forcing the patient to actively initiate expiration causes discomfort and respiratory distress. Many ICU ventilators now

(continued)

enable the inspiratory to expiratory cycling threshold to be adjusted between 10% and 90% of peak flow rate to enable optimal setting for the individual patient. A value greater than 50% of peak flow is likely to be indicated in patients with COPD.

✪ Learning point Role of non-invasive ventilation to support weaning

Initial attempts to wean using a phased reduction in pressure support ventilation often fail in patients with COPD. One approach is to extubate the patient onto NIV as soon as spontaneous breathing is established and not to attempt traditional weaning of pressure support or unsupported periods on tracheostomy mask.

A Cochrane review in 2013 highlighted the benefits of NIV as a weaning technique in patients with COPD where it is associated with a significantly improved mortality (relative risk 0.36; 95% confidence interval 0.24–0.56) and rates of ventilator-acquired pneumonia (relative risk 0.25; 95% confidence interval 0.15–0.43) [36].

Role of tracheostomy

Some may consider performing an early tracheostomy in patients with COPD in order to assist weaning. However prospective trials do not support this approach. The TracMan trial, a multicentre randomized clinical trial which assessed early versus late tracheostomy in a heterogeneous ICU population with 70% having pulmonary pathology, found no benefit from undertaking tracheostomy before 10 days. The evidence implies that tracheostomy should be considered in patients with COPD only after failed attempts to wean using NIV [37].

Managing heart failure

Left ventricular failure is a common factor impairing weaning in COPD and may be precipitated by the significant increase in cardiac afterload that occurs during the transition from positive pressure ventilation to spontaneous breathing. Judicious use of diuretics to achieve a negative fluid balance combined with angiotensin-converting enzyme inhibitors to reduce afterload can be very effective. A fluid management strategy guided by B-type natriuretic peptide measurements has been associated with a reduced time to extubation [38].

❝ Expert comment

'Delayed weaning' has been defined as unsuccessful weaning after 2 weeks of attempts, with 'weaning failure' occurring after 3 weeks. A trial undertaken in a long-term ventilation unit reported that classic weaning with once-daily periods of spontaneous breathing with complete ventilatory rest in between was associated with improved weaning outcomes compared to gradual reduction in pressure support [39].

Outcomes from specialist weaning centres suggest that up to 50% of patients referred with weaning failure will be successfully liberated from assisted ventilation with 35% requiring some form of long-term ventilatory support and 15% not surviving [40]. However, long-term survival was less good with less than 50% surviving 12 months and few patients surviving 5 years (see also Case 16).

✪ Learning point Treatment limitations and end of life care

In many patients with severe and advanced chronic respiratory disease, initiating or continuing to provide mechanical ventilatory support may be considered inappropriate when the clinician considers that there is no realistic chance that it will result in long-term survival. There is usually a degree of uncertainty with such decisions and the balance of risks and benefits needs to be considered. Consultation with colleagues may provide useful second opinions.

Clinicians may therefore be presented with several ethical challenges such as making treatment limitation decisions, often in patients who lack mental capacity, managing withdrawal of ventilatory

(continued)

support, and instituting end of life care. The Mental Capacity Act 2005 provides a clear framework for the legal and ethical management of these issues in England and Wales. In Scotland, decision-making in this area is covered by the Adults with Incapacity (Scotland) Act 2000. In Northern Ireland, decision-making is governed by the common law though the Northern Ireland assembly is working towards statutory regulation. The General Medical Council has produced guidance for the care of patients without capacity in the UK. Legal frameworks will differ in other countries, as may ethical perspectives. These include different legislation and arrangements around decision-making in those who lack mental capacity and around end of life care. These arrangements also vary over time. The following section relates to the UK at the time of writing.

Ideally, all patients with chronic respiratory failure who have limited life expectancy should have discussions about the appropriateness and effectiveness of interventions such as mechanical ventilation before they become acutely ill and potentially lose the mental capacity to be involved in their decision-making. Patient's wishes may have been recorded by means of an advance directive and clinicians may be presented with such a document in the acute situation. Advance decisions to refuse treatment are legally binding and should be followed as long as they relate to the specific circumstances.

✪ **Learning point Advance decisions**

Advance decisions may be legally binding in the UK and are described in the Mental Capacity Act 2005.

An *advance decision to refuse medical treatment* is a legally binding document that is very specific with regards to the treatments refused. It may not encompass the complex array of physiological support that may be provided in an ICU. It is legally binding as long as:

- the patient had capacity when they made it
- they have made the advance decision of their own accord
- they specify clearly which treatments they wish to refuse
- they explain the circumstances in which they wish to refuse them
- the decision applies to the current situation
- it is signed by the patient and by a witness
- they have not said or done anything that would contradict the advance decision since they made it (e.g. changing their mind).

An *advance statement* is not legally binding, but should be taken into account when determining the patient's view. An advance statement is intended to communicate the patient's wishes, feelings, and preferences to anyone involved in their care if they lose capacity. It does not need to be signed nor does it need to be witnessed.

✪ **Learning point Assessing capacity using the Mental Capacity Act 2005**

In the acute setting, patients may have lost mental capacity and are unable to be involved in decision-making. The Mental Capacity Act 2005 was developed to provide guidance in such settings. A key component of the Act is that a person may have capacity to make some decisions but not others, known as 'decision-specific capacity'. It recommends that the more serious the decision, for example, not to undergo tracheal intubation and ventilation, the more formal the capacity assessment.

A patient should always be assumed to have capacity unless they cannot do one or more of the following:

- Understand information given to them about the decision.
- Retain the information for long enough to make the decision.
- Weigh up the information as part of the decision-making process.
- Communicate their decision by any means.

(continued)

The Mental Capacity Act 2005 allows people with capacity over 18 years of age to give lasting power of attorney (LPA) for health and welfare to one or more people to make health and personal welfare decisions when capacity is lost. This is not covered by a LPA for financial affairs. Registration takes up to 10 weeks but once complete it will give the attorney(s) the power to make decisions about the patient's medical care, including life-sustaining treatment. It can be used only when the patient loses capacity.

It is still relatively unusual for patients to have given LPA for health and welfare to someone close to them. Clinicians must then make decisions that are judged to be in the patient's best interests and must consult others to find out what the patient's views would be. Anyone who has an interest in the welfare of the patient should be consulted including close family, carers, and friends. If there is no one who can be consulted then the advice of an Independent Mental Capacity Advocate (IMCA) should be sought.

✪ Learning point Independent Mental Capacity Advocate (IMCA)

IMCAs have a role created by the Mental Capacity Act 2005 to represent people who lack capacity to make decisions and have no family, friends, or other advocate who it is appropriate to consult. Most IMCAs are based in the community to act on behalf of a person with limited capacity, for example, an adult with learning difficulties needing to make decisions about long-term accommodation. Intensive care physicians are more likely to encounter non-instructed IMCAs (i.e. employees of a local authority who of necessity are appointed to act for a patient who they have not previously met) who act on behalf of a person who is unable to give a clear indication of their views or wishes in a specific situation.

IMCAs have the power to gather information, including reading the patient's notes, to gain an idea of what they might choose to do should they have capacity. They also have the power to request a second medical opinion if they believe it to be necessary. IMCAs act as an advocate for the patient's wishes in the same way as family or friends would if they were present. The IMCA assists the medical team in making decisions for the patient but it is not their position to make decisions for the medical team. The IMCA service is not available outside of office hours, at weekends, or during public holidays.

✪ Learning point Determining a patient's best interests.

A checklist devised by the Mental Capacity Act 2005 states:

- Does the patient lack the capacity to make this decision?
- Does the patient have an LPA or court-appointed deputy who has the power to make this decision?
- Should an IMCA be involved?
- Is there an advance decision to refuse treatment?
- Can the decision wait until the patient regains capacity?
- Has the person been involved in the decision-making process as effectively as possible?

Management of conflict

Clinicians should aim to obtain a consensus from all those with an interest in the patient's welfare as to what treatment and care are in the patient's best interests if they lack capacity. Occasionally, disagreements may arise within the clinical team or within those close to the patient. These can usually be resolved with a number of approaches including giving time to reflect, open and honest discussion, organizing a case conference, or offering a second opinion from an appropriately experienced and independent clinician. This could be a clinician from a different specialty or from a neighbouring ICU. If there remains serious disagreement despite these measures then legal advice will need to be taken in order to apply to the appropriate court for an independent ruling.

> ✪ **Learning point** Withdrawal of assisted ventilation
>
> If a decision is made to withdraw assisted ventilation in a ventilator-dependent patient, it must be well managed in order to prevent distress and discomfort to the patient and those close to the patient. The Association for Palliative Medicine's guidelines for the withdrawal of assisted ventilation in patients with motor neuron disease are relevant to withdrawal of ventilation in other patient groups. Anticipate symptoms of breathlessness and distress and treat with opioids and benzodiazepines. Sedate patients who are highly ventilator dependent before ventilation is discontinued otherwise they will quickly become distressed.
>
> Consider whether the patient would wish to be an organ donor. Discuss with the family and a specialist nurse in organ donation (see Case 18).

A final word from the expert

Patients with an acute exacerbation of chronic respiratory failure may present many clinical and ethical challenges. Unless there is clear evidence that the patient has terminal respiratory failure or there is a relevant advance directive, admission to ICU is usually appropriate. Treatment should involve controlled oxygen therapy, optimizing underlying and associated medical conditions, and NIV. Careful consideration needs to be given before embarking on invasive ventilation and although weaning may be protracted, the outcome is often better than many would predict.

References

1. Donald K, Simpson T, Mcmichael J, Lennox B. Neurological effects of oxygen. *Lancet.* 1949;254:1056–7.
2. Abdo WF, Heunks LM. Oxygen-induced hypercapnia in COPD: myths and facts. *Crit Care.* 2012;16:323.
3. O'Driscoll BR, Howard LS, Davison AG, British Thoracic Society. BTS guideline for emergency oxygen use in adult patients. *Thorax.* 2008;63 Suppl 6:vi1–68.
4. Department of Health and Social Care. *An Outcomes Strategy for COPD and Asthma: NHS Companion Document.* London: Department of Health and Social Care; 2012.
5. National Institute for Health and Care Excellence. *Chronic Obstructive Pulmonary Disease.* Clinical guideline [CG101]. London: National Institute for Health and Care Excellence; 2010. Available from: https://www.nice.org.uk/guidance/cg101.
6. Seemungal T, Harper-Owen R, Bhowmik A, et al. Respiratory viruses, symptoms, and inflammatory markers in acute exacerbations and stable chronic obstructive pulmonary disease. *Am J Respir Crit Care Med.* 2001;164:1618–23.
7. Garcha DS, Thurston SJ, Patel ARC, et al. Changes in prevalence and load of airway bacteria using quantitative PCR in stable and exacerbated COPD. *Thorax.* 2012;67:1075–80.
8. Aleva FE, Voets LWLM, Simons SO, de Mast Q, van der Ven AJAM, Heijdra YF. Prevalence and localization of pulmonary embolism in unexplained acute exacerbations of COPD. A systematic review and meta-analysis. *Chest.* 2017;151:544–54.
9. Abroug F, Ouanes-Besbes L, Nciri N, et al. Association of left-heart dysfunction with severe exacerbation of chronic obstructive pulmonary disease. *Am J Respir Crit Care Med.* 2012;174:990–6.

10. Ram FS, Picot J, Lightowler J, Wedzicha JA. Non-invasive positive pressure ventilation for treatment of respiratory failure due to exacerbations of chronic obstructive pulmonary disease. *Cochrane Database Syst Rev.* 2004;1:CD004104.

11. Roberts CM, Brown JL, Reinhardt AK, et al. Non-invasive ventilation in chronic obstructive pulmonary disease: management of acute type 2 respiratory failure. *Clin Med.* 2008;8:517–21.

12. Vital FMR, Ladeira MT, Atallah AN. Non-invasive positive pressure ventilation (CPAP or bilevel NPPV) for cardiogenic pulmonary oedema. *Cochrane Database Syst Rev.* 2013;5:CD005351.

13. National Clinical Guideline Centre (UK). *Acute Heart Failure: Diagnosing and Managing Acute Heart Failure in Adults.* London: National Institute for Health and Care Excellence; 2014.

14. Wang YC, McPherson K, Marsh T, Gortmaker SL, Brown M. Health and economic burden of the projected obesity trends in the USA and the UK. *Lancet.* 2011;378:815–25.

15. Mokhlesi B. Obesity hypoventilation syndrome: a state-of-the-art review. *Respir Care.* 2010;55:1347–5.

16. Carrillo A, Ferrer M, Gonzalez Diaz G, et al. Noninvasive ventilation in acute hypercapnic respiratory failure caused by obesity hypoventilation syndrome and chronic obstructive pulmonary disease. *Am J Respir Crit Care Med.* 2012;186:1279–85.

17. Glossop AJ, Shephard N, Shepherd N, Bryden DC, Mills GH. Non-invasive ventilation for weaning, avoiding reintubation after extubation and in the postoperative period: a meta-analysis. *Br J Anaesth.* 2012;109:305–14.

18. Ireland CJ, Chapman TM, Mathew SF, Herbison GP, Zacharias M. Continuous positive airway pressure (CPAP) during the postoperative period for prevention of postoperative morbidity and mortality following major abdominal surgery. *Cochrane Database Syst Rev.* 2014;8:CD008930.

19. Kaul S, Pearson M, Coutts I, Lowe D, Roberts M. Non-invasive ventilation (NIV) in the clinical management of acute COPD in 233 UK hospitals: results from the RCP/BTS 2003 National COPD Audit. *COPD.* 2009;6:171–6.

20. Frat J-P, Thille AW, Mercat A, et al. High-flow oxygen through nasal cannula in acute hypoxemic respiratory failure. *N Engl J Med.* 2015;372:2185–96.

21. Kilger E, Möhnle P, Nassau K, et al. Noninvasive mechanical ventilation in patients with acute respiratory failure after cardiac surgery. *Heart Surg Forum.* 2010;13:E91–5.

22. Hernández G, Vaquero C, González P, et al. Effect of postextubation high-flow nasal cannula vs conventional oxygen therapy on reintubation in low-risk patients: a randomized clinical trial. *JAMA.* 2016;315:1354–61.

23. Plant PK, Owen JL, Elliott MW. Early use of non-invasive ventilation for acute exacerbations of chronic obstructive pulmonary disease on general respiratory wards: a multicentre randomised controlled trial. *Lancet.* 2000;355:1931–5.

24. Funk GC, Bauer P, Burghuber OC, et al. Prevalence and prognosis of COPD in critically ill patients between 1998 and 2008. *Eur Respir J.* 2013;41:792–9.

25. Esteban A, Anzueto A, Frutos F, et al. Characteristics and outcomes in adult patients receiving mechanical ventilation: a 28-day international study. *JAMA.* 2002;287:345–55.

26. Wildman MJ, Sanderson C, Groves J, et al. Implications of prognostic pessimism in patients with chronic obstructive pulmonary disease (COPD) or asthma admitted to intensive care in the UK within the COPD and asthma outcome study (CAOS): multicentre observational cohort study. *BMJ.* 2007;335:1132.

27. Burney PGJ, Patel J, Newson R, Minelli C, Naghavi M. Global and regional trends in COPD mortality, 1990–2010. *Eur Respir J.* 2015;45:1239–47.

28. Steer J, Gibson GJ, Bourke SC. Predicting outcomes following hospitalization for acute exacerbations of COPD. *QJM.* 2010;103:817–29.

29. Steer J, Gibson J, Bourke SC. The DECAF Score: predicting hospital mortality in exacerbations of chronic obstructive pulmonary disease. *Thorax.* 2012;67:970–6.

30. Chailleux E, Fauroux B, Binet F, Dautzenberg B, Polu JM. Predictors of survival in patients receiving domiciliary oxygen therapy or mechanical ventilation. A 10-year analysis of ANTADIR Observatory. *Chest*. 1996;109:741–9.

31. Rabinovich RA, Bastos R, Ardite E, et al. Mitochondrial dysfunction in COPD patients with low body mass index. *Eur Respir J*. 2007;29:643–50.

32. Plataki M, Tzortzaki E, Rytila P, Demosthenes M, Koutsopoulos A, Siafakas NM. Apoptotic mechanisms in the pathogenesis of COPD. *Int J Chron Obstruct Pulmon Dis*. 2006;1:161–71.

33. Blackwood B, Alderdice F, Burns KE, Cardwell CR, Lavery G, O'Halloran P. Protocolized versus non-protocolized weaning for reducing the duration of mechanical ventilation in critically ill adult patients. *Cochrane Database Syst Rev*. 2010;5:CD006904.

34. Butler R, Keenan SP, Inman KJ, Sibbald WJ, Block G. Is there a preferred technique for weaning the difficult-to-wean patient? A systematic review of the literature. *Crit Care Med*. 1999;27:2331–6.

35. McClave SA, Taylor BE, Martindale RG, et al. Guidelines for the provision and assessment of nutrition support therapy in the adult critically ill patient: Society of Critical Care Medicine (SCCM) and American Society for Parenteral and Enteral Nutrition (A.S.P.E.N.). *JPEN J Parenter Enteral Nutr*. 2016;40:159–211.

36. Burns KEA, Meade MO, Premji A, Adhikari NKJ. Noninvasive positive-pressure ventilation as a weaning strategy for intubated adults with respiratory failure. *Cochrane Database Syst Rev*. 2013;12:CD004127.

37. Young D, Harrison DA, Cuthbertson BH, Rowan K. Effect of early vs late tracheostomy placement on survival in patients receiving mechanical ventilation: the TracMan randomized trial. *JAMA*. 2013;309:2121–9.

38. Dessap AM, Roche-Campo F, Kouatchet A, et al. Natriuretic peptide-driven fluid management during ventilator weaning. *Am J Respir Crit Care Med*. 2012;186:1256–63.

39. Jubran A, Grant BJB, Duffner LA, et al. Effect of pressure support vs unassisted breathing through a tracheostomy collar on weaning duration in patients requiring prolonged mechanical ventilation: a randomized trial. *JAMA*. 2013;309:671–7.

40. Rose L, Fraser IM. Patient characteristics and outcomes of a provincial prolonged-ventilation weaning centre: a retrospective cohort study. *Can Respir J*. 2012;19:216–20.

Multiple organ support in an ageing population

Matt Oliver

❶ **Expert Commentary** Dave Murray

Case history

An 82-year-old man was brought to the emergency department by ambulance with severe abdominal pain. He had been housebound for 3 days, and had been eating and drinking very little over the preceding week due to increasing pain. His neighbours were concerned and had contacted the emergency services.

The patient lived alone but was frail, requiring assistance in self-care, cleaning, and shopping. He had to stop at least once on the short flight of stairs up to his bedroom to catch his breath. He had ischaemic heart disease (coronary stent inserted 5 years previously), controlled hypertension, and chronic obstructive pulmonary disease. He took ramipril 10 mg once daily, atorvastatin 40 mg once daily, clopidogrel 75 mg once daily, and Symbicort (400/12) one actuation twice daily. His previous hospital records indicated he did not tolerate beta blockers.

Examination by the emergency medicine registrar identified abdominal rigidity, guarding, and rebound tenderness; he was profoundly dehydrated. Observations on presentation are shown in Table 9.1 and initial blood results in Table 9.2. An electrocardiogram showed a sinus tachycardia without any other abnormalities.

> ✪ **Learning point**
> **Interpretation of observations and blood results**
>
> His clinical presentation includes hypotension and evidence of organ dysfunction. He has all three of the criteria on a quick Sequential (Sepsis-Related) Organ Failure Assessment for high risk of sepsis (systolic blood pressure <100 mmHg, respiratory rate >22 breaths/min, and altered mental state) (see Case 1). His initial investigations show evidence of a normocytic anaemia, acute kidney injury, and raised markers of inflammation.

Table 9.1 Observations on presentation to the emergency department

Variable	Observation
Heart rate (beats/min)	120
Blood pressure (mmHg)	90/65
Arterial blood oxygen saturation (on air) (%)	94
Respiratory rate (breaths/min)	22
Glasgow Coma Scale score	14
Temperature (°C)	38.2

> ❶ **Expert comment**
>
> The delayed presentation and clinical findings are not atypical in an elderly patient presenting with an acute abdominal problem and subsequently needing an emergency laparotomy. The observations reveal the effects of both dehydration and sepsis.

Table 9.2 Initial blood results

Variable	Value (reference range)
Haematology	
Haemoglobin (g/L)	105 (130–180)
MCV (fL)	85 (85–97)
Platelets (× 10⁹/L)	350 (150–400)
WCC (× 10⁹/L)	18.2 (4–11)
Neutrophils (× 10⁹/L)	15.8 (2–7)

(continued)

Table 9.2 Continued

Variable	Value (reference range)
HCT (%)	38 (40–52)
INR	1.2 (0.9–1.4)
APTT	28 (30–40)
Biochemistry	
Na (mmol/L)	144 (135–145)
K (mmol/L)	5.4 (3.5–5.5)
Urea (mmol/L)	18.3 (2.5–6.7)
Cr (µmol/L)	220 (60–110)
Bilirubin (µmol/L)	18 (<22)
ALT (IU/L)	35 (5–40)
AST (IU/L)	29 (5–45)
Alkaline phosphatase (IU/L)	144 (40–129)
Albumin (g/L)	38 (34–48)
Glucose (mmol/L)	7.5 (3.5–8.5)
C-reactive protein (mg/L)	320 (<10)
Lactate (mmol/L)	4.2 (0.0–1.8)

ALT, alanine aminotransferase; APTT, activated partial thromboplastin time; AST, aspartate transaminase; Cr, creatinine; HCT, haematocrit; INR, international normalized ratio; K, potassium; MCV, mean cell volume; Na, sodium; WCC, white cell count.

The patient was referred to the surgical team for immediate senior review. In the meantime, referring to the hospital's emergency laparotomy pathway, the following actions were undertaken:

- Facemask oxygen (5 L/min) was administered.
- A 16-gauge intravenous (IV) cannula was sited.
- Blood samples (including peripheral blood cultures and venous blood gas) were taken.
- A urethral catheter was inserted with institution of hourly urine output measurements.
- A litre of crystalloid fluid was administered.
- Tazocin (4.5 g) IV was administered IV as per the local microbiology guidelines.
- An urgent abdominal computed tomography (CT) scan was requested.

> **Expert comment**
>
> CT scanning can be extremely helpful in defining the underlying surgical pathology and its extent. It may help distinguish between benign and malignant disease, including the presence of metastases. The value of CT scanning is significantly enhanced if not only is it reported by a specialist radiologist, but also the findings are discussed with the surgical team.
>
> Hospitals need to ensure there is a pathway in place that guarantees urgent CT scanning for this group of patients. Urgent radiology should not delay emergency surgery.

> **⊕ Clinical tip Clinical pathways**
>
> The use of clinical pathways that prescribe investigation, treatment, and referral points can aid delivery of prompt care. They improve reliability of care ensuring that all elements of care are considered and delivered consistently to all patients. Prompt administration of antibiotics is essential in patients with signs of sepsis. Arterial or venous blood lactate is helpful in judging the severity of any shock. In this case, the high lactate suggests the start of organ dysfunction caused by both septic shock and dehydration.

The CT scan was performed within 30 min and reported by a consultant radiologist. The findings were discussed directly with the surgical team. The provisional CT report identified findings consistent with a large bowel perforation. There was evidence of a mass suggestive of an erosive colonic tumour (Figure 9.1).

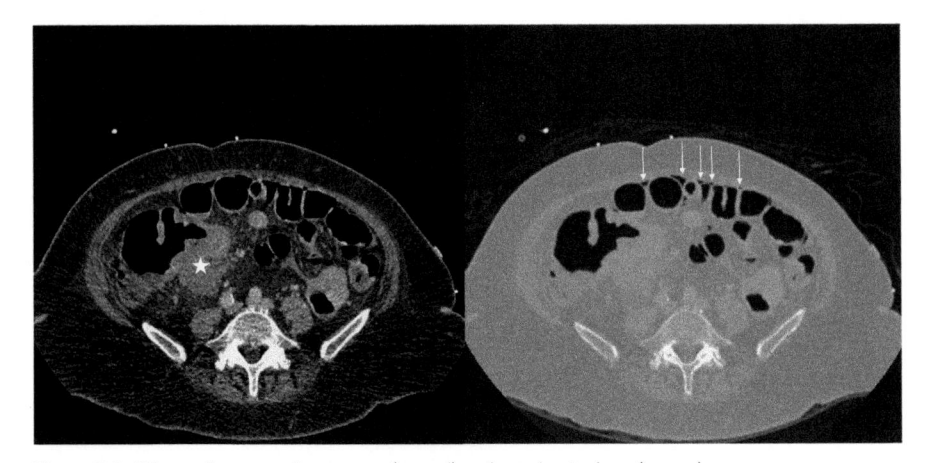

Figure 9.1 CT scan demonstrating tumour (starred) and extraluminal gas (arrows).

✪ Learning point Emergency laparotomy: incidence and patient outcomes

Emergency laparotomy describes a wide range of invasive abdominal operations that are performed commonly across the globe for potentially life-threatening conditions. An estimated 1:1100 of the population undergo emergency laparotomy each year [1].

In developed counties, mortality at 1 month exceeds 10% and major morbidity 30%. Sequelae may represent a significant burden to patients and healthcare systems long after the operative period [2]. Morbidity and mortality rates are substantially higher in certain subgroups: 30-day mortality is approximately 25% in patients aged 80 years or older and in those requiring immediate surgery, and approximately 75% in patients with severe liver disease [3, 4]. Associations between frailty syndromes and postoperative outcomes are currently poorly understood.

Currently, intra-abdominal malignancies are common precipitants of emergency laparotomy and the incidence of colorectal cancers in older people is increasing [5, 6]. In the next two decades, the proportion of the population aged over 65 years will markedly increase and around 10% of patients will be aged at least 80 years. According to the Office for National Statistics, by mid-2039, more than 13% of the population will be 75 years and older [7]. The number and complexity of emergency laparotomies performed is therefore anticipated to increase dramatically over coming decades.

✪ Learning point Perioperative care pathways in emergency laparotomy

Evidence supports the use of care bundles comprising:

- risk assessment
- early antibiotics
- maintaining the interval between decision and operation at less than 6 hours
- goal-directed fluid therapy (GDFT)
- postoperative admission to an intensive care unit (ICU) [8].

Standards of care support:

- sepsis bundles including prompt administration of broad-spectrum antibiotics and timely source control
- review by a senior surgeon within 14 hours of admission
- prompt imaging and timely reporting by a consultant radiologist
- assessment and documentation of risk of death
- arrival in the operating room (OR) in a time commensurate with operative urgency
- the presence of a consultant surgeon and anaesthetist in the OR if estimated risk of death is 5% or greater
- postoperative level 2 or level 3 care if estimated risk of death is 5% or greater
- involvement of a care of the elderly physician in the postoperative care of older patients [9].

> **⑥ Expert comment**
>
> Frailty describes the global deterioration in strength (and physiological reserve) that occurs with ageing. It may also occur with chronic illness and particularly with advanced cancer. Frailty includes loss of muscle bulk and power, termed sarcopenia, in the elderly. It is an area of considerable clinical importance and research interest, but at present, while it is recognized as a clinical entity, there is a lack of clinical consensus on definition, diagnosis, or gradation. An example of a grading system is the Clinical Frailty Scale [10].
>
> Frailty is particularly important in critical illness as it is a predictor of a poor outcome. Surgery is associated with a 15–25% loss of muscle power in the early postoperative phase and this will be dramatically worsened by complications that prevent mobilization and increase catabolism. Muscle weakness impacts mobilization, effective coughing, and weaning from mechanical ventilation. Frail survivors of critical illness experience greater impairment in health-related quality of life compared with those who are not frail [11].
>
> While considerable efforts are being made to address concerns around frailty, there are currently no established treatments to lessen its impact in the perioperative period. Preoperative exercise training (for elective patients), early mobilization, prompt reintroduction of nutrition, simple respiratory exercises, and avoidance of complications (especially delirium) are likely to be of benefit [12].

> **✪ Learning point** **National Emergency Laparotomy Audit and care pathways**
>
> National Emergency Laparotomy Audit (NELA) is a continuous national audit programme in England and Wales that was started in 2012. It was commissioned following evidence of high rates of mortality and variations in organization of care and outcomes. The programme combines an audit of structure, process, and outcome measures for all hospitals in these countries performing emergency laparotomy. It gained evidence from approximately 60,000 emergency laparotomies in its first 2 years.
>
> The first two NELA reports identified poor delivery of key processes of care in a substantial minority of cases; this included those patients for whom risk was not documented preoperatively [3, 9]. A principal recommendation of the NELA reports was the routine use of care pathways to reduce variation and improve patient outcomes.

The surgical trainee used the P-POSSUM (Portsmouth Physiological and Operative Severity Score for the Enumeration of Mortality and Morbidity) and SORT (Surgical Outcomes Risk Tool) tools to risk assess the patient [13–15]. Although these risk tools were developed to calculate risk within populations and not for individual patient decision-making, they were used here to alert the team that they were dealing with a patient at high risk of perioperative morbidity and mortality. P-POSSUM estimated the 30-day mortality for this patient at 91% and SORT at 28%.

The patient was discussed with the consultant surgeon, consultant anaesthetist, and consultant intensivist so that the risks and benefits could be assessed before the patient was offered surgery. The patient had capacity and the high risk of potential complications, including death and chronic deterioration in health quality, was discussed at length with him. Palliative care was also explained as an alternative to surgery. The patient wanted to pursue all active treatment options. Their next of kin was contacted to inform them of the patient's decision, rationale for surgery, and the potential risks involved. The patient was consented and booked for an emergency laparotomy.

In the OR, the patient's data were entered into the NELA web tool.

ⓘ Expert comment

The legal framework for consent differs between countries but good practice requires a patient-centred approach. That implies that a patient is informed of all the risks that they would consider pertinent before undergoing a procedure and that all relevant alternatives (including no treatment) are also discussed. This approach is established in UK law [16, 17]. For patients such as this with a high mortality risk, and also a high risk of survival with a poorer quality of life than before admission, this may require considerable explanation and discussion, and should be led by appropriately senior members of the team, including intensivists. The clinical condition of the patient may make such discussions difficult and it requires careful judgement to balance adequate provision of information against overload of information in an acutely ill patient. Surgery will not be an appropriate solution in all cases and as it is poor practice to offer futile treatments. Risk assessment and discussion of an appropriate course of action should take place before surgery is offered.

★ Learning point Quantifying risk

Tools for assessing risk incorporate two or more variables into a score or equation, to stratify or estimate the likelihood of an adverse outcome, often short-term mortality. Component variables are independent predictors of the outcome, usually identified through an iterative process of multivariable regression. Many are now available online as smart phone apps.

The American Society of Anesthesiologists (ASA) physical status tool is widely used, easily understood, and of practical value. However, it is highly subjective, takes little account of patient age, and wide inter-observer variability is reported [18].

SORT uses six routinely measured variables to estimate the likelihood of 30-day mortality [15]. These are ASA physical status, operation type, severity and urgency, presence of malignancy, and age. It was developed in response to recommendations from the 2011 National Confidential Enquiry into Patient Outcome and Death study on perioperative care, 'Knowing the Risk' [19]. Data from 16,788 patients in this study were used to develop and internally validate SORT. It may require external validation in high-risk populations, including emergency laparotomy.

P-POSSUM was derived from the original POSSUM risk prediction tool that was developed in 2002 [13, 14]. It uses 12 physiological and 6 operative variables for its calculation. It requires operative findings to be included, which reduces its value preoperatively, as these must be entered based on anticipated surgical findings. It is widely used and has been validated for use in emergency laparotomy [20], demonstrating moderate performance in this setting. Predicted P-POSSUM mortality has now been compared to observed mortality in over 40,000 patients in the NELA database. This has demonstrated that P-POSSUM over-predicts mortality almost twofold at higher mortality rates (e.g. >25–30%). It does show good correlation below 15% predicted mortality, and is therefore useful for stratification of risk in order to better define high-risk patients (predicted mortality >5%) and the need for critical care and presence of a consultant.

Data from NELA has now been used to develop a bespoke risk prediction tool for patients undergoing emergency laparotomy [21]. It is more accurate than P-POSSUM, which has now been removed from NELA in favour of the NELA risk prediction model.

ⓘ Expert comment

Estimation of risk of death constitutes a standard of care for all patients undergoing surgery in the UK. It serves two purposes: to help inform patients of the risk of surgery, and to help plan subsequent care and the need for resources such as consultant input and critical care.

Importantly, risk tools use population data to predict mortality (or morbidity) in patient populations. Results from risk prediction tools therefore describe how a large population of patients with the inputted characteristics might be predicted to behave, but cannot accurately predict the outcome for an individual patient—which in terms of mortality is dichotomous (i.e. they survive or die). As such, they are of value for risk stratification but applying specific outputs of risk assessments to individual patients as the sole means of decision-making is discouraged. Risk prediction tools should be used to support clinical decision-making in conjunction with discussion with the patient and their family.

(continued)

High-risk patients mandate the presence of senior decision-makers. Emergency laparotomy patients are frequently very sick and can deteriorate quickly, requiring prompt decision-making which is best provided by experienced clinicians. This can include changing the surgical plan mid operation, depending on changes in the patient's condition. For instance, in a patient with escalating inotrope requirements, it may be appropriate to abandon plans to anastomose the bowel, and instead provide an end stoma. Intraoperative findings such as the presence of metastases or extensive ischaemic bowel may make limitations on care appropriate.

The patient remained oligoanuric despite fluid resuscitation. A further fluid bolus was prescribed and the patient was transferred urgently to the OR.

Within 4 hours of presentation in the emergency department the patient arrived in the OR. He was transferred directly onto the operating table. He remained tachycardic (heart rate 130 beats/min), hypotensive (blood pressure 85/60 mmHg), tachypnoeic (respiratory rate 28 breaths/min), and hypoxaemic (SpO$_2$ 92% breathing 15 L/min of oxygen). He had now become delirious.

⚕ Expert comment

Given the patient's dehydration and lack of urine output, it may be tempting to delay surgery to enable fluid resuscitation. However, this must be balanced with the overriding requirement for prompt source control to manage his septic shock. It is easier to infuse fluids rapidly in the OR than it is on the ward and where necessary such resuscitation is best performed in the OR or ICU.

Critically ill patients should have anaesthesia induced in the OR rather than in the anaesthetic room. This avoids moving a potentially unstable patient soon after induction and the 'monitoring gap' that otherwise occurs during transfer.

The anaesthetic team, led by a consultant, thoroughly pre-oxygenated the patient while a third litre of crystalloid was infused rapidly and a radial arterial line sited. In view of recent antiplatelet medication and the likely need for level 3 postoperative care, an epidural catheter was not inserted preoperatively; instead, rectus sheath catheters were to be sited by the surgical team before wound closure. Anaesthesia was induced with 150 mcg fentanyl (2 mcg/kg), 70 mg ketamine (1 mg/kg), and 70 mg suxamethonium (1 mg/kg).

Volume-controlled ventilation was commenced with a lung protective strategy: tidal volume 420 mL (6 mL/kg ideal body weight), rate 16 bpm, inspiratory:expiratory ratio 1:2, positive end-expiratory pressure 5 cmH$_2$O. His plateau pressure was maintained at 30 cmH$_2$O or less. Anaesthesia was maintained using sevoflurane titrated to bispectral index values of 40–60 and neuromuscular blockade with boluses of atracurium. He was intubated with an 8.0 mm inner diameter tracheal tube, with subglottic suction, as postoperative ventilation on ICU was anticipated. After induction of anaesthesia, an infusion of metaraminol and intermittent boluses (0.5 mg) were required to maintain the 70 mmHg predefined mean arterial pressure (MAP) target. An antibiotic-impregnated, five-lumen right internal jugular central line was inserted using full asepsis and ultrasound guidance. A noradrenaline infusion was started and the metaraminol stopped. Cardiac output monitoring using oesophageal Doppler showed a corrected flow time less than 450 ms, which suggested hypovolaemia.

A midline laparotomy incision extending above the umbilicus was made. There was extensive faecal contamination with pockets of pus. The bowel had perforated just proximal to a suspected colonic tumour. A Hartmann's procedure was performed.

Intravascular filling (with crystalloid and blood products) and titration of noradrenaline was guided by blood pressure and cardiac output monitoring and lactate clearance. His noradrenaline requirements escalated and hydrocortisone 50 mg four times daily was started to potentially enable a dose reduction in noradrenaline. Intraoperatively, the metabolic acidosis worsened, accompanied by increasing lactate value, hyperkalaemia, and deranged clotting. Only 50 mL of urine had been passed since catheterization. It was anticipated that renal replacement therapy would be required so a right internal jugular dialysis catheter was inserted under ultrasound guidance.

The surgeons anticipated postoperative ileus was likely. Before surgical closure, a fine-bore feeding tube was passed nasally and with the help of the surgeons was placed in the jejunum, to facilitate post-pyloric feeding on the ICU.

✆ Expert comment

Currently, evidence for the use of cardiac output monitoring to guide GDFT in emergency laparotomy is derived primarily from elective surgical populations. In major elective gastrointestinal surgery, GDFT may reduce postoperative complication rates but has not been shown to reduce mortality [22]. A UK multicentre, randomized controlled trial of GDFT in emergency laparotomy populations was underway in the UK in 2017 (http://www.floela.org.uk).

Patients undergoing high-risk emergency laparotomy, such as this patent, are likely to require organ support and level 3 care on ICU and preparations for this can be started in the OR. In patients likely to require controlled ventilation, cardiovascular support, renal replacement therapy, or enteral feeding (especially with prolonged gastroparesis or ileus), this will include placing a tracheal tube with subglottic suction, a central venous catheter, an enteral feeding tube (especially nasojejunal), and possibly a dialysis catheter.

✪ Learning point **Epidemiology and burden of sepsis**

Sepsis is defined as life-threatening organ dysfunction caused by a dysregulated host response to infection. Septic shock is a subset of sepsis involving profound circulatory, cellular, and metabolic abnormalities. Patients with septic shock require a vasopressor to maintain a MAP of 65 mmHg or greater and a serum lactate level greater than 2 mmol/L in the absence of hypovolaemia. This combination is associated with hospital mortality rates greater than 40% and is even higher in older patients [23]. Organ failure is the commonest cause of short-term mortality in surgical patients.

Timeline

18.00	Arrival at hospital
+30 min	Seen in emergency department resuscitation
+45 min	Anaesthetic review
+1.00 hour	CT scan
+1:25 hours	Senior surgical review
+1:45 hours	Senior anaesthetist, intensivist, and surgeon review. Discussion with patient. Booked for theatre
+3:00 hours	Arrival in emergency theatre
+3:45 hours	Surgery
+6:30 hours	End of surgery
+7:15 hours	Admission to ICU

> ❂ **Learning point** Pre-existing susceptibility to sepsis
>
> Sepsis is more common with increasing age [24] and increased age and multimorbidity are associated with an increased likelihood of developing multiple organ dysfunction [25]. Risk factors include pre-existing organ impairment and immunosuppression, including diabetes mellitus and hepatic cirrhosis [26].
>
> **Iatrogenic component**
>
> Medical therapies, such as use of inappropriately high tidal volumes during mechanical ventilation, have been implicated in the development of the acute respiratory distress syndrome and acute kidney injury. The 'two-hit' hypothesis proposes that in the presence of predisposing acute or chronic disease, a trigger (such as mechanical ventilation or vasopressor drugs) precipitates organ failure.

The patient remained sedated and mechanically ventilated at the end of surgery and was admitted to the ICU. Sedation and analgesia were maintained with propofol and fentanyl infusions and noradrenaline continued targeting a MAP greater than 70 mmHg. Lung protective ventilation continued.

Cardiac output monitoring continued and this indicated a reduced stroke volume and normovolaemia. A dobutamine infusion was started to improve myocardial contractility. Despite an adequate MAP, metabolic acidosis worsened in the hour after ICU admission and the patient remained oliguric, so continuous renal replacement therapy was started.

Regular gastroprotection with omeprazole was prescribed, but thromboprophylaxis was delayed pending review of clotting function. Tazocin was continued and metronidazole added as per local microbiology policy. The patient was nursed using ventilator-associated pneumonia, central line, and pressure care bundles. Enteral nutrition was started via the nasojejunal tube but he did not absorb this.

> ⑥ **Expert comment**
>
> Emergency laparotomy is a high-risk procedure: 30-day mortality is greater than 15% rising to greater than 20% for those over 80 years of age [3, 27–29]. A disproportionate number of patients are elderly—approximately two-thirds of patients are aged over 60 years and approximately 85% of deaths occur in this group. As many as half of patients may not return to their original place of residence after surgery [30]. Increased mortality extends beyond the hospital stay and more than one-third of deaths occur after 1 month [28]. Despite this, ICU admission is not mandated and varies markedly between countries (24% Denmark, 60% UK) [3, 28].
>
> Complications occurring after surgery are associated with prolonged admission and increased hospital mortality [31]. Patients experiencing postoperative complications have increased mortality for several years, compared to patients who do not experience complications [32]. More patients undergoing emergency laparotomy will experience complications that delay discharge than after elective surgery, but evidence suggests it is the patient's and the hospital's response to complications that impacts outcome more than the number of complications itself [33]. Hospitals with better outcomes do not have lower rates of complications but rather are better at detecting and managing those patients who are deteriorating and at managing serious complications [34]. Older patients may not experience more complications, but are more likely to die from them and to experience death between 3 and 30 days postoperatively [28]. While respiratory, gastrointestinal and infective morbidity is common, cardiovascular complications may be more important in determining outcome [30, 33].
>
> Admission to ICU postoperatively provides the opportunity to manage the patient in an area with higher nurse–patient and doctor–patient ratios, to provide optimal monitoring, and to provide monitoring, expertise, and advanced treatments that cannot be provided on the wards. Although there is a lack of definitive evidence that critical care admission reduces mortality in this group of patients, it seems logical. Regular senior multidisciplinary review, physiological optimization, early detection and treatment of deterioration, and, where feasible, early mobilization and intensive rehabilitation
>
> *(continued)*

are the mainstay of treatment. Supportive evidence of the benefit of ICU includes the observation that hospitals with better outcomes from emergency surgery have more ICU beds [35]. In one small study, the risk-adjusted standardized mortality rate of patients admitted to the ICU after emergency laparotomy was substantially lower than that of the patients who were sent directly to the ward [36]. Several studies have observed that the highest mortality occurs in patients who are initially discharged to the wards and are subsequently admitted to the ICU [27].

Quality improvement projects that include bundles of care—including increasing the proportion of patients admitted to the ICU—after emergency laparotomy have had success in reducing the length of stay and mortality in this high-risk group [37]. Several national bodies recommend ICU admission for emergency laparotomy patients with a predicted mortality of greater than 5 or 10% [38] and that hospitals should have the capacity to admit all such cases to the ICU. In practice, this includes all patients aged older than 60 years, all those with comorbidities, and all patients with an elevated lactate. A strong argument therefore can be made for defaulting to admission of all patients to critical care after emergency laparotomy, thereby making admission to the wards the exception.

On days 1–3, the patient remained on multiorgan support (sedated, ventilated, renal replacement therapy, vasopressors, and inotrope support).

By day 3, persistently elevated inflammatory markers and haemodynamic instability suggested failure of source control. Exploration in the OR demonstrated four-quadrant purulent fluid. An abdominal washout was performed and a large-bore drain inserted.

After a further return to the OR for abdominal washout, inflammatory markers began to decline and haemodynamic support was weaned off. However, despite lung protective ventilation, by 72 hours the patient fulfilled the criteria for acute respiratory distress syndrome.

After his second return to the OR, parenteral nutrition was started via a dedicated peripherally inserted central catheter line (see Case 13). On day 6, a percutaneous tracheostomy was sited to aid with weaning. On day 10, he developed ventilator-associated pneumonia with a resistant *Pseudomonas* infection.

❻ Expert comment

It is not unusual for patients to need to return to theatre. Data from NELA suggest this ranges from 2% to 20%, and is associated with increased mortality and longer hospital stay. In some case this may be planned, particularly if 'damage control' surgery has been performed, when the patient has been too unstable for an initial definitive procedure, or to close a laparostomy. Unplanned returns for complications are also likely. This may be due to a remaining source of sepsis, anastomotic breakdown, bowel ischaemia, or to assess stoma viability.

The timing of a return to theatre can be problematic as patients may be unstable due to ongoing sepsis and multiple organ failure. Instability may preclude performing further CT scans, requiring surgery to be undertaken with diagnostic intent.

The patient spent a long time in the ICU. Over the next 2 months, his recovery and rehabilitation was complicated by a protracted wean from ventilatory support because of a combination of underlying chronic lung disease, acute pathology, and critical illness myoneuropathy.

Routine investigations excluded intrinsic and postrenal causes of his acute kidney injury and this was attributed to sepsis. Continuous renal replacement therapy was provided for the first month of his stay.

His intra-abdominal sepsis settled slowly and enteral nutrition was re-established after 2 weeks. He remained weak and required intensive chest and rehabilitative physiotherapy.

Almost 2 months after his initial surgery, the patient's tracheostomy was decannulated, and he was discharged to a medicine for the care of older people ward where he remained an inpatient for a further 2 months. Despite intensive multidisciplinary rehabilitation, he did not regain his previous level of mobility and could walk only short distances and under close supervision. Due to increased frailty and ongoing complex medical needs, he was discharged to a nursing home. Four months after hospital discharge and 8 months after his initial presentation the patient died.

Discussion

Development of multiple organ dysfunction is common in patients admitted to ICUs. The number of impaired organ systems and severity of their impairment may be used to quantify the severity of illness and likelihood of subsequent morbidity and mortality.

Sepsis is the commonest cause of multiple organ dysfunction, and in this setting outcomes are poor. Survival of older people with multiple organ dysfunction is likely to involve a complicated and prolonged period of recovery and often leads to a subsequent reduction of functional ability. The relatively poor prognosis necessitates monitoring of clinical progress and assessment of quality of survival.

In this case, pre-existing frailty and multiple morbidity not only predisposed to the development of multiorgan failure, but also resulted in a critical loss of functional ability, such that the patient required nursing care following hospital discharge [39, 40].

It is preferable for individuals to have discussed their wishes in advance of such a scenario, whether with health professionals, friends, and family or by formal documentation. Where possible, this information should be actively sought out to inform these decisions and in particular to support limitation of treatment when clinically appropriate (see Case 8).

A final word from the expert

The outcome of this case is not surprising given the systemic impact of emergency laparotomy in an elderly patient whose pre-existing reserve was already very limited. At present, there is very limited data available on longer-term outcomes and quality of life following emergency laparotomy. This can make informed discussion with patients and family challenging. It is hoped that this may be answered by ongoing research.

The urgent nature of emergency laparotomy means that there may be limited time to consider some of these aspects, but it is important to do so. These discussions impact subsequent care, and may avoid prolonged and distressing treatment for a patient if there is a limited chance of a successful outcome and good quality of life. These decisions need to be individualized to each patient, and are best made when senior clinicians from all relevant specialties are involved.

References

1. Shapter SL, Paul MJ, White SM. Incidence and estimated annual cost of emergency laparotomy in England: is there a major funding shortfall? *Anaesthesia*. 2012;67:474–8.

2. Oliver M, Grocott M, Anderson I, Murray D. The problem with emergency laparotomies. *Br J Hosp Med (Lond)*. 2015;76:498–9.

3. NELA Project Team. *Second Patient Audit Report of the National Emergency Laparotomy Audit*. London: Royal College of Anaesthetists; 2016.

4. Hoteit MA, Ghazale AH, Bain AJ, et al. Model for end-stage liver disease score versus Child score in predicting the outcome of surgical procedures in patients with cirrhosis. *World J Gastroenterol*. 2008;14:1774–80.

5. Faiz O, Warusavitarne J, Bottle A, et al. Nonelective excisional colorectal surgery in English National Health Service trusts: a study of outcomes from hospital episode statistics data between 1996 and 2007. *J Am Coll Surg*. 2010;210:390–401.

6. Kesisoglou I, Pliakos I, Sapalidis K, Deligiannidis N, Papavramidis S. Emergency treatment of complicated colorectal cancer in the elderly. Should the surgical procedure be influenced by the factor 'age'? *Eur J Cancer Care*. 2010;19:820–6.

7. Office for National Statistics. National Population Projections: 2014-Based Statistical Bulletin [Internet]. Office for National Statistics; 2015 [cited 2 April 2017]. Available from: https://www.ons.gov.uk/peoplepopulationandcommunity/populationandmigration/populationprojections/bulletins/nationalpopulationprojections/2015-10-29.

8. Huddart S, Mowat I, Sanusi S, et al. Introduction of an integrated care pathway for emergency laparotomies saves lives. *Anaesthesia*. 2012;67:20.

9. NELA Project Team. *First Patient Report of the National Emergency Laparotomy Audit*. London: Royal College of Anaesthetists; 2015.

10. Rockwood K, Song X, MacKnight C, et al. A global clinical measure of fitness and frailty in elderly people. *CMAJ*. 2005;173:489–95.

11. Bagshaw SM, Stelfox HT, Johnson JA, et al. Long term association between frailty and health related quality of like among adult survivors of critical illness: a prospective multicentre cohort study. *Crit Care Med*. 2015;43:973–82.

12. Cassidy MR, Rosenkranz P, McCabe K, Rosen JE, McAneny D. iCough: reducing postoperative pulmonary complications with a multidisciplinary patient care program. *JAMA Surg*. 2013;148:740–5.

13. Copeland GP, Jones D, Walters M. POSSUM: a scoring system for surgical audit. *Br J Surg*. 1991;78:355–60.

14. Prytherch DR, Whiteley MS, Higgins B, Weaver PC, Prout WG, Powell SJ. POSSUM and Portsmouth POSSUM for predicting mortality. Physiological and Operative Severity Score for the enUmeration of Mortality and morbidity. *Br J Surg*. 1998;85:1217–20.

15. Protopapa KL, Simpson JC, Smith NCE, Moonesinghe SR. Development and validation of the Surgical Outcome Risk Tool (SORT). *Br J Surg*. 2014;101:1774–83.

16. Yentis SM, Hartle AJ, Barker IR, et al. Consent for anaesthesia. Association of Anaesthetists of Great Britain and Ireland. *Anaesthesia*. 2017;72:93–105.

17. Montgomery *v* Lanarkshire Health Board [2015]. UKSC 11.

18. Haynes SR, Lawler PG. An assessment of the consistency of ASA physical status classification allocation. *Anaesthesia*. 1995;50:195–9.

19. Findlay GP, Goodwin APL, Protopapa K, Smith NCE, Mason M. *Knowing the Risk. A Review of the Peri-Operative Care of Surgical Patients*. London: National Confidential Enquiry into Patient Outcome and Death; 2011. Available from:http://www.ncepod.org.uk/2011report2/downloads/POC_fullreport.pdf.

20. Oliver CM, Walker E, Giannaris S, Grocott MPW, Moonesinghe SR. Risk assessment tools validated for patients undergoing emergency laparotomy: a systematic review. *Br J Anaesth*. 2015;115:849–60.

21. Eugene N, Oliver CM, et al. Development and internal validation of a novel risk adjustment model for adult patients undergoing emergency laparotomy surgery: The National Emergency Laparotomy Audit risk model. *Br J Anaesth*. 2018;121:739–48.

22. Pearse RM, Harrison DA, MacDonald N, et al. Effect of a perioperative, cardiac output-guided hemodynamic therapy algorithm on outcomes following major gastrointestinal surgery: a randomized clinical trial and systematic review. *JAMA*. 2014;311:2181–90.

23. Singer M, Deutschman C, Seymour C, et al. The Third International Consensus Definitions for Sepsis and Septic Shock (Sepsis-3). *JAMA*. 2016;315:801–10.

24. Martin GS, Mannino DM, Moss M. The effect of age on the development and outcome of adult sepsis. *Crit Care Med*. 2006;34:15–21.

25. Perl TM, Dvorak LA, Hwang T, Wenzel RP. Long-term survival and function after suspected gram-negative sepsis. *JAMA*. 1995;274:338–45.

26. Martin G, Brunkhorst FM, Janes JM, et al. The international PROGRESS registry of patients with severe sepsis: drotrecogin alfa (activated) use and patient outcomes. *Crit Care*. 2009;13:R103.

27. Vester-Andersen M, Lundstrøm LH, Møller MH, et al. Mortality and postoperative care pathways after emergency gastrointestinal surgery in 2904 patients: a population-based cohort study. *Br J Anaesth*. 2014;112:860–70.

28. Tengberg LT, Cihoric M, Foss NB, et al. Complications after emergency laparotomy beyond the immediate postoperative period—a retrospective, observational cohort study of 1139 patients. *Anaesthesia*. 2017;72:309–16.

29. Saunders DI, Murray D, Pichel AC, Varley S, Peden CJ; UK Emergency Laparotomy Network. Variations in mortality after emergency laparotomy: the first report of the UK Emergency Laparotomy Network. *Br J Anaesth*. 2012;109:368–75.

30. McGillicuddy EA, Schuster KM, Davis KA, Longo WE. Factors predicting morbidity and mortality in emergency colorectal procedures in elderly patients. *Arch Surg*. 200;144:1157–62.

31. Khuri SF, Henderson WG, DePalma RG, et al. Determinants of long-term survival after major surgery and the adverse effect of postoperative complications. *Ann Surg*. 2005;242:326–41.

32. Moonesinghe SR, Harris S, Mythen MG, et al. Survival after postoperative morbidity: a longitudinal observational cohort study. *Br J Anaesth*. 2014;113:977–84.

33. Howes TE, Cook TM, Corrigan LJ, Dalton SJ, Richards SK, Peden CJ. Postoperative morbidity survey, mortality and length of stay following emergency laparotomy. *Anaesthesia*. 2015;70:1020–7.

34. Ghaferi AA, Birkmeyer JD, Dimick JB. Variation in hospital mortality associated with inpatient surgery. *N Engl J Med*. 2009;361:1368–75.

35. Ozdemir BA, Sinha S, Karthikesalingam A, et al. Mortality of emergency general surgical patients and associations with hospital structures and processes. *Br J Anaesth*. 2016;116:54–62.

36. Clarke A, Murdoch H, Thomas MJ, Cook TM, Peden CJ. Mortality and postoperative care after emergency laparotomy. *Eur J Anaesthesiol*. 2011;28:16–9.

37. Huddart S, Peden CJ, Swart M, et al. Use of a pathway quality improvement care bundle to reduce mortality after emergency laparotomy. *Br J Surg*. 2015;102:57–66.

38. The Royal College of Surgeons of England. *The Higher Risk General Surgical Patient: Towards Improved Care for a Forgotten Group. Report of the Royal College of Surgeons of England/Department of Health Working Group on Peri-operative Care of the Higher-Risk General Surgical Patient*. London: The Royal College of Surgeons of England; 2011. Available from: http://patientsafety.health.org.uk/resources/higher-risk-general-surgical-patient-towards-improved-care-forgotten-group.

39. Barnett K, Mercer SW, Norbury M, Watt G, Wyke S, Guthrie B. Epidemiology of multimorbidity and implications for health care, research, and medical education: a cross-sectional study. *Lancet*. 2012;380:37–43.

40. Bagshaw SM, Stelfox HT, McDermid RC, et al. Association between frailty and short- and long-term outcomes among critically ill patients: a multicentre prospective cohort study. *CMAJ*. 2014;186:E95–102.

10 Sedation and delirium

Nim Pathmanathan

⊕ Expert Commentary Paul Nixon

Case history

A 45-year-old, 80 kg male was admitted by the emergency department (ED) trauma team following a road traffic collision. He was intoxicated with alcohol, and had lost control while driving a car, hitting a tree at approximately 50 miles/hour. Injuries identified in emergency department assessment included fractured ribs 5–11 on the right with a flail segment and haemopneumothorax, an unstable pelvic fracture, and open fractures of the right femur, distal ulna and radius. He had an intercostal chest drain inserted with an initial output of 500 mL of blood. Haemodynamic stability was achieved after resuscitation with 1 L of Hartmann's solution, 3 units of red blood cells, and placement of a pelvic binder (see also Case 4). He underwent a trauma series computed tomography (CT) scan and was then transferred to the operating room.

The patient was admitted to the intensive care unit (ICU) at 20:00 following a 4-hour operation, which involved external fixation of the pelvis, femur, and forearm. Intraoperatively, he received paracetamol 1 g and morphine 20 mg. His last dose of neuromuscular blocker was 2 hours before ICU admission. In the operating room, he had been transfused 8 units of red blood cells, 4 units of fresh frozen plasma, and one adult therapeutic dose of platelets. Low-pressure suction was applied to the intercostal chest drain and output was 400 mL for the previous 4 hours. The trauma surgeons planned to internally fix the pelvis, femur and forearm in 2 days.

The patient returned to ICU intubated, his lungs were mechanically ventilated (synchronized intermittent mandatory ventilation tidal volume 480 mL (6 mL/kg ideal body weight), respiratory rate 18 breaths/min, positive end-expiratory pressure (PEEP) 8 cmH$_2$O, pressure support 15 cmH$_2$O), and his arterial blood oxygen saturation was 98% (fraction of inspired oxygen (FiO$_2$) 0.5). His heart rate was 110 beats/min, blood pressure 102/56 mmHg, supported by 0.1 mcg/kg/min noradrenaline. Urine output was 220 mL over the past 4 hours and his temperature was 36.0°C. He was sedated with propofol 200 mg/hour and morphine 6 mg/hour. The Richmond Agitation–Sedation Scale (RASS) score was − 5. Initial blood gas values were pH 7.32, partial pressure of carbon dioxide (PaCO$_2$) 5.8 kPa, partial pressure of oxygen (PaO$_2$) 14.7 kPa, bicarbonate (HCO$_3^-$) 18.1 mmol/L, haemoglobin 88 g/L, and lactate 2.6 mmol/L.

⊙ Clinical tip Sedation after transfer

Attend to the sedation strategy as soon as the patient is admitted to the ICU. A recent longitudinal study suggested an association between early deep sedation (within 48 hours) and increased mortality and duration of mechanical ventilation [1]. Deep sedation is often used following intubation in the ED or operating room in order to facilitate safe transfer to the ICU but is often then unnecessarily

(continued)

continued on admission to ICU. Examine the sedation strategy in the ED and again on admission to ICU; stipulate and regularly review the target level of sedation. Despite the use of sedation scales, sedation protocols, and emerging evidence of harm from deep sedation, patients commonly remain over-sedated [2, 3].

⊗ **Learning point Sedation scoring tools**

Sedation can be assessed by clinical scoring systems and by objective measures such as bispectral index (BIS) or auditory evoked potentials. Objective measures are no substitute for clinical scoring systems, but are useful in assessing the depth of sedation when neuromuscular blockade is being used, making clinical scoring systems impractical.

There are numerous clinical scoring systems in use. The RASS (Table 10.1) and Riker Sedation Agitation Scale (SAS; Table 10.2) are reliable, validated in adult ICU patients, and used widely [3]. They are the most frequently used scales in Australasia whereas the Ramsay Sedation Scale (Table 10.3) is the most frequently used in the UK [4]. The particular tool used is less important than familiarity with it and the quality of its implementation. Staff training is essential to maintain adherence to sedation scoring.

Table 10.1 Richmond Agitation–Sedation Scale (RASS)

Score	Scale	Description
+4	Combative	Violent, combative, immediate danger
+3	Very agitated	Pulls or removes tubes/lines, aggressive
+2	Agitated	Non-purposeful movements, fights ventilator
+1	Restless	Anxious, not aggressive
0	Alert and calm	
−1	Drowsy	Not alert, opens eyes and makes eye contact to verbal stimulation for ≥10 seconds
−2	Light sedation	Not alert, opens eyes and makes eye contact to verbal stimulation for <10 seconds
−3	Moderate sedation	Not alert, briefly opens eyes but no eye contact to verbal stimulation
−4	Deep sedation	Not alert, opens eyes to physical stimulation
−5	Unrousable	No response to verbal or physical stimulation

RASS +1 to +4 = agitated; RASS 0 = awake and calm; RASS −1 to −2 = lightly sedated; RASS −3 to −5 = deeply sedated.

Procedure for RASS assessment [5]:

1. Observe patient:
   • Patient is alert, restless, or agitated   Score 0 to +4
2. If not alert, state patient's name and instruct to open eyes and look at speaker:
   • Patient awakens with sustained eye opening and eye contact   Score −1
   • Patient awakens with eye opening and eye contact but not sustained   Score −2
   • Patient has any movement in response to voice but no eye contact   Score −3
3. When no response to verbal stimulation, physically stimulate patient by shaking shoulders and/or rubbing sternum:
   • Patient has any movement to physical stimulation   Score −4
   • Patient has no response to any stimulation   Score −5

(continued)

Table 10.2 Riker Sedation–Agitation Scale (SAS)

Score	Term	Descriptor
7	Dangerous agitation	Pulling at tracheal tube, trying to remove catheters, climbing over bedrail, striking at staff, thrashing side to side
6	Very agitated	Requiring restraint and frequent verbal reminding of limits, biting tracheal tube
5	Agitated	Anxious or physically agitated, calms to verbal instructions
4	Calm and cooperative	Calm, easily rousable, follows commands
3	Sedated	Difficult to rouse but awakens to verbal stimuli or gentle shaking, follows simple commands but drifts off again
2	Very sedated	Arouses to physical stimuli but does not communicate or follow commands, may move spontaneously
1	Unrousable	Minimal or no response to noxious stimuli, does not communicate or follow commands

Table 10.3 Ramsay Sedation Scale

Score	Description
1	Anxious, agitated or restless
2	Cooperative, oriented, tranquil
3	Responds only to verbal commands
4	Asleep, brisk response to light stimulation
5	Asleep, sluggish response to stimulation
6	Unrousable

Clinical tip Bolus doses

Use bolus doses of drugs before starting analgesic and sedative infusions. Bolus doses enable rapid achievement of analgesia and optimal sedation. Conversely, a change in an infusion rate may take many hours to achieve a stable plasma level (and clinical effect). By loading the patient with bolus doses, the subsequent infusion can often be at a lower rate, which may prevent excessive drug administration. This requires regular sedation assessment.

The ICU plan was for stabilization overnight and consideration of extubation in the morning. The propofol and morphine were discontinued to target a RASS score of 0 to −2. Two hours later, the noradrenaline infusion had been weaned off and the patient's RASS score was −2. However, he was grimacing and localizing to the tracheal tube and appeared to be in pain. A 5 mg morphine bolus was administered. Pain was regularly assessed during the subsequent hour and he required two further boluses of morphine and subsequently an infusion at 5 mg/hour. At 03:00 there was no evidence of pain, but he now appeared agitated, with a RASS score of +1. A 30 mg bolus of propofol was given followed by an infusion at 50 mg/hour. The RASS score at 04:00 was −1.

Learning point Sedation protocols

Sedation protocols are most likely to be effective when packaged with assessment of pain and delirium.

Key points of any sedation protocol include:

- staff training in the use of the protocol
- a target sedation score is set regularly (e.g. twice daily)
- a light sedation target (e.g. RASS score 0 to −2) is the default unless clinically contraindicated
- regular assessment of sedation scores—minimum four times per day
- administration of boluses of sedatives and titration of infusions accordingly
- regular audit of sedation management.

Expert comment

Analgesics, such as an opioid, form the mainstay of sedation protocols. Address the patient's pain first and then target an appropriate sedation level. Many analgesics sedate and this secondary effect may limit the requirements of other sedative hypnotics. If an intubated patient is pain free, alert, and calm, additional sedation is of little benefit.

⊕ **Learning point**
Strategies to minimize sedation

Acceptable ways to minimize sedation include the use of a protocolized light sedation policy or daily sedation interruptions. A daily sedation interruption is the reduction or cessation of sedation to wake the patient, with the aim of reducing sedation accumulation. Sedation interruptions are not suitable for patients receiving neuromuscular blockers or those receiving high-level respiratory or cardiovascular support.

🕐 **Expert comment**

The pharmacokinetics and pharmacodynamics of drugs are often difficult to predict in the ICU setting. Institutional and practitioner preferences lead to widespread variation in sedation management. Sedation protocols improve sedation practice by providing a framework to standardize sedation strategies and by incorporating regular patient assessment, with an algorithm for titration of analgesic and sedative drugs.

Sedation scoring tools are most effective when they are used in conjunction with a targeted sedation protocol. Targets are set by the medical team or default targets applied depending on the presenting case. Bedside nursing staff can then titrate analgesic and sedative drugs to meet the desired sedation target. Assess frequently, up to hourly if possible, until stability at the target level is achieved. Frequent assessment leads to earlier achievement of the target and may prevent excessive drug accumulation.

⊕ **Learning point** **Light versus deep sedation**

ICU patients receiving mechanical ventilation often require sedation and analgesia for a variety of reasons including the treatment of pain, tolerance of the tracheal tube and mechanical ventilation, to permit invasive procedures, to reduce physiological stress, and to enable respite from a noisy and often distressing environment.

Historically deep sedation (e.g. RASS score − 5 to − 3) was thought to be most suitable to achieve these goals and to avert longer-term psychological consequences. However, studies have shown that deep sedation results in prolonged duration of mechanical ventilation and ICU length of stay [6–9]. The reason for this is not clear but may be related to complications such as ventilator-associated pneumonia, barotrauma, airway complications, delirium, and adverse effects of the sedating drugs including hypotension, bradycardia, reduced gastric motility, respiratory depression, and suppression of the cough reflex [9].

The aim for most patients is a RASS score of − 2 to 0 (or equivalent in other scoring systems), whereby patients are comfortable, orientated, alert or easily rousable, have good sleep architecture, and can cooperate with interventions such as physiotherapy.

In some patients, light sedation may be harmful. Examples include patients with intracranial injury and high intracranial pressures, severe acute respiratory distress syndrome, or status epilepticus. These patients require deeper sedation (e.g. RASS score of − 3 to − 5 or equivalent). Ensure adequate levels of sedation are maintained if neuromuscular blocking drugs are administered. Potential side effects of under and over sedation are shown in Table 10.4.

✔ **Evidence base** **Daily interruption of sedative infusions in critically ill patients undergoing mechanical ventilation [7]**

- Randomized controlled trial (RCT) in 128 patients in a medical ICU.
- Daily sedation interruption until patients were awake versus routine care.
- Median duration of mechanical ventilation reduced from 7.3 days in the control group to 4.9 days in the intervention group (P = 0.004).
- Median ICU length of stay reduced from 9.9 to 6.4 days (P = 0.02).
- In the intervention group, 9% versus 27% in the control group underwent radiological imaging to assess neurological status (P = 0.02).
- No difference in complications (e.g. unintended tracheal tube/central venous catheter removal).

Table 10.4 Potential adverse effects of under- and oversedation

Light sedation (RASS score at or above − 2)	Deep sedation (RASS score − 3 to − 5)
Pain/discomfort	Increased length of mechanical ventilation
Anxiety	Increased length of admission
Agitation	Increased vasopressor requirements
Risk to patient/carer safety	Decreased cooperation with physiotherapy
Increased oxygen consumption	Reduced cough and secretion clearance
Increased energy expenditure	Unnecessary radiological investigations
Decreased tolerance of invasive procedures	Increased delirium
Risk of dislodgement of devices including airway and vascular access devices	Disorders of sleep architecture
	Pressure sores
Awareness of pain during invasive procedures	Post-traumatic stress disorder

Day 2

The patient remained lightly sedated at 08:00 with a RASS score of − 1. His oxygen requirements, however, had increased: FiO_2 was 0.6, PEEP was 12 cmH_2O, with pressure support of 15 cmH_2O. Tidal volumes were in the range of 300–400 mL but he was limited by pain when asked to take deep breaths. The intercostal chest drain remained on suction and had drained 250 mL of haemoserous fluid over 12 hours. Repeat chest X-ray, showed a small residual right pneumothorax and increasing opacification throughout the right lung field. A sedation interruption was not undertaken as extubation was not appropriate. Cardiovascular, renal, and liver function were stable and unsupported. Delirium was assessed as negative via the Confusion Assessment Method for the Intensive Care Unit (CAM-ICU) tool. Pain was assessed using a numeric rating scale, scoring 8 out of 10. A bolus of morphine 5 mg was given and the infusion was increased to 8 mg/hour. His pain score reduced to 4 increasing to 7 on deep inspiration. Following discussion with the acute pain service a paravertebral catheter was sited and a bolus of 0.125% bupivacaine was given followed by an infusion; his pain subsided significantly and respiratory variables gradually improved. His RASS score at 18:00 was − 3 and the propofol and morphine infusions were reduced to 30 mg/hour and 4 mg/hour respectively.

✪ Learning point Delirium screening tools

Delirium in ICU patients is common with an incidence of up to 83% [10]. As delirium can lead to an increased hospital length of stay, morbidity, and even 6-month mortality [11], it is recommended that patients are routinely monitored for delirium to enable early detection, investigation, and treatment. However, screening for delirium is surprisingly uncommon, only 3.7% in Canadian ICUs surveyed in 2006 [12].

Validated methods of screening are available such as the CAM-ICU [10] and the Intensive Care Delirium Screening Checklist (ICDSC) [13]. On completion of both scales, delirium is either present or absent, but no severity marker is indicated. Undertake the assessment at least once per nursing shift or more frequently if the patient's behaviour changes (Figure 10.1).

CAM-ICU Assessment
- If RASS is − 5 to − 4, stop and reassess when more awake.
- If RASS − 3 to +4, proceed to delirium assessment.

(continued)

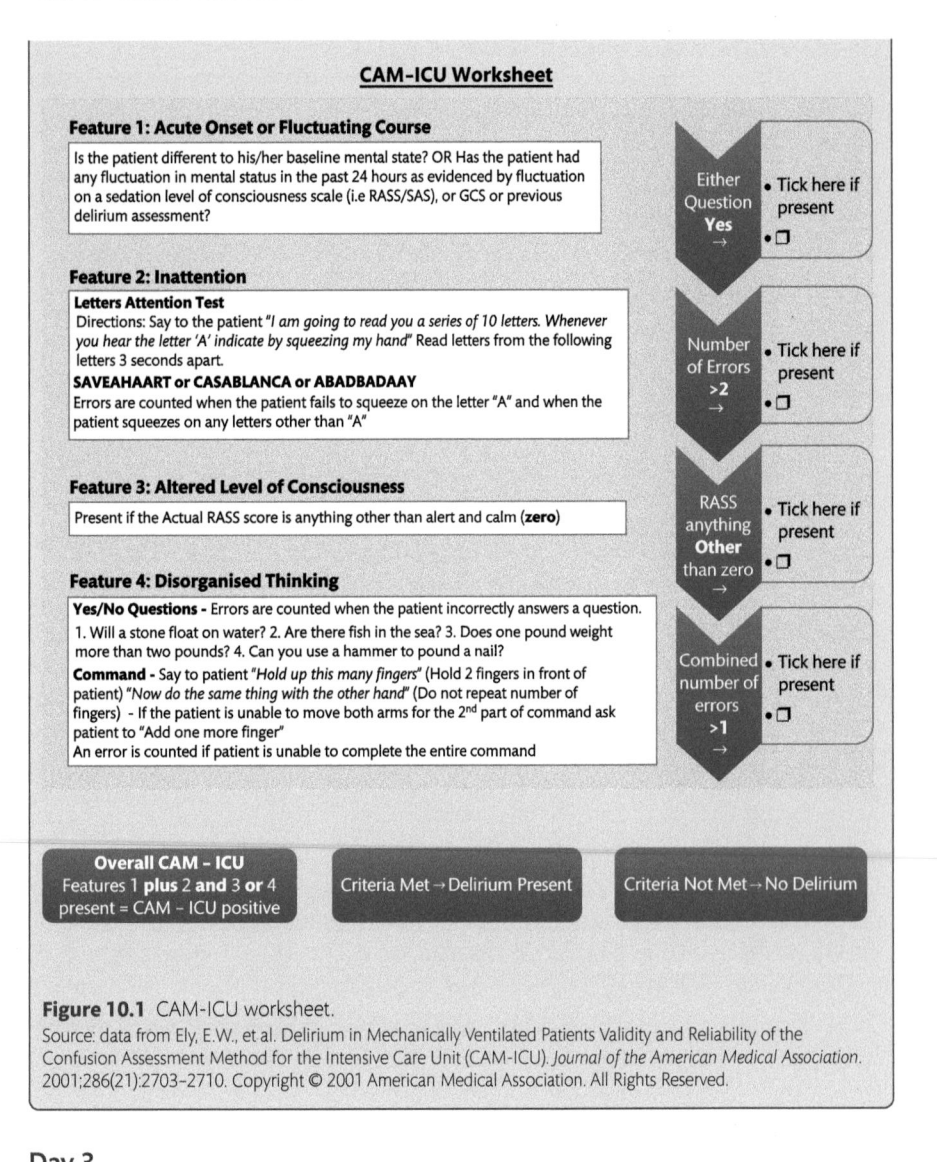

Figure 10.1 CAM-ICU worksheet.
Source: data from Ely, E.W., et al. Delirium in Mechanically Ventilated Patients Validity and Reliability of the Confusion Assessment Method for the Intensive Care Unit (CAM-ICU). *Journal of the American Medical Association.* 2001;286(21):2703–2710. Copyright © 2001 American Medical Association. All Rights Reserved.

Day 3

The patient's respiratory condition improved overnight. The FiO_2 was weaned to 0.4, PEEP was 8 cmH_2O, with pressure support of 10 cmH_2O. During that morning, a family meeting was undertaken and a collateral history was obtained: the patient drank approximately 60 units of alcohol per week, used cannabis and methamphetamine regularly, and smoked 15 cigarettes each day. Pabrinex supplements, thiamine 300 mg intravenously (IV) three times daily, and a 21 mg nicotine patch were started.

He returned to theatre and underwent open reduction and internal fixation of the pelvis, right femur, and forearm. After 6 hours of surgery he returned intubated and ventilated without cardiovascular support. He was sedated with propofol 200 mg/hour and analgesia was provided by morphine 10 mg/hour and the paravertebral infusion of bupivacaine. His RASS score was − 5.

Day 4

The patient's respiratory condition improved again overnight (FiO_2 of 0.3, PEEP 8 cmH_2O, and pressure support 8 cmH_2O) and his sedation was weaned to morphine

5 mg/hour and propofol 50 mg/hour. His RASS score was +2. He denied any pain but was restless and appeared agitated. The propofol infusion was stopped, while continuing the morphine to assess suitability for extubation.

> **✪ Learning point Pain assessment and scoring**
>
> Pain is not confined to the surgical cohort of ICU patients and assessment is vital when addressing the patient's analgesic and sedation requirements. Pain can lead to tachycardia and hypertension, and agitation, delirium, and symptoms of acute psychological distress. Patients with pain may be agitated and can pose a threat to themselves and the staff caring for them.
>
> Pain can be difficult to assess in a mechanically ventilated ICU patient. Vital signs can be an aid, but should not be used alone to monitor pain [3]. There are many scoring systems to help clinicians assess pain, an example being the Behavioural Pain Scale. These scoring systems can be used in medical, postoperative patients and trauma patients (except for the head injured). As with the assessment of sedation, pain assessment should be performed regularly and treated accordingly.

During the next 30 min he became very agitated and was pulling at his tracheal tube and intravenous lines. He was tachycardic and tachypnoeic. Arterial blood gas analysis showed pH 7.46, $PaCO_2$ 4.0 kPa, PaO_2 12.3 kPa, HCO_3^- 27.3 mmol/L, and lactate 1.3 mmol/L. CAM-ICU screening was positive for delirium. Extubation was deemed unsafe and he was administered propofol 30 mg and the infusion restarted at 50 mg/hour. A delirium screen (see Table 10.5) was started to seek a modifiable cause. There were no signs of infection and no modifiable causes of delirium other than possible alcohol and drug withdrawal. Diazepam 10 mg via a nasogastric (NG) tube was prescribed 6-hourly as per the local alcohol withdrawal regimen. The agitation persisted, however, and he remained CAM-ICU positive. Quetiapine 25 mg twice daily NG was prescribed. His infusions remained relatively unchanged over the day: propofol 40 mg/hour and morphine 4 mg/hour.

> **✚ Clinical tip**
>
> Pay attention to procedures such as suctioning and mobilization that can cause pain in the ICU. Consider giving a bolus of analgesic drug before these procedures. Opioids are the analgesic of choice in the critically ill.

Table 10.5 Delirium risk factors

Past medical history	Acute illness	Environmental	Medication	Social history
Age >70 years	Sepsis	Catheters/tubes/drains	Benzodiazepines	Smoker
Cardiac failure	Fever	Visual/hearing impairment	Opioids	Alcohol abuse
Hepatic failure	Hypoxia		Corticosteroids	Malnutrition
Renal failure	Hypotension	Absence of visible daylight	Tricyclic antidepressants	Lack of visitors
Hypertension	APACHE II score >15	Physical restraints	Anticholinergics	
Dementia	Hypo/hypernatraemia	Sleep deprivation	Antiemetics	
Epilepsy	Hypo/hyperglycaemia	Loss of diurnal rhythm	Drug/medication withdrawal	
Depression	Hypocalcaemia			
	Thyroid dysfunction			
	Acute kidney injury			
	Pain			

APACHE II, Acute Physiology, Age, Chronic Health Evaluation II.

> **✚ Clinical tip Treating delirium**
>
> Treat reversible causes of delirium and optimize non-pharmacological treatments before treating with drugs. Exclude withdrawal states (e.g. alcohol, recreational drugs, antidepressants, and nicotine) and, if appropriate, reintroduce the drug or substitutes. A commonly overlooked cause of delirium is the abrupt cessation of prolonged infusions of sedative medication such as benzodiazepine, opioids, or alpha agonists. A slower tapering of the sedative medication should be considered and alternative medications, such as clonidine, may be instituted to dampen down the withdrawal effect.

> **✪ Learning point Non-pharmacological management of delirium**
>
> Non-pharmacological management is an integral part of the management of delirium. Ensure visual aids are available and hearing aids are in place and switched on. Enhance communication, where appropriate, using aids such as word charts. Orientation should occur including the establishment of day–night orientation and the use of clocks. Reduce ambient lighting during night-time and keep sound to a minimum; consider using quiet bins and reducing the volume of telephones and avoid non-essential interventions during rest periods. Ear plugs and eye pads may be useful as may night time melatonin to improve sleep pattern. These non-pharmacological measures may also lead to less sedative medication being required.

> **✪ Learning point Pharmacological management of delirium**
>
> Despite lacking a strong evidence base, the mainstay of pharmacological management of delirium is antipsychotic medication. Examples of medications used for the treatment of delirium include the following:
>
> - Antipsychotics:
>   - Quetiapine 12.5–25 mg orally/NG twice daily plus 12.5–25 mg as required (PRN) (can be titrated up to a maximum of 200 mg/day in divided doses).
>   - Olanzapine: 2.5–5 mg orally/NG every night plus 2.5–5 mg twice daily PRN (can be titrated to 10 mg twice daily and a maximum daily dose of 30 mg).
>   - Haloperidol: if oral route not available or patient is acutely agitated/delirious; 0.5–2.5 mg IV repeated after 15 min if required. Can also be given intramuscularly if no IV access available. For elderly/frail patients, start at half the recommended dose and titrate slowly.
> - Alpha agonists
>   - Dexmedetomidine: infusion of 0.2–1.5 mcg/kg/hour.
>   - Clonidine: 1–4 mcg/kg/hour.
>
> Antipsychotics can all cause the long QT syndrome and neuroleptic malignant syndrome. The newer atypical drugs (quetiapine, olanzapine) cause these side effects less commonly than the traditional drugs such as haloperidol. They are contraindicated in patients with pre-existing long QT syndrome and in Parkinson's disease which they exacerbate. Long-term treatment is not usually required; stop these drugs when the delirium resolves.

> **⑪ Expert comment**
>
> There is no clear evidence guiding the optimal medication for the treatment of delirium in the ICU. Studies have shown an association between benzodiazepines and delirium and they should be avoided if possible (except in the case of benzodiazepine for alcohol withdrawal or as dose-sparing drugs in deep sedation). Based on limited data, antipsychotics (e.g. quetiapine or haloperidol) and alpha$_2$-receptor agonists (e.g. clonidine and dexmedetomidine) are useful [3, 14, 15].

Day 5

Following a settled night, the patient was again assessed for suitability for extubation. He was calm and cooperative with a RASS score of −1. The CAM-ICU remained positive and quetiapine doses were continued. The propofol was stopped and the patient was extubated successfully to humidified oxygen. He was discharged to the ward the following day. The quetiapine and diazepam were weaned off over the following 5 days.

Discussion

Both protocolized sedation and daily sedation interruptions are acceptable strategies to minimize sedation use. In one study, the addition of a daily sedation interruption to routine care reduced sedative use, the duration of mechanical ventilation, and ICU length of stay [7]. More recent trials have documented inconsistent results when daily sedation interruptions were compared to protocolized sedation [16, 17] and there has been concern about patient comfort and safety and increasing nursing workload [18].

Numerous studies have shown that the introduction of a sedation protocol or package can reduce the duration of mechanical ventilation, ICU length of stay, and hospital length of stay [6, 19–21]. Other studies have been unable to reproduce these benefits [22, 23]. The reasons for this are unclear but may be due to nursing intensity, prior experience of sedation management, or studies being underpowered.

✪ Learning point Analgesia-first sedation

A study using daily sedation interruptions compared analgesia-only sedation in the form of morphine with sedation using propofol or midazolam [24]. In the analgesia-only arm, there was an increased number of ventilator-free days and a decreased ICU and hospital length of stay. However, more patients in the analgesia-only group developed agitated delirium. While the results of this study do not advocate a purely analgesia-based sedation protocol, the study shows potential benefits of an analgesia-first protocol. By prioritizing the treatment of pain, the reduction of co-administered hypnotic drugs may improve outcomes.

✔ Evidence base Awakening and Breathing Controlled (ABC) trial [25]

- Multicentre RCT.
- Included 336 patients who underwent either daily sedation interruption plus a daily spontaneous breathing trial (SBT) or a daily SBT alone.
- Patients in the daily sedation interruption plus SBT group were discharged earlier from ICU (9.1 vs 12.9 days; P = 0.01) and hospital (median 14.9 vs 19.2 days; P = 0.04).
- There was an increase in self-extubation events in the daily sedation interruption plus SBT group but no increase in the rates of reintubation.
- One-year survival showed a mortality benefit in the daily sedation interruption plus SBT group (Hazard ratio 0.68; 95% confidence interval 0.50–0.92; P = 0.01).

While light sedation increases oxygen consumption, energy expenditure, and catecholamine release [27, 28], there is no evidence this translates into increased rates of myocardial ischaemia or infarction [29, 30]. Similarly, there is no evidence of psychological harm from light sedation. There is an association between amnesia in critical illness and the development of post-traumatic stress disorder symptoms [31]; these symptoms may be related to having delusional memories without factual recall [32, 33]. An RCT evaluating the effect of light or deep sedation on mental health showed that post-traumatic stress disorder symptoms were more common in the deep sedation cohort but this was not statistically significant. This cohort had increased rates of disturbing memories with lower rates of factual recall [8]. Two large RCTs have also shown no evidence of long-term psychological harm from daily sedation interruptions [34, 35].

Patients who are administered neuromuscular blockade are obviously unsuitable for light sedation. Clinical scoring systems are of no use to assess depth of sedation; monitors such as the BIS may have a role in monitoring sedation depth and titrating sedation. There is, however, a poor correlation of depth of sedation when assessed by clinical scoring tools and by BIS (in patients who were not being administered neuromuscular blockade) [36]. Furthermore, BIS is not validated in ICUs and there is uncertainty about the level that indicates deep sedation.

There is insufficient evidence to suggest that a particular drug or sedation strategy is superior to any other and sedation management is often guided by individual or

---

❝ Expert comment

Introducing sedation scoring protocols into an ICU requires a complex change management process. Stakeholder buy-in is required and education of all team members involved is essential. Staff must be well supported and educated regularly. Regular audits and reinforcement are required until the unit culture is adjusted.

✔ Evidence base

Sedation Lightening and Evaluation of A Protocol (SLEAP) trial [26]

- Multicentre RCT.
- Included 430 patients who underwent daily sedation interruption plus protocolized sedation or protocolized sedation alone.
- No difference in time to extubation, or ICU or hospital length of stay.
- Higher mean doses of sedation used in the daily sedation interruption cohort.

✪ Learning point

Analgesia and anaesthesia for procedures

Light sedation is used to tolerate invasive ventilation and enable respite from a distressing environment. However, this level of sedation is often not adequate for procedures. Suctioning and mobilization are examples that may require a prior bolus of sedation. More invasive procedures such as percutaneous tracheostomy require analgesia and anaesthesia to ensure comfort and prevent awareness. This is imperative when using neuromuscular blockade to avoid the distress of unintended awareness during paralysis, not infrequently identified in the ICU population [37].

institutional preferences including factors such as familiarity and cost. The commonly used medications include propofol, benzodiazepines, and opioid analgesics. Worldwide, an opioid plus a hypnotic such as propofol or midazolam is the most commonly used combination. Other frequently used medications include clonidine, dexmedetomidine, and ketamine. As sedation involves elements of analgesia and hypnosis, combining an opioid with a hypnotic is often beneficial. The different mechanisms of action of the drugs reduce overall dosage and dose-dependent side effects. An overview of sedation options is given in Table 10.6.

Benzodiazepines are cheap and the most commonly used class of sedatives worldwide. However, the American Pain, Agitation, and Delirium Guidelines 2013 advocate using non-benzodiazepine medication in mechanically ventilated ICU patients because benzodiazepines prolong the duration of ventilation and ICU length of stay and increase the incidence of delirium [3]. Benzodiazepines retain a role in alcohol withdrawal and as dose-sparing drugs in deep sedation.

Opioids are used in most sedation regimens. There is no evidence to suggest better outcomes for a particular opioid; morphine and fentanyl are most commonly used. Remifentanil may offer advantages over other opioids because it has a sedative-sparing effect, metabolism independent of organ function, and a context-insensitive half-life where the half-life remains at 3–4 min irrespective of infusion duration. This fast, predictable offset time facilitates rapid neurological assessment. One of the disadvantages of remifentanil is the rapid and total lack of analgesia once the infusion is stopped. It is also more expensive than other opioids.

Propofol is commonly used in the ICU. It has a fast onset and a faster offset than benzodiazepines. It has no analgesic properties and is therefore often used in combination with an opioid. It can make blood more lipaemic, which can interfere with some blood tests. A rare adverse consequence is propofol infusion syndrome (PRIS).

✪ Learning point Propofol infusion syndrome

- PRIS is a rare life-threatening condition caused by impairment of mitochondrial oxidative phosphorylation and free fatty acid utilization [38].
- The true incidence of PRIS is unknown, but it is much higher in children and for this reason propofol is not licensed for sedation in ICU patients aged less than 16 years
- Features include new or unexplained metabolic acidosis, cardiac dysfunction, rhabdomyolysis, renal failure, hypertriglyceridaemia, hepatomegaly, and lipaemia.
- Risk factors include young age, increasing dose and duration, severe head injuries, sepsis, high exogenous or endogenous catecholamine and glucocorticoid levels, and a low carbohydrate to high lipid intake [38].
- Mortality is 18–30% in suspected cases [39, 40].
- PRIS persists after stopping the drug; prevention is imperative and a high index of suspicion is required as only supportive treatment is available.
- Propofol is not recommended for sedation at a dose of greater than 4 mg/kg/hour. However, there are case reports of PRIS at lower doses.
- Daily monitoring of creatine kinase and triglycerides has been proposed as surveillance when propofol is used for over 24 hours.

Dexmedetomidine is a relatively recent addition to the choice of ICU sedatives, which can be used as a sole sedative drug for light to moderate sedation and is thought to lead to a more cooperative patient with less respiratory depression. The main adverse effects are bradycardia and hypotension.

Dexmedetomidine has been compared with traditional sedatives in several RCTs including MENDS [41] (comparator lorazepam), SEDCOM [42] (comparator midazolam),

Table 10.6 Overview of sedation options

	Examples	Mechanism of action	Pharmacokinetics	Pharmacodynamics	Useful properties	Adverse effects
Propofol		Thought to be due to positive modulation of GABA at the GABA$_A$ receptor leading to hyperpolarization following chloride influx	Highly protein bound to albumin (98%)	Decreased systemic vascular resistance, cardiac output, and blood pressure	Due to rapid clearance, can be used for frequent neurological assessment of patients	Propofol infusion syndrome
			Fast onset and offset due to high clearance			Pain on injection (bolus)
				Respiratory depressant	Anticonvulsant	Hyperlipidaemia
			Accumulation in tissue stores when used in prolonged infusions (without use of targeted light sedation)	Antitussive	Antiemetic	
					Anxiolysis	
					Amnesia	
Benzodiazepines	Lorazepam, midazolam, diazepam	Modulate the effect of GABA at GABA$_A$ receptors	Midazolam is oxidized by the cytochrome P450 enzyme system to form water-soluble metabolites which can accumulate in renal failure and have central nervous system depressant effects	Dose-dependent respiratory depression	Anticonvulsant	Unpredictable and prolonged effect in hepatic and renal failure and critical illness
				Decreased heart rate and systemic vascular resistance	Anxiolytic	
					Potentiate the effects of opioids	Risk of toxicity from propylene glycol (carrier for lorazepam)
			Lorazepam is primarily metabolized by glucuronidation to inactive metabolites			May prolong the duration of ventilation, intensive care stay, and hospital stay
			Midazolam has a higher clearance than lorazepam			May increase the incidence of delirium
						Risk of withdrawal with prolonged use
Opioids	Morphine	Agonist at opioid receptors	Mainly metabolized in the liver to both inactive and active compounds that are excreted in urine and bile	Respiratory depression	Analgesia	Tolerance and risk of withdrawal with prolonged use
	Alfentanil	Alfentanil is 10 times more potent than fentanyl which is 100 times more potent than morphine		Bradycardia	Sedation at higher doses	Prolonged effect in hepatic/renal dysfunction
	Fentanyl			Antitussive	May reduce dose of co-administered sedatives	
					Generally cheap and familiar	
	Remifentanil	Selective mu agonist	Ultrashort-acting opioid due to metabolism by plasma esterases	Bradycardia and hypotension (when used at higher doses)	Potent analgesic	Cost
			Displays a context-insensitive half-time; half-life of drug remains at 3–4 min irrespective of duration of infusion	Respiratory depression	Renal/hepatic dysfunction does not prolong the duration	Chest wall rigidity (bolus)
					Sedative-sparing effect	
					Easily titratable	

(continued)

Table 10.6 Continued

	Examples	Mechanism of action	Pharmacokinetics	Pharmacodynamics	Useful properties	Adverse effects
Alpha$_2$ receptor agonists	Dexmedetomidine	Centrally acting alpha$_2$ agonist at the locus coeruleus Affinity for alpha$_2$:alpha$_1$ 1600:1 Active d-stereoisomer of medetomidine	Highly protein bound (94%) Metabolized by glucuronidation and hydroxylation in the liver and excreted predominantly by the kidneys	Sedation Analgesia Bradycardia Hypotension	Minimal respiratory depression	Bradycardia Reduced clearance in hepatic failure Cost
	Clonidine	Centrally acting postsynaptic alpha$_2$ agonist at the lateral reticular nucleus of the medulla. Leads to reduced intracellular cAMP and increases potassium ion conductance Stimulates alpha$_2$ receptors in the spinal cord leading to increased endogenous opiate release Affinity for alpha$_2$:alpha$_1$ 200:1	Metabolized by the liver to inactive metabolites that are excreted by the kidneys	Sedation Analgesia Bradycardia Hypotension	Minimal respiratory depression Not commonly used as a first-line agent. May have a role as an adjunct when sedation is difficult to manage or wean Useful drug in the setting of recreational substance abuse	May cause initial hypertension via alpha$_1$ stimulation prior to the hypotensive alpha$_2$ effects Bradycardia Can cause rebound hypertension on sudden cessation of the drug
Ketamine		Non-competitive antagonism at the NMDA receptor	Metabolized by the liver to the active norketamine prior to further conjugation to inactive metabolites which are excreted in the urine	Analgesic Increased heart rate, maintains blood pressure and cardiac output Bronchodilator	Laryngeal reflexes usually intact when used for sedation	Hallucinations Uncertain effect on intracranial pressure No studies supporting its use in sedation in intensive care Hypersalivation

MIDEX [43] (comparator midazolam), PRODEX [43] (comparator propofol), and DESIRE [44, 45] (comparator mixed sedatives). In summary, dexmedetomidine was non-inferior to all these traditional sedatives and led to reduced rates of delirium when compared to lorazepam [41] and midazolam [42] and a modest reduction in mechanical ventilation time compared to midazolam [42, 43]. There was no difference in the duration of mechanical ventilation when compared to propofol [43]. It also allowed patients to communicate pain more effectively when compared to both propofol and midazolam [43].

Dexmedetomidine is not suitable for use when deep sedation is required [44]. It is also substantially more expensive than traditional sedatives and until there is a clear benefit or a reduction in cost, it will remain a second-line drug. It has a role in weaning sedation when sedation management or delirium is problematic.

Clonidine has a role as an adjunct when sedation is difficult to manage or wean and may have a role as an adjunct in the management of alcohol withdrawal.

Ketamine is used primarily as an analgesic adjunct. Analgesia occurs at much lower concentrations than required for sedation. It is not widely used for sedation in ICU, nor supported by evidence. Ketamine causes transient sympathetic nervous system stimulation and bronchodilation with preservation of the cough reflex. It causes a degree of muscle rigidity and is associated with distressing dreaming or hallucinations, which may be ameliorated by co-administration of benzodiazepines.

Analgesics that are often used as adjuncts in ICU include paracetamol, tramadol, gabapentinoids, ketamine, and clonidine. Non-steroidal anti-inflammatory drugs are often avoided in many patients in the ICU because of the potential for upper gastrointestinal ulceration and renal injury. Consider using regional anaesthetic techniques such as epidural and paravertebral analgesia when applicable.

Delirium

Delirium is a syndrome of acute onset characterized by a fluctuation of mental state, inattention, and either disorganized thinking or an altered level of consciousness. It can be classified into three subtypes: hyperactive (where patients appear agitated, restless, or paranoid), hypoactive (where patients appear lethargic, inattentive, or apparently pleasantly confused), and mixed (where patients fluctuate between the two). While the symptoms of hyperactive delirium are the most synonymous with a diagnosis of delirium, this subtype is the least common form [46]. The pathophysiology of delirium remains poorly understood, but current theories include an imbalance of neurotransmitters with gamma-aminobutyric acid (GABA), acetylcholine, and dopamine playing a role.

The incidence of delirium in ICU is as high as 83 % depending on the screening tool used and population studied [10]. Delirium was thought to be a relatively benign sign of the severity of critical illness, but has been found to be an independent predictor of increased ICU and hospital length of stay, increased 6-month and 1-year mortality [11, 47], and it is linked to longer-term neurocognitive disturbance in survivors [48]. The duration of delirium also has an effect on 6-month and 1-year mortality [49]. In the US in 2006, delirium was estimated to cost $6.9 billion per year [50].

There is currently no conclusive evidence to support the use of prophylactic antipsychotics to reduce the incidence of delirium and the cornerstone of the prevention of delirium is the minimization of risk factors [51, 52]. Limited evidence suggests that light sedation reduces the rates of delirium and enables early assessment and detection of delirium. It also enables early mobilization, which may reduce rates of delirium and has numerous other benefits.

Expert comment

Without the use of validated assessment tools such as the CAM-ICU, hypoactive delirium is often missed by clinicians. Hypoactive delirium causes the same degree of morbidity and mortality as hyperactive delirium, and may even be worse [11]. Identification of risk factors and non-pharmacological management are the mainstay of treatment. It is unclear whether medications (e.g. antipsychotics) are beneficial in the management of hypoactive delirium.

A final word from the expert

Management of sedation in the ICU requires a team-based approach. Validated assessment tools are available and are best used in conjunction with a protocolized sedation algorithm. Prioritize analgesia in any sedation process even if the patient is assumed to have minimal discomfort. Active sedation management begins on admission of the patient to the ICU so that unnecessary accumulation of drugs and their subsequent side effects are prevented.

Delirium in the ICU is challenging to treat and is associated with patient morbidity and mortality. It is important to attempt to prevent delirium and to identify its presence early. Seek risk factors and causes and treat appropriately. There is only limited evidence to indicate that treatment of delirium with drugs is effective. This topic requires further research.

References

1. Shehabi Y, Bellomo R, Reade MC, et al. Early intensive care sedation predicts long-term mortality in ventilated critically ill patients. *Am J Respir Crit Care Med.* 2012;186:724–31.
2. Watson PL, Shintani AK, Tyson R, Pandharipande PP, Pun BT, Ely EW. Presence of electroencephalogram burst suppression in sedated, critically ill patients is associated with increased mortality. *Crit Care Med.* 2008;36:3171–7.
3. Barr J, Fraser GL, Puntillo K, et al. Clinical practice guidelines for the management of pain, agitation, and delirium in adult patients in the intensive care unit. *Crit Care Med.* 2013;41:263–306.
4. Shehabi Y, Botha JA, Boyle MS, et al. Sedation and delirium in the intensive care unit: an Australian and New Zealand perspective. *Anaesth Intensive Care.* 2008;36:570–8.
5. Ely EW, Truman B, Shintani A, et al. Monitoring sedation status over time in ICU patients. Reliability and validity of the Richmond Agitation-Sedation Scale (RASS). *JAMA.* 2003;289:2983–11.
6. Brook AD, Ahrens TS, Schaiff R, et al. Effect of a nursing-implemented sedation protocol on the duration of mechanical ventilation. *Crit Care Med.* 1999;27:2609–15.
7. Kress JP, Pohlman AS, O'Connor MF, Hall JB. Daily interruption of sedative infusions in critically ill patients undergoing mechanical ventilation. *N Engl J Med.* 2000;342:1471–7.
8. Treggiari MM, Romand JA, Yanez ND, et al. Randomized trial of light versus deep sedation on mental health after critical illness. *Crit Care Med.* 2009;37:2527–34.
9. Kollef MH, Levy NT, Ahrens TS, Schaiff R, Prentice D, Sherman G. The use of continuous IV sedation is associated with prolongation of mechanical ventilation. *Chest.* 1998;114:541–8.
10. Ely EW, Inouye SK, Bernard GR, et al. Delirium in mechanically ventilated patients: validity and reliability of the Confusion Assessment Method for the Intensive Care Unit (CAM-ICU). *JAMA.* 2001;286:2703–10.
11. Ely EW, MD, Shintani A, Truman B, et al. Delirium as a predictor of mortality in mechanically ventilated patients in the intensive care unit. *JAMA.* 2004;291:1753–62.
12. Mehta S, Burry L, Fischer S, et al. Canadian survey of the use of sedatives, analgesics, and neuromuscular blocking agents in critically ill patients. *Crit Care Med.* 2006;34:374–80.
13. Bergeron N, Dubois MJ, Dumont M, et al. Intensive Care Delirium Screening Checklist: evaluation of a new screening tool. *Intensive Care Med.* 2001;27:859–64.
14. Rubino AS, Onorati F, Caroleo S, et al. Impact of clonidine administration on delirium and related respiratory weaning after surgical correction of acute type-A aortic dissection: results of a pilot study. *Interact Cardiovasc Thorac Surg.* 2010;10:58–62.

15. Reade MC, O'Sullivan K, Bates S, Goldsmith D, Ainslie WR, Bellomo R. Dexmedetomidine vs haloperidol in delirious, agitated, intubated patients: a randomised open-label trial. *Crit Care*. 2009;13:R75.

16. De Wit M, Gennings C, Jenvey WI, Epstein SK. Randomized trial comparing daily interruption of sedation and nursing-implemented sedation algorithm in medical intensive care unit patients. *Critical Care*. 2008;12:R70.

17. Nassar JAP, Park M. Daily sedative interruption versus intermittent sedation in mechanically ventilated critically ill patients: a randomized trial. *Ann Intensive Care*. 2014;4:1–2.

18. Devlin JW, Tanios MA, Epstein SK. Intensive care unit sedation: waking up clinicians to the gap between research and practice. *Crit Care Med*. 2006;34:556–7.

19. Brattebo G, Hofoss D, Flaatten H, Muri AK, Gjerde S, Plsek PE. Effect of a scoring system and protocol for sedation on duration of patients' need for ventilator support in a surgical intensive care unit. *Qual Saf Health Care*. 2004;13:203–5.

20. Quenot JP, Ladoire S, Devoucoux F, et al. Effect of a nurse-implemented sedation protocol on the incidence of ventilator-associated pneumonia. *Crit Care Med*. 2007;35:2031–6.

21. Marshall J, Finn CA, Theodore AC. Impact of a clinical pharmacist-enforced intensive care unit sedation protocol on duration of mechanical ventilation and hospital stay. *Crit Care Med*. 2008;36:427–33.

22. Bucknall TK, Manias E, Presneill JJ. A randomized trial of protocol directed sedation management for mechanical ventilation in an Australian intensive care unit. *Crit Care Med*. 2008;36:1444–50.

23. Elliott R, McKinley S, Aitken LM, et al. The effect of an algorithm-based sedation guideline on the duration of mechanical ventilation in an Australian intensive care unit. *Intensive Care Med*. 2006;32:1506–14.

24. Strøm T, Martinussen T, Toft P. A protocol of no sedation for critically ill patients receiving mechanical ventilation: a randomised trial. *Lancet*. 2010;375:475–80.

25. Girard TD, Kress JP, Fuchs BD, et al. Efficacy and safety of a paired sedation and ventilator weaning protocol for mechanically ventilated patients in intensive care (Awakening and Breathing Controlled trial): a randomised controlled trial. *Lancet*. 2008;371:126–34.

26. Mehta S, Burry L, Cook D, et al. Daily sedation interruption in mechanically ventilated critically ill patients cared for with a sedation protocol: a randomized controlled trial. *JAMA*. 2012;308:1985–92.

27. Terao Y, Miura K, Saito M, Sekino M, Fukusaki M, Sumikawa K. Quantitative analysis of the relationship between sedation and resting energy expenditure in postoperative patients. *Crit Care Med*. 2003;31:830–3.

28. Plunkett JJ, Reeves JD, Ngo L, et al. Urine and plasma catecholamine and cortisol concentrations after myocardial revascularization. Modulation by continuous sedation. *Anesthesiology*. 1997;86:785–96.

29. Hall RI, Maclaren C, Smith MS, et al. Light versus heavy sedation after cardiac surgery: myocardial ischemia and the stress response. *Anesth Analg*. 1997;85:971–8.

30. Kress JP, Vinayak AG, Levitt J, et al. Daily sedative interruption in mechanically ventilated patients at risk for coronary artery disease. *Crit Care Med*. 2007;35:365–71.

31. Granja C, Gomes E, Amaro A, et al. Understanding posttraumatic stress disorder-related symptoms after critical care: the early illness amnesia hypothesis. *Crit Care Med*. 2008;36:2801–9.

32. Jones C, Griffiths RD, Humphris G, Skirrow PM. Memory, delusions, and the development of acute posttraumatic stress disorder-related symptoms after intensive care. *Crit Care Med*. 2001;29:573–80.

33. Larson MJ, Lindell KW, Hopkins RO. Cognitive sequelae in acute respiratory distress syndrome patients with and without recall of the intensive care unit. *J Int Neuropsychol Soc*. 2007;13:595–605.

34. Jackson JC, Girard TD, Gordon SM, et al. Long-term cognitive and psychological outcomes in the Awakening and Breathing Controlled trial. *Am J Respir Crit Care Med*. 2010;182:183–91.

35. Kress JP, Gehlbach B, Lacy M, Pliskin N, Pohlman AS, Hall JB. The long-term psychological effects of daily sedative interruption on critically ill patients. *Am J Respir Crit Care Med*. 2003;168:1457–61.

36. Nasraway SA, Wu EC, Kelleher RM, Yasuda CM, Donnelly AM. How reliable is the Bispectral Index in critically ill patients? A prospective, comparative, single-blinded observer study. *Crit Care Med*. 2002;30:1483–7.

37. Cook TM, Andrade J, Bogod DG, et al. 5th National Audit Project (NAP5) on accidental awareness during general anaesthesia: patient experiences, human factors, sedation, consent, and medicolegal issues. *Br J Anaesth*. 2014;113:560–74.

38. Loh NW, Nair P. Propofol infusion syndrome. *Continuing Educ Anaesth Crit Care Pain*. 2013;13:200–2.

39. Roberts RJ, Barletta JF, Fong JJ, et al. Incidence of propofol-related infusion syndrome in critically ill adults: a prospective, multicentre study. *Crit Care*. 2009;13:R169.

40. Fong JJ, Sylvia L, Ruthazer R, Schumaker G, Kcomt M, Devlin JW. Predictors of mortality in patients with suspected propofol infusion syndrome. *Crit Care Med*. 2008;36:2281–7.

41. Panharipande PP, Pun BT, Herr DL, et al. Effect of sedation with dexmedetomidine vs lorazepam on acute brain dysfunction in mechanically ventilated patients: the MENDS randomized controlled trial. *JAMA*. 2007;298:2644–53.

42. Riker RR, Shehabi Y, Bokesch PM, et al. Dexmedetomidine vs midazolam for sedation of critically ill patients: a randomised trial. *JAMA*. 2009;301:489–99.

43. Jakob SM, Ruokenen E, Grounds RM, et al. Dexmedetomidine vs midazolam or propofol for sedation during prolonged mechanical ventilation. *JAMA*. 2012;307:1151–60.

44. Kawazoe Y, Miyamoto K, Morimoto T, et al. Effect of dexmedetomidine on mortality and ventilator-free days in patients requiring mechanical ventilation with sepsis: a randomized clinical trial. *JAMA*. 2017;317:1321–8.

45. Ruokonen E, Parviainen I, Jakob SM, et al. Dexmedetomidine versus propofol/midazolam for long-term sedation during mechanical ventilation. *Intensive Care Med*. 2009;35:282–90.

46. Peterson JF, Pun BT, Dittus RS, et al. Delirium and its motoric subtypes: a study of 614 critically ill patients. *J Am Geriatr Soc*. 2006;54:479–84.

47. Pisani MA, Kong SY, Kasl SV, Murphy TE, Araujo KL, Van Ness PH. Days of delirium are associated with 1-year mortality in an older intensive care unit population. *Am J Respir Crit Care Med*. 2009;180:1092–7.

48. Girard TD, Jackson JC, Pandharipande PP, et al. Delirium as a predictor of long-term cognitive impairment in survivors of critical illness. *Crit Care Med*. 2010;38:1513–20.

49. Shehabi Y, Riker RR, Bokesch PM, et al. Delirium duration and mortality in lightly sedated, mechanically ventilated intensive care patients. *Crit Care Med*. 2010;38:2311–18.

50. Inouye SK, Ferrucci L. Elucidating the pathophysiology of delirium and the interrelationship of delirium and dementia. *J Gerontol A Biol Sci Med Sci*. 2006;61:1277–80.

51. Page VJ, Ely EW, Gates S, et al. Effect of intravenous haloperidol on the duration of delirium and coma in critically ill patients (Hope-ICU): a randomised, double-blind, placebo-controlled trial. *Lancet Respir Med*. 2013;1:515–23.

52. Wang W, Hong-Liang L, Wang D, et al. Haloperidol prophylaxis decreases delirium incidence in elderly patients after noncardiac surgery: a randomized controlled trial. *Crit Care Med*. 2012;40:731–9.

Acute-on-chronic liver failure

Tasneem Pirani

ⓘ **Expert Commentary** Julia Wendon

Case history

A 55-year-old female presented with a 10-day history of painless jaundice and abdominal distension. She had continued to work as a nurse until the week before when colleagues had commented on her conjunctival discolouration. She denied weight loss or change in bowel habit. She reported normal coloured but loose stools and dark urine. In the last few days her urge to pass urine had reduced and she had not passed urine for more than 12 hours.

She had a past medical history of hypertension and mild asthma. She had no history of chronic liver disease. Her medications included irbesartan 150 mg once daily, bendroflumethiazide 2.5 mg once daily, verapamil 120 mg three times a day, and a salbutamol inhaler as required. She had no allergies. She was a lifelong non-smoker but reported a 50 units/week alcohol history for at least the last 15 years (Table 11.1) [1]. She denied significant family history, recent travel, and use of illicit or recreational drugs. She denied use of new prescribed or over-the-counter medications (including paracetamol and salicylates) and could not recall any courses of antibiotics in the preceding 6 months. She had not consumed herbal medication or nutritional/weight loss supplements.

⭐ Learning point Calculating units

Table 11.1 Calculating alcohol units

Wine		Beer/lager/cider			Other drinks	
Quantity	Units	Strength	Units (can)	Units (pint glass)	Drink	Units
Small 125 mL	1.6	Regular	1.8	2.3	25 mL single spirit/mixer (40% ABV)	1
Standard 175 mL	2.3	Strong	2.2	3		
Large 250 mL	3.3	Extra-strong	3.5	4	275 mL bottle of alcopop (5.5% ABV)	1.5
Bottle	10					

One unit equals 10 mL or 8 g of pure alcohol. The number of units in a drink is based on the size of the drink as well as its alcohol strength. Most alcohol will have an alcohol by volume (ABV) percentage on the container (ABV = how much of the total volume is alcohol). Therefore: units = strength (ABV) × volume (mL) ÷ 1000.
Source: data from NHS. (2012) *Change4life: Alcohol units and guidance*. Copyright © 2012 NHS. Contains public sector information licensed under the Open Government Licence v3.0.

⊕ Expert comment

It is always important to maintain an open mind about the cause of acute liver dysfunction—considering presenting features, clinical history, examination, and diagnostics. The basics of pre-hepatic, hepatic and post-hepatic aetiologies should always be considered in a systematic fashion.

✪ Learning point History and investigations

The initial meeting may be the best or only time to obtain details before the patient deteriorates from hepatic encephalopathy (HE). Social, medication (all antibiotics in the preceding 6 months, new over-the-counter or prescription medication, nutritional supplements, anabolic steroids, and recreational drugs), drug and alcohol history, and psychiatric history are often overlooked. A full history is especially important when a transplant centre considers feasibility for transplantation.

It is prudent to investigate for all potential causes of acute liver failure (ALF) (Table 11.2) [2] in a patient with no known prior history of cirrhosis or chronic liver disease, albeit investigations may subsequently suggest an acute-on-chronic process.

Table 11.2 Investigations

Haematology	FBC, blood film
Biochemistry	Renal (urea, creatinine, potassium, sodium, corrected calcium, phosphate) Liver (ALT, AST, GGT, ALP, conjugated and unconjugated bilirubin, albumin), vitamin B_{12}, folate, thyroid function tests, ferritin, lipid profile, creatine kinase, amylase, lactate dehydrogenase, and glucose
Coagulation	INR, prothrombin time (used in many scoring systems), and fibrinogen
Arterial blood sample	Lactate and ammonia
Toxicology	Paracetamol and salicylate levels and additional screen if indicated
Viral screen	HIV, EBV, CMV, HSV, HAV IgM, and IgG (if travel to endemic area), HBsAg, anti-HB core IgM, anti-HEV IgM, adenovirus, parvovirus B19, and leptospirosis serology (if history relevant)
Metabolic screen	Serum copper and caeruloplasmin (if age appropriate)
Autoimmune screen	Immunoglobulins, liver autoantibodies (smooth muscle antibody, antimitochondrial antibody, liver/kidney microsomal antibody), antinuclear antibody, and antineutrophil cytoplasmic antibody
Radiology	Liver ultrasound scan with focus on liver parenchyma, vascular patency (hepatic artery, hepatic veins and portal vein), and spleen size as well as presence or absence of ascites (signs of portal hypertension)
	CT scan and/or MRI /MRCP to further characterize the hepatic parenchyma and patency of vessels (e.g. recanalization of the umbilical vein suggesting a chronic disease process). Also to assess for pancreatitis (often reported in cases of paracetamol overdose) [2], visualize the bile ducts, and rule out any contraindications to transplantation such as metastatic malignancy

ALP, alkaline phosphatase; ALT, alanine transaminase; AST, aspartate transaminase; CMV, cytomegalovirus; EBV, Epstein–Barr virus; FBC, full blood count; GGT, gamma-glutamyltransferase; HAV, hepatitis A virus; HB, hepatitis B; HEV, hepatitis E virus; HIV, human immunodeficiency virus; HSV, herpes simplex virus; IgM, immunoglobulin M (recent infection); IgG, immunoglobulin G (recent or past infection); MRCP, magnetic resonance cholangiopancreatography; MRI, magnetic resonance imaging.

⊕ Expert comment

Elevated transaminases greater than 5000 IU/L raise the possibility of hypoxic hepatitis or paracetamol-induced toxicity, while elevated alkaline phosphatase should raise the concern of infiltrative processes. Liver biopsy is required occasionally (guided by hepatological input) but only rarely alters treatment. An enlarged liver may be seen in those with severe acute alcoholic hepatitis (AH) but should again raise concern of infiltration.

On examination, she was obese (estimated body mass index of 43 kg/m^2). She was alert but weak and lethargic. Her Glasgow Coma Scale (GCS) score was 15. She had a blood pressure of 98/60 mmHg and heart rate of 130 beats/min in sinus rhythm. Her jugular venous pulse was visible 2 cm above the sternal notch. The electrocardiogram showed sinus tachycardia and left ventricular hypertrophy. She was cool to the elbows with a central capillary refill time of 4 seconds. Capillary blood glucose was 4.5 mmol/L and tympanic temperature was 37.9°C.

She was clinically jaundiced and had conjunctival pallor. She had spider naevi over her anterior chest, upper back, and face. She had no rash but did have bruises over her arms and feet. Her cardiorespiratory examination was grossly normal, but she

Table 11.3 Initial investigations

Arterial blood gas (FiO₂ 0.21)	Full blood count	Liver enzymes	Coagulation	Urea and electrolytes
pH 7.30 (7.35–7.45)	Hb (g/dL) 10.1 (130–165)	ALT (IU/L) 135 (10–40)	INR 2.2 (0.9–1.4) PT (sec)	Na (mmol/L) 129 (135–145)
PaO₂ (kPa) 12.1 (>10.5)	MCV (fL) 109 (77–95)	AST (IU/L) 270 (10–50)	30 (30–40) Fibrinogen (g/L)	K (mmol/L) 3.3 (3.5–5.0)
PaCO₂ (kPa) 3.2 (4.5–6.3)	Plt (× 10⁹/L) 61 (150–450)	ALP (IU/L) 203 (30–130)	4.1 (1.5–4.5)	Urea (mmol/L) 4.2 (3.3–6.7)
HCO₃ (mmol/L) 16.4 (22–28)	WCC (× 10⁹/L) 18.2 (4.0–11.0)	GGT (IU/L) 447 (1–55)		Cr (µmol/L) 168 (45–120)
BE (mmol/L) –10.1 (+2–2)	Neut (10⁹/L) 16.9 (2.0–6.3)	Bili (µmol/L) 651 (3–20)		Corr Ca (mmol/L) 2.1 (2.15–2.6)
Glucose (mmol/L) 4.8 (3.9–7.2)		Amy (IU/L) 70 (<100)		Albumin (g/L) 26 (35–50)
Lactate (mmol/L) 3.2 (<2.0)				PO₄ (mmol/L) 0.61 (0.8–1.4)
				CRP 80 (<5)

ALT, alanine transaminase; Amy, amylase; AST, aspartate transaminase; ALP, alkaline phosphatase; BE, base excess; Bili, bilirubin; Corr Ca, calcium corrected for albumin; Cr, creatinine; CRP, C-reactive protein; GGT, gamma glutamyl transferase; Hb, haemoglobin; HCO₃, bicarbonate; INR, international normalized ratio; K, potassium; MCV, mean corpuscular volume; Na, sodium; Neut, neutrophils; PCO₂, partial pressure of carbon dioxide; Plt, platelets; PaO₂, partial pressure of oxygen; PaO₄, phosphate; PT, prothrombin time; WCC, white cell count.

could not lie flat because of shortness of breath. Her abdomen was grossly distended, with shifting dullness and minimal tenderness in the right upper quadrant, but no organomegaly. She had peripheral oedema to the knees.

The clinical impression was that of an index presentation with decompensated cirrhosis secondary to alcohol. However, with no prior history of cirrhosis, ALF or subacute liver failure were potential differentials requiring exploration and exclusion.

Large-bore intravenous access was established and blood tests (Table 11.3), including blood cultures, sent. A urinary catheter was inserted and urinalysis revealed trace blood but no evidence of infection. The urine was sent for culture. The chest radiograph was normal.

The clinical history and initial investigations (temperature, white cell count (WCC), C-reactive protein, lactate, sinus tachycardia, and relative hypotension) raised the possibility of sepsis-related decompensation of cirrhosis with jaundice, coagulopathy, and ascites. AH was also within the differential diagnoses.

She was commenced on broad-spectrum antibiotics (piperacillin–tazobactam 4.5 g three times daily) and intravenous fluid, initially as 250 mL boluses to assess the haemodynamic response. Following approximately 2 L of 0.9% sodium chloride, an infusion of 100 mL/hour was started. A diagnostic paracentesis was not performed because of the risk of bleeding, but antibiotics were continued for presumed spontaneous bacterial peritonitis (SBP). The renal impairment was initially treated as prerenal in origin. A non-contrast CT confirmed the presence of cirrhosis with portal hypertension and a large amount of ascites. The hepatic vasculature appeared patent (Figure 11.1).

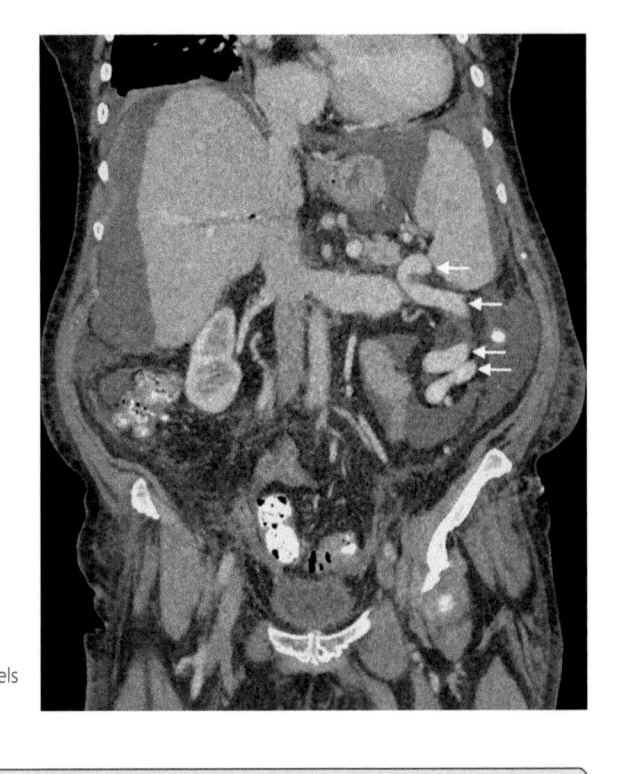

Figure 11.1 A coronal reconstruction CT image, after intravenous contrast, showing a small liver with an irregular margin in keeping with cirrhosis, generalized large volume ascites, and splenomegaly. The labelled lienorenal/splenorenal shunt vessels are due to portal hypertension.

⭐ **Learning point** Nutritional deficiencies and alcohol withdrawal syndrome

Prophylactic parenteral thiamine (3 days) followed by oral thiamine is recommended for dependent drinkers if they are malnourished, at risk of malnourishment, or have decompensated liver disease. Do not give intravenous dextrose before high-dose parenteral thiamine because of the risk of precipitating Wernicke's encephalopathy.

Alcohol withdrawal syndrome is a severe medical condition that can affect alcohol-dependent patients who suddenly stop drinking. The symptoms can occur as early as 6 hours after discontinuation and patients admitted to hospital must be monitored for this.

The revised Clinical Institute Withdrawal Assessment of Alcohol (CIWA-Ar) scale [3] is a 10-point score that enables clinical quantitation of the severity of the alcohol withdrawal syndrome and treatment tailored accordingly. Benzodiazepines are considered the gold standard treatment for alcohol withdrawal syndrome.

In patients with advanced cirrhosis or acute AH, consider short-acting benzodiazepines (e.g. lorazepam or oxazepam) instead of chlordiazepoxide to avoid oversedation or worsening of HE.

💬 **Expert comment**

In the clinical context of altered GCS, neurology, or worsening delirium, always consider metabolic causes, sepsis, dehydration, or drug-related neurotoxicity—recognizing especially the increased sensitivity of cirrhotic patients to opiates and benzodiazepines.

💬 **Expert comment**

International normalized ratio (INR) does not reflect risk of bleeding in ALF or acute-on-chronic liver failure (ACLF) as there are balanced changes in procoagulants and anticoagulant levels. Low platelet count and fibrinogen, usually in association with prolonged APTT identify those at risk of bleeding. There is no evidence that prophylactic use of coagulation support is beneficial.

⭐ **Learning point** Clotting in liver disease

The liver plays a central role in the haemostatic system as it synthesizes most coagulation factors and proteins involved in fibrinolysis [4]. Clotting dysfunction in liver disease has been extensively studied.

The haemostatic alterations that occur in acute and chronic liver failure affect both procoagulant (elevated factor VIII, low plasminogen, decreased protein C and S, and reduced antithrombin levels) and anticoagulant (vitamin K deficiency, dysfibrinogenaemia, and thrombocytopenia) pathways. This means that patients with chronic liver failure are at risk of complications of both thrombosis and bleeding.

Routine correction of coagulation abnormalities may not be necessary for standard intensive care unit (ICU) procedures. Functional tests for clotting (e.g. thromboelastography) are more useful as they measure the dynamics of thrombin production, provide a global assessment of coagulation, and can guide clinical management.

Over the following 48 hours she received treatment for SBP, until an ascitic tap showed no evidence of this. Her renal function continued to deteriorate despite intravenous fluid resuscitation (urine output < 500 mL/day, creatinine 230 µmol/L, urea 21 mmol/L), so terlipressin and albumin (20 % human albumin solution, 100 mL twice daily) was started for type 1 hepatorenal syndrome (HRS).

The viral screen and microbiology yielded negative results. She developed signs of confusion and agitation. She was treated for HE with lactulose 20 mL three times daily via nasogastric tube and supportive management.

Within 72 hours of admission, her GCS score decreased acutely to 3/15. She was intubated for airway protection and transferred to the ICU via a computed tomography (CT) scan to rule out an acute intracranial bleed or ischaemic event. The CT head was normal.

> **Expert comment**
>
> Moderate decreases in GCS score can result in microaspiration and increase the risk of chest sepsis.

> **Learning point** Fluids in cirrhosis
>
> Hyponatraemia is common in cirrhosis as portal hypertension causes the release of potent arteriolar vasodilators, such as nitric oxide, which affect the splanchnic circulation predominantly [5, 6]. This causes a drop in the central effective circulating volume which causes relative hypotension and activation of the renin–angiotensin–aldosterone, antidiuretic hormone, and sympathetic nervous systems [7]. The net outcome of this is increased renal salt and water reabsorption (total body salt and water overload), and accumulation of extracellular fluid. The hyponatraemia is therefore a dilutional hyponatraemia and total body sodium is not reduced.
>
> Normal saline and sodium-containing crystalloids have traditionally been avoided in patients with cirrhosis because of concerns about simply expanding the extravascular volume and reducing renal perfusion without a net positive effect on effective circulating volume. In haemodynamically unstable patients, certainly in severely ill patients (Child–Turcotte–Pugh class B and C cirrhosis), volume expansion reduces plasma levels of renin, suggesting some degree of effective circulating volume expansion [8]. However, it is important to recognize hyponatraemia and avoid crystalloids such as 5% dextrose that worsen hyponatraemia and risk precipitation of HE.

> **Expert comment**
>
> Always assess the circulating volume in patients with cirrhosis. Oedema and ascites are not reflective of central blood volume, some patients will be under-filled and respond to fluid therapy while others will show central volume overload with pulmonary venous hypertension. Giving fluids to the latter subgroup will potentially worsen renal function through increasing renal venous pressure and decreasing perfusion pressure.
>
> Albumin for resuscitation and replacement of intravascular volume deficit has been debated extensively over the years. In liver disease, albumin has an established role in three situations:
>
> 1. Prevention of (large volume) paracentesis-induced circulatory dysfunction.
> 2. Prevention of renal failure during SBP.
> 3. Treatment of HRS, in addition to vasoconstrictors.
>
> There have been two recent randomized controlled trials that showed no survival benefit in using albumin in cirrhotic patients with sepsis other than SBP [9]. The smaller study (100 patients) did show improved circulatory function and less kidney injury [10].

> **Learning point** The kidneys in cirrhosis
>
> Up to 20% of hospitalized patients with decompensated cirrhosis have renal complications [11]. The most common causes are prerenal, acute tubular necrosis, and HRS, but other causes such as glomerulonephritis, diuretic or non-steroidal anti-inflammatory drug toxicity, and abdominal
>
> (continued)

compartment syndrome from tense ascites also occur [11]. Many patients with cirrhosis have underlying parenchymal renal disease.

Despite the common misconception, renal dysfunction in the context of cirrhosis is not automatically a diagnosis of HRS: rather, HRS is a diagnosis of exclusion with a defined set of diagnostic criteria. It can only be diagnosed when all other causes of renal failure have been ruled out [12, 13].

Type 1 HRS is a rapidly progressive (i.e. <2 weeks) acute renal impairment that frequently develops following a precipitating factor that causes deterioration of liver function and other organ dysfunction.

Type 2 HRS occurs in patients with refractory ascites and there is a moderate but steady degree of renal impairment which is now categorized as chronic kidney injury.

The diagnosis of type 1 HRS, previously required fulfilment of stringent creatinine-based criteria, often delaying treatment with vasopressor therapy. Patients with renal dysfunction and cirrhosis who do not fulfil the diagnostic criteria of type 1 HRS have similarly poor outcomes as those with HRS [14], so a consensus definition of what constitutes acute kidney injury (AKI) in cirrhosis is necessary.

Serum creatinine level is a poor biomarker of renal dysfunction in patients with cirrhosis, especially in those with ascites and muscle wasting [15], and patients may have AKI despite normal creatinine.

The prognostic importance of small changes in serum creatinine in cirrhosis [16] led to the International Club of Ascites defining AKI in patients with cirrhosis as an increase in serum creatinine of at least 26.5 μmol/L within 48 hours or at least a 50% rise from a known or presumed baseline within the preceding 7 days [17].

🕕 Expert comment

Always consider AKI when there is a rise in creatinine. A protein:creatinine ratio that is only moderately elevated predicts progression and is potentially a marker for earlier interventions. Earlier treatment with vasoactive agents, prior to profound oliguria and marked elevation in creatinine, is more likely to preserve renal function.

✪ Learning point Acute on chronic liver failure (ACLF)

ACLF occurs in patients with pre-existing chronic liver disease (CLD) or cirrhosis (compensated or decompensated) who develop hepatic *and* extrahepatic organ failure. There are numerous identifiable precipitants for ACLF but in up to 40% of cases no precipitant is identified [18, 19]. Infection is the commonest precipitant, with viruses, drugs, ischaemia, alcohol, surgery, and sepsis all common. When no obvious cause is identified, treatment for sepsis is appropriate.

Recognition of ACLF as a clinically and pathophysiologically distinct syndrome from acute decompensation (AD) of compensated CLD is important in order to initiate prompt management and reduce the associated high 28-day mortality (Tables 11.4 and 11.5).

Table 11.4 ACLF grade as proposed by the CANONIC study

ACLF grade 1	ACLF grade 2	ACLF grade 3
Three subgroups: 1. Kidney failure solely 2. Single non-renal organ failure (liver, coagulation, circulation, or respiration) and a serum creatinine 132–176 μmol/L (1.5–1.9 mg/dL) and/or mild to moderate hepatic encephalopathy 3. Single cerebral failure and a serum creatinine 132–176 μmol/L (1.5–1.9 mg/dL)	2 organ failures as defined by CLIF-SOFA score	≥3 organ failures as defined by CLIF-SOFA score

Note: renal failure = creatinine ≥177 μmol/L (≥2mg/dL).

Source: data from Moreau, R., et al. CANONIC Study Investigators of the EASL–CLIF Consortium: Acute-on-chronic liver failure is a distinct syndrome that develops in patients with acute decompensation of cirrhosis. *Gastroenterology.* 44(7), 1426–37. Copyright © 2013 Elsevier Inc. All rights reserved.

Table 11.5 Mortality according to ACLF grade

ACLF grade	28-day mortality (%)	90-day mortality (%)
Grade 0 (no organ failure)	4.7	11
Grade 1	22.1	40.7
Grade 2	32	52.3
Grade 3	76.7	79.1

✔ **Evidence base CLIF Acute-on-Chronic Liver Failure in Cirrhosis (CANONIC) study**

The landmark CANONIC study [20] showed a clear difference in mortality between simple AD (manifesting as ascites, encephalopathy, gastrointestinal haemorrhage, and SBP) and ACLF (with additional organ failure). The Chronic Liver Failure–Sequential Organ Failure Assessment (CLIF-SOFA) score and definition of ACLF have been validated in various studies internationally and are thought to be good independent predictors of short-term mortality in patients with ACLF [21–23]; the CLIF-SOFA may be useful in assessing response to ICU treatment [24].

On arrival in ICU, she was anuric, with a GCS of 4T (E1, VT, M3). She swiftly developed circulatory shock with a lactate level of 6.4 mmol/L and this was treated with noradrenaline 0.5 mcg/kg/min and terlipressin 0.2 mg/hour. She was noted to have an ammonia level of 180 µmol/L, and continuous venovenous haemofiltration was started at 35 mL/kg/hour exchange. A septic screen was repeated and antibiotics were escalated by addition of amikacin (an aminoglycoside thought to be less nephrotoxic than gentamicin). However, there was no clear source of sepsis to explain the systemic inflammatory response and a diagnosis of AH was thought to be the overall underlying precipitant of ACLF.

The Maddrey score [25] was 77.3 and as a result steroid therapy was started (hydrocortisone 50 mg 6-hourly), with a planned review in 7 days in combination with results of the Lille score [26]. At this stage, she had established liver, coagulation, cardiovascular, renal, and neurological failure.

Her Child–Turcotte–Pugh score was C [12] with a Model for End-stage Liver Disease (MELD) score of 35, suggesting a 52.6% 3-month mortality without transplantation.

❝ Expert comment

Kidneys contribute to 20% of ammonia clearance and thus AKI will decrease ammonia clearance and increase the risk of HE.

✪ **Learning point Definition and diagnosis of alcoholic hepatitis**

AH is a distinct clinical syndrome caused by chronic alcohol abuse and has a poor prognosis: 28-day mortality ranges from 30% to 50% [25]. Although AH is an acute condition, approximately 50% of patients with AH have established cirrhosis [27].

Patients have a history of alcohol excess leading up to presentation, but a period of abstinence (up to 4 weeks) before presentation is not uncommon, possibly due to development of symptoms. Abstinence for longer than 3 months should raise the suspicion of cirrhosis and/or decompensation.

The diagnosis is based on history and a high index of suspicion. Patients typically present with non-specific symptoms such anorexia, nausea, vomiting, and malaise. They are jaundiced and can have features of ACLF and a systemic inflammatory response with tachycardia and fever. Superimposed bacterial and fungal infections are common in AH and often contribute to multiorgan failure [28].

> ### ✪ Learning point Prognostic scores used in cirrhosis and ACLF
>
> Scores such as the King's College criteria [29] and others are specifically used to prognosticate in ALF and determine which patients might be considered for emergency transplantation. However, these scoring systems do not apply to patients with cirrhosis and ACLF.
>
> Of note, none of the scores are reliable indicators of futility and their use early in the clinical course to determine admission to the ICU is not appropriate. Patients with cirrhosis and organ dysfunction or failure often warrant a trial of critical care [23].
>
> #### Child–Turcotte–Pugh score
>
> The Child–Turcotte–Pugh score was developed in 1964 to predict the outcome after portocaval shunting surgery in patients with cirrhosis [30] and later modified to include prothrombin time which replaced 'nutritional status' [19] (Table 11.6).
>
> **Table 11.6** Variables included in the Child–Turcotte–Pugh score and associated 1- and 2-year mortality
>
> | Measure | 1 point | 2 points | 3 points |
> |---|---|---|---|
> | Albumin g/L (g/dl) | >35 (3.5) | 28–35 (2.8–3.5) | <28 (<2.8) |
> | Bilirubin µmol/L (mg/dl) | 34 (<2) | 34–51 (2–3) | >51 (>3) |
> | Ascites | None | Controlled | Refractory |
> | Hepatic encephalopathy | None | 1–2 | 3–4 |
> | Prothrombin time prolongation (sec) | <4 | 4–6 | >6 |
> | International normalized ratio | <1.7 | 1.7–2.3 | >2.3 |
>
> | Score | Class | 1-year survival (%) | 2-year survival (%) |
> |---|---|---|---|
> | 5–6 | A | 100 | 85 |
> | 7–9 | B | 81 | 57 |
> | 10–15 | C | 45 | 35 |
>
> A weakness of the Child–Turcotte–Pugh score is the inclusion of variables based on subjective clinical assessment.
>
> #### Model for End-stage Liver Disease score
>
> $$\text{MELD} = 3.8 \times \log_e(\text{serum bilirubin}\,[\mu\text{mol}/\text{L}]) + 11.2 \times \log_e(\text{INR})$$
> $$+ \ 9.6 \times \log_e(\text{serum creatinine}\,[\mu\text{mol}/\text{L}]) + 6.4$$
>
> Bilirubin 17.1 µmol/L = 1 mg/dL; creatinine 88.4 µmol/L = 1 mg/dL.
>
> MELD score-associated mortality at 3 months:
>
> - 30–39: 52.6% mortality
> - 20–29: 19.6% mortality.
> - 10–19: 6.0% mortality.
>
> The minimum score is 6 and maximum 40. Bias against people on long-term renal replacement therapy (RRT) is taken away by a maximum creatinine (354 µmol/L).
>
> The MELD score [31] has been used in numerous clinical settings including assisting decisions on referral, listing, and prioritizing for transplantation [32] and to guide management of AH [33].
>
> In patients with cirrhosis, an increasing MELD score indicates worsening hepatic dysfunction and increased 3-month mortality risk.
>
> The MELD score may be modified by inclusion of serum sodium (UKELD, MELD-NA scores) to reflect the impact of hyponatraemia on mortality and neurological dysfunction [34, 35].
>
> #### CLIF SOFA/CLIF-C OF, CLIF-C ACLF, and CLIF-AD scores
>
> The CLIF-SOFA score was devised to diagnose ACLF in the CANONIC study [20] and is a simple validated organ function scoring system that predicts 28-day and 90-day mortality. The CLIF SOFA score replaces platelets with INR and GCS score with grade of HE in the original SOFA score [36] (Table 11.7).
>
> *(continued)*

Table 11.7 Components of the original SOFA score compared with the CLIF-SOFA score

SOFA score (scored 0-4)	CLIF-SOFA score (scored 0-4)
• PaO_2/FiO_2	• PaO_2/FiO_2
• GCS	• HE grade
• MAP or use of vasopressors/inotropes	• MAP or use of vasopressors/inotropes/terlipressin
• Bilirubin	• Bilirubin
• Platelets	• INR (platelets <20 = score 4)
• Creatinine or urine output/24 hours	• Creatinine or use of RRT
Minimum score 0 and maximum 24	Minimum score 0 and maximum 24

FiO_2, fraction of inspired oxygen; HE, hepatic encephalopathy; INR, international normalized ratio; MAP, mean arterial pressure; PaO_2, partial pressure of oxygen; RRT, renal replacement therapy.

Age and WCC were identified as independent prognostic markers by the study and have been included in an updated scoring system, the CLIF-C ACLF score. This score predicts 28-day mortality significantly better at 48 hours, 3-7 days, and 8-15 days after ACLF diagnosis than at diagnosis [37] and is therefore useful in tracking patients' progress.

Numerous trials have evaluated prognostic scores for cirrhotic patients admitted to ICU. The SOFA score [36] predicts ICU mortality better than liver-specific scores such as Child-Turcotte–Pugh and MELD scores [38, 39]. For cirrhotic patients with AD, but without ACLF, the CLIF Consortium Acute Decompensation score (CLIF-C ADs) is more accurate than other liver scores in predicting prognosis [40].

The Liver Injury Failure Evaluation score

Recently, the Liver Injury Failure Evaluation (LiFe) score [41] was developed from a large international retrospective cohort study of 1916 patients with CLD admitted to the ICU. The score is easily calculated from arterial lactate, total bilirubin, and INR. It predicts short-term mortality in ACLF almost as well as SOFA and CLIF SOFA scores.

Scores specific to alcoholic hepatitis

Maddrey discriminant function

This is used to estimate disease severity and mortality in acute AH [25]:

$$\text{Maddrey discriminant function} = (4.6 \times [\text{prothrombin time (sec)} - \text{control prothrombin time (sec)}]) \\ + (\text{serum bilirubin} (\mu mol / L) / 17.1)$$

A score of 32 or greater has a predicted 1-month mortality rate of 25–45% compared with less than 10% at up to 3 months for milder AH.

Glasgow Alcoholic Hepatitis Score

See Table 11.8 [42].

Table 11.8 Variables for calculating the Glasgow Alcoholic Hepatitis Score (GAHS). A score of 9 or greater is associated with a higher mortality

Variable	Score		
	1	2	3
Age	<50	≥50	–
White cell count (10^9/L)	<15	≥15	–
Urea (mmol/L)	<5	≥5	–
INR	<1.5	1.5–2.0	>2.0
Bilirubin (μmol/L)	<125	125–250	>250

INR, international normalized ratio.
The results of this score are categorized into <9 or ≥9. Corticosteroids improve survival in patients with a Maddrey score ≥32 and a GAHS ≥9, (59% vs 38% at 84 days), but there is no survival benefit with a GAHS <9 [43].

(continued)

Lille model

Lille score = 3.19 − 0.101 × (age in years) + 0.147 × (albumin day 0 in g/L) + 0.0165 × (day 7 bilirubin level in μmol/L) − (0.206 × creatinine day 0 in μmol/L) − 0.0065 × (bilirubin day 0 in μmol/L) − 0.0096 × (INR or prothrombin time in seconds)

The Lille score [26] is used to determine response to steroids in AH at 7 days of treatment: a score greater than 0.45 indicates non-response. Mortality at 6 months is notably higher with a score greater than 0.45 (75% vs 15%).

⊕ **Clinical tip Prognostic scoring in liver failure**

All the liver scores can be calculated on calculators found on various websites and smartphone applications.

The patient's clinical condition remained precarious for the first week on the ICU. Despite standard medical treatment for HE (treatment of precipitating cause, ensuring bowels were opening regularly, and avoidance of sedation after initial stabilization), she remained grade 4 encephalopathic. Three days after the initiation of parenteral l-ornithinine l-aspartate (LOLA), her neurological condition improved, although she remained myopathic. Optimal feeding was established early into her ICU admission ensuring adequate calorie and protein provision to avoid muscle loss.

On day 7, her Lille score was 0.38, confirming steroid response, and prednisolone 40 mg once daily was continued for 28 days. By day 10, her GCS was consistently 15/15, she had weaned off vasopressor support, was undergoing ventilation wean, but still required continuous renal replacement therapy (CRRT).

On day 16 she developed persistent pyrexia of at least 38°C, tachycardia, and hypotension (mean arterial pressure 50 mmHg) and soon her GCS dropped to 6, requiring reintubation. A diagnostic paracentesis confirmed SBP (WCC 1570 cells/microL, 90% neutrophils). Fluid resuscitation, antibiotics, and vasopressor support were recommenced. In view of the use of steroids and the high risk of fungal sepsis, antifungal cover using the echinocandin, anidulafungin, was commenced. Serum beta-d-glucan was requested while awaiting culture results.

✪ **Learning point Hepatic encephalopathy**

HE is a brain dysfunction caused by liver insufficiency and/or portosystemic shunting, causing a wide spectrum of neurological or psychiatric abnormalities ranging from subclinical alterations to coma [44]. Psychomotor abnormalities in overt HE can be detected by bedside clinical tests.

Diagnosis and management of HE is a challenge. Classification is based on four aspects: type of hepatic abnormality, time course, presence or absence of precipitating factors, and characteristics of neurological manifestation (Table 11.9). The presence or absence of ACLF has been proposed as a fifth domain [45].

In patients with cirrhosis, HE is an event that defines decompensation, similar to variceal bleed and ascites. Patients with cirrhosis or CLD admitted to the ICU must be screened for alterations in mental state at repeated intervals. HE must be distinguished from other causes of altered mental state and neurology. Common differentials are included in Table 11.10. Hyponatraemia and hyperammonaemia affect neurological function synergistically and hyponatraemia with HE has a poor prognosis [46]. HE affects 30–45% of patients with cirrhosis and its occurrence is associated with increased mortality: median survival with decompensated cirrhosis and HE is approximately 2 years, compared with at least 12 years in patients with compensated cirrhosis without HE [47].

(continued)

Table 11.9 Classification of hepatic encephalopathy [48]

HE type	Description	Subcategory	Subdivisions	Clinical manifestation
A	HE associated with Acute liver failure	–	–	–
B	HE associated with portosystemic Bypass or shunts and no evidence of intrinsic liver disease	Episodic	Precipitated Spontaneous[a] Recurrent[b]	GCS or according to West Haven criteria
C	HE associated with Cirrhosis and portal hypertension/or portosystemic shunts	Persistent	Mild Severe Treatment dependent	GCS or according to West Haven criteria
		Minimal (MHE)[c]	–	Not detected clinically, needing complex neuropsychiatric and psychometric testing

[a] No obvious precipitating factor; [b] repeated episodes with a time interval of 6 months or less; [c] abnormal results of established psychometric or neuropsychological tests without clinical manifestations.
Source: data from Ferenci, P., et al. Hepatic encephalopathy - Definition, nomenclature, diagnosis, and quantification: Final report of the Working Party at the 11th World Congresses of Gastroenterology, Vienna, 1998. *Hepatology*. 35(3), 716–21. Copyright © 2002 American Association for the Study of Liver Diseases.

Table 11.10 Common differentials to be considered when faced with the non-specific symptoms of hepatic encephalopathy

Drugs and toxins	Metabolic	Infection	Endocrine	Vascular	Inflammatory	Others
Alcohol withdrawal or intoxication	Diabetic ketoacidosis	Encephalitis	Hyponatraemia	Intracranial haemorrhage	Autoimmune encephalitis	Dementia
Benzodiazepines	Hypoglycaemia	Septic encephalopathy	Hypercalcaemia	Hypoxic encephalopathy	Sarcoidosis	Status epilepticus
Opioids	Hyperosmolar hyperglycaemic state	Cerebral abscess	Hypothyroidism	Ischaemic stroke	Systemic lupus erythematosus	Inherited urea cycle disorders causing raised ammonia
Wernicke's encephalopathy	Uraemia					Space-occupying lesions
Recreational drug use						Hypercarbia (sleep apnoea)

> ⭐ **Learning point** How to diagnose hepatic encephalopathy
>
> A thorough history, examination, and a high clinical suspicion on the basis of known CLD is key to making the diagnosis. There is no specific test for HE, and exclusion of other conditions may require CT scanning, magnetic resonance imaging, lumbar puncture, electroencephalography, and blood biochemistry. Seek and treat any precipitants of HE. A response to treatment can be used to confirm the diagnosis.
>
> Ammonia has been postulated in the pathophysiology of HE and circulating values can be elevated in patients with CLD, ACLF, and ALF, as well as AD cirrhosis. Measuring ammonia concentrations remains controversial but a normal ammonia value in a patient with overt HE should encourage a diagnostic re-evaluation. Conversely, an elevated ammonia alone should not be used to make the diagnosis of HE, but it is contributory. It does not provide staging or prognostic information for HE in
>
> *(continued)*

patients with CLD [49]. In ALF, by contrast, ammonia is an independent risk factor for development of high-grade HE and intracranial hypertension secondary to cerebral oedema [50], and treatment to lower ammonia, such as RRT, is established practice. Despite cerebral oedema being a more common occurrence in ALF (approximately 25% [51]), sudden increases in ammonia may be observed alongside an inflammatory response in ACLF patients resulting in neurological disturbances [52, 53]; a common scenario being that of insertion of a new transjugular intrahepatic portosystemic shunt, sepsis, and concurrent hyponatraemia. Epileptiform activity should always be sought and treated.

There is a significant risk of intracranial haemorrhage in patients with ACLF and high-grade HE and this diagnosis is considered in ACLF patients with new focal neurology, or poor neurological recovery in ICU upon sedation withdrawal [54].

Potential precipitants for HE include:

- infections (commonest precipitant)—chest, urinary tract, SBP, and unidentified
- gastrointestinal bleed—variceal or non-variceal
- hypovolaemia
- transjugular intrahepatic portosystemic shunt procedure
- constipation
- electrolyte abnormalities—new diuretic
- alcohol binge
- sedatives or antidepressants/antipsychotics
- hepatocellular carcinoma
- acute portal vein thrombus
- recent surgery causing acute decompensation
- non-compliance with medication
- unknown.

✪ Learning point Management of hepatic encephalopathy in ACLF

Management depends on the classification and severity of HE. Management of HE in ALF is very distinct and will not be covered in this chapter.

In HE, the aim is to induce remission and maintain remission. The first step is to provide supportive care in a safe environment. This may include one-to-one nursing with frequent monitoring of mental status. Appropriate (often nasogastric) enteral feed avoids protracted energy restriction, especially when neurology prevents normal feeding. ICU admission for intubation and ventilation is often required when the GCS falls and airway safety is compromised.

Specific management is focused on managing the precipitant to prevent progression of HE, and to reduce the duration of high-grade HE. This may include stopping implicated medication, treating sepsis, correcting electrolytes and dehydration, and in the case of a recently inserted portosystemic shunt for ascites or variceal haemorrhage, consideration of downsizing the shunt. Often, no specific cause is identified and patients receive empirical antibiotics, intravenous hydration, and vitamin replacement in addition to supportive care.

Therapies specifically targeting HE are then initiated.

🟊 Expert comment

None of the therapies for HE have been examined in the context of critical illness. One study has demonstrated that in high-grade encephalopathy, enteral nutrition was not harmful; while treatment with albumin did not alter resolution of encephalopathy. For other treatments, the evidence must be extrapolated from evidence gained in other settings.

✪ Learning point Therapies targeting hepatic encephalopathy

Non-absorbable disaccharides

Lactulose (beta galactosidofructose) and lactitol (beta galactosidosorbitol) are metabolized to lactic and acetic acid in the colon, thereby reducing the pH which results in the conversion of ammonia to ammonium and passage of ammonia from tissues to the colonic lumen. Colonic flora shifts from urease- to non-urease-producing bacterial species. Their cathartic effects reduce colonic bacterial load and may also reduce ammonia. A meta-analysis did not support its routine use in clinical practice [55], but newer studies suggest improved neuropsychometric and quality of life scores [56]. Current

(continued)

guidelines still favour the use of lactulose. The initial dose recommendation is 25 mL orally or via nasogastric tube 4-hourly, until soft stools, followed by further titration in order to achieve three soft stools/day. Over-dosage can lead to severe ileus, diarrhoea and dehydration, electrolyte imbalances such as hypernatraemia, and even precipitation of HE [57]. Lactulose can be administered as an enema (300 mL lactulose with 700 mL water, as a retention enema every 4 hours as needed) if the enteral route is unavailable.

Enemas do not confer additional benefit if oral/enteral purgatives are maintaining more than three soft motions/day.

Antibiotics

Rifaximin is used in addition to lactulose to prevent HE. It is a semisynthetic antibiotic derived from rifamycin that has gained popularity due to its tolerability and safe side effect profile. The National Institute for Health and Care Excellence has recommended rifaximin on the evidence of a large, well-conducted randomized controlled trial [58] which showed fewer and shorter hospitalizations related to HE in patients taking rifaximin. Plasma values of rifaximin are negligible and the risk of bacterial resistance appears to be lower with rifaximin than with systemic antibiotics. Rifaximin is recommended as secondary prophylaxis for persistent HE in patients who have had episodes of overt HE while on lactulose alone.

In patients on ICU receiving high doses of broad-spectrum antibiotics, there is no evidence for adding rifaximin.

L-Ornithine L-aspartate

LOLA is a compound salt of the amino acids ornithine and aspartate. These amino acids activate the urea cycle enzymes that convert ammonia into urea. LOLA also stimulates glutamate transaminase, increasing glutamate levels. Ammonia is used in the conversion to glutamate to glutamine in skeletal muscle by glutamine synthetase. The net effect is reduction of ammonia.

LOLA (oral or intravenous) has improved ammonia values, and various HE parameters in settings outside critical care and in low grades of HE [59]. Some benefit has also been reported in higher grades of HE, such as those seen in ACLF, and LOLA was safe and associated with shorter hospital stay [60]. In the setting of ACLF, LOLA may be considered as an adjunctive therapy if the patient does not respond to conventional therapy. The usual dose is one 20 g infusion/day for 7 days. Oral LOLA (6 g three times daily) can also be used in grade 1–2 HE that persists despite resolution of the precipitant.

CRRT with haemofiltration

In patients with ACLF, CRRT is often required for treatment of concomitant AKI. Approximately 20% of ammonia load is excreted renally, so AKI may increase ammonia values in liver disease [61] and haemofiltration may improve ammonia clearance [62]. There is a linear relationship between increasing ultrafiltration rates and ammonia clearance, and a close correlation between ammonia and urea clearance. Urea clearance can therefore be used as a surrogate marker for ammonia clearance.

The use of ultra-high-volume CRRT (40–60 mL/kg/hour) has been explored in several settings, but is generally of little benefit over conventional CRRT (30–35 mL/kg/hour).

> ### ✚ Clinical tip Anticoagulation for renal replacement therapy
>
> Anticoagulation of RRT circuits may be achieved with prostacyclin, heparin, or citrate. ACLF patients appear to tolerate citrate well although those with profound elevation of aspartate transaminase, INR, or lactate should be closely monitored to ensure appropriate citrate metabolism. There was no difference in rates of severe disturbance in pH or calcium in patients with normal, mild, or severe liver failure in a recent multicentre prospective observational study [63].

> ### ★ Learning point Molecular adsorbent recirculating system
>
> The molecular adsorbent recirculating system (MARS) is an extracorporeal liver support system based on albumin dialysis. Blood is dialysed across an albumin-impregnated membrane using 20% albumin as dialysate. Charcoal and anion exchange resin columns in the circuit cleanse and regenerate the albumin dialysate. MARS does not replace the synthetic function of the liver. It does, however, remove albumin-bound toxins such as bilirubin, bile acids, nitric oxide, and endogenous benzodiazepines, as well as exogenous drugs and toxins and water-soluble ammonia. These effects can improve HE, systemic haemodynamics, and renal function. As such, it is a promising treatment for management of liver failure in patients who simply require additional time for recovery or potentially as a bridge to liver transplantation.
>
> In the ICU setting, MARS has been used for various clinical situations (Table 11.11) [66].
>
> *(continued)*

> ### Learning point Nutrition
>
> Traditional low-protein diets to reduce intestinal ammonia production are not needed. A normal protein diet is safe, and avoids protein malnutrition that contributes to muscle wastage [64, 65]. Daily targets of 35–45 kcal/g and 1.2–1.5 g/kg of protein are appropriate.
>
> Early specialist dietetic input is vital in AD cirrhosis or ACLF to avoid deterioration in nutritional status, which will negatively impact recovery.

Table 11.11 The main indications for MARS

Acute liver failure	
Acute-on-chronic liver failure complicated by:	• Jaundice • Hepatic encephalopathy • Renal dysfunction
Acute intoxication or overdose with albumin-bound and other protein-bound substances	• E.g. benzodiazepines, carbamazepine, phenytoin, and valproate
Intractable pruritus in cholestatic liver conditions	
Acute liver failure after major hepatectomy	
Post transplant	• Primary non-function • Secondary liver failure or multiorgan failure • Disease recurrence in graft

Source: data from Saliba, F. The Molecular Adsorbent Recirculating System (MARS®) in the intensive care unit: a rescue therapy for patients with hepatic failure. *Critical Care.* 10(1), 118. Copyright © 2006 BioMed Central Ltd.

A large trial comparing MARS with standard medical therapy in ACLF showed MARS to be safe but it did not improve 90-day liver transplant-free survival [67]. It continues to be used throughout the world for various indications.

Overall, MARS and other artificial liver systems do not improve mortality in ALF or ACLF but may improve HE and other biochemical indices. American and European guidelines do not recommend MARS for the treatment of resistant HE [44]. However, carefully chosen patients may benefit from extracorporeal liver support either as a bridge to transplantation or instead of transplantation.

Despite advances in the understanding of ALF and ACLF, no specific medical treatments have been developed and liver transplantation remains the only definitive treatment.

The prospect of liver transplantation was raised by the patient's next of kin due to persistent deterioration. The current evidence for this was provided to them.

Over the following 8 days she received full supportive treatment for multiorgan failure and eventually began making a recovery. She was eventually discharged to the ward after a protracted 50-day ICU admission.

Discussion

ACLF is a distinct clinical entity that carries a high mortality. Early recognition of the condition and intensive management in order to prevent progression to multiorgan failure may improve the short-term prognosis.

Despite full supportive care, and a marked improvement in the understanding of the pathophysiology of ACLF, limitations of treatment modalities persist. The mainstay of management is currently supportive, and, in a small minority of carefully selected cases, transplantation.

AH is a cause of ACLF and carries a high short-term mortality. Use of steroids in patients with more severe disease (Maddrey score ≥32, GAHS ≥9) has been reported to improve short-term mortality; however, ongoing studies aim to clarify its role in long- and short-term mortality and morbidity.

The use of extracorporeal liver support and high-volume plasmapheresis for ACLF varies within and between different countries. Its role as a bridge to recovery remains unclear [71].

Transplantation has been performed on patients with ACLF with encouraging results; given the narrow window of opportunity for success, further understanding of the pathophysiology may make ACLF an indication for emergency transplantation.

> ★ **Learning point**
> **Alternatives to transplantation**
>
> **Plasma exchange and high-volume plasmapheresis**
>
> Plasma exchange is a form of extracorporeal support that simulates some functions of the liver by removing toxic metabolites and mediators of multiorgan failure (proinflammatory cytokines) while replenishing potentially beneficial factors.
>
> To date there are no large studies evaluating plasma exchange using the current definition of ACLF and it is therefore not undertaken routinely.

A final word from the expert

AH can be a cause of ACLF. Timely diagnosis, recognition of the syndrome, and early intervention is the key to successful outcomes. Scoring systems have been developed but should not be used to determine who would benefit from ICU treatment, but more to monitor progress while in critical care. Liver transplantation remains the definitive treatment of decompensated cirrhosis; however, timing for transplantation, patient selection, and ultimately the scarcity of organs means that further research into pathophysiology of ACLF and other supportive treatments is required.

References

1. National Health Service. (2012) Change4life: Alcohol Units and Guidance [Internet]. Available from: http://www.nhs.uk/Change4Life/Pages/alcohol-lower-risk-guidelines-units.aspx.
2. Sy-Jou C, Chin-Sheng L, Chin-Wang H, Cheng-Li L, Chia-Hung K. Acetaminophen poisoning and risk of acute pancreatitis: a population-based cohort study. *Medicine (Baltimore)*. 2015;94:e1195.
3. Sullivan JT, Sykora K, Schneiderman J, Naranjo CA, Sellers EM. Assessment of alcohol withdrawal: the revised Clinical Institute Withdrawal Assessment for Alcohol Scale (CIWA-Ar). *Br J Addict*. 1989;84:1353–7.
4. Lisman T, Porte RJ. Rebalanced hemostasis in patients with liver disease: evidence and clinical consequences. *Blood*. 2010;116:878–85.
5. Schrier RW, Arroyo V, Bernardi M, et al. Peripheral arterial vasodilation hypothesis: a proposal for the initiation of renal sodium and water retention in cirrhosis. *Hepatology*. 1988;8:1151–7.

6. Henriksen JH, Bendtsen F, Sorensen TI, et al. Reduced central blood volume in cirrhosis. *Gastroenterology*. 1989;97:1506–13.

7. Schrier RW. Body fluid volume regulation in health and disease: a unifying hypothesis. *Ann Intern Med*. 1990;113:155–9.

8. Brinch K, Moller S, Bendtsen F, et al. Plasma volume expansion by albumin in cirrhosis. Relation to blood volume distribution, arterial compliance and severity of disease. *J Hepatol*. 2003;39:24–31.

9. Thévenot T, Bureau C, Oberti F, et al. Effect of albumin in cirrhotic patients with infection other than spontaneous bacterial peritonitis. A randomized trial. *J Hepatol*. 2015;62:822–30.

10. Guevara M, Terra C, Nazar A, et al. Albumin for bacterial infections other than spontaneous bacterial peritonitis in cirrhosis. A randomized, controlled study. *J Hepatol*. 2012;57:759–65.

11. Garcia-Tsao G, Parikh CR, Viola A. Acute kidney injury in cirrhosis. *Hepatology*. 2008;48:2064–77.

12. Salerno F, Gerbes A, Ginès P, Wong F, Arroyo V. Diagnosis, prevention and treatment of hepatorenal syndrome in cirrhosis. *Gut*. 2007;56:1310–18.

13. Ginès P, Guevara M, Arroyo V, Rodés J. Hepatorenal syndrome. *Lancet*. 2003;362:1819–27.

14. Salerno F, Cazzaniga M, Merli M, et al. Diagnosis, treatment and survival of patients with hepatorenal syndrome: a survey on daily medical practice. *J Hepatol*. 2011;55:1241–8.

15. Sherman, DS, Fish DN, Teitelbaum I. Assessing renal function in cirrhotic patients: problems and pitfalls. *Am J Kidney Dis*. 2003;41:269–78.

16. Cholongitas E, Calvaruso V, Senzolo M, et al. RIFLE classification as predictive factor of mortality in patients with cirrhosis admitted to intensive care unit. *J Gastroenterol Hepatol*. 2009;24:1639–47.

17. Angeli P, Gines P, Wong F, et al. Diagnosis and management of acute kidney injury in patients with cirrhosis: revised consensus recommendations of the International Club of Ascites. *Gut*. 2015;64:531–7.

18. Bernal W, Jalan R, Quaglia A, Simpson K, Wendon J, Burroughs A. Acute on chronic liver failure. *Lancet*. 2015;386:1576–87.

19. Pugh R, Murray-Lyon I, Dawson J, Pietroni MC, Williams R. Transection of the esophagus in bleeding oesophageal varices. *Br J Surg*. 1973;60:648–52.

20. Moreau R, Jalan R, Gines P, et al. CANONIC Study Investigators of the EASL–CLIF Consortium. Acute-on-chronic liver failure is a distinct syndrome that develops in patients with acute decompensation of cirrhosis. *Gastroenterology*. 2013;44:1426–37.

21. Lee M, Oh S, Jang Y, et al. CLIF-SOFA scoring system accurately predicts short-term mortality in acutely decompensated patients with alcoholic cirrhosis: a retrospective analysis. *Liver Int*. 2015;35:46–57.

22. Soares e Silva P, Lazzarotto C, Ronsoni M, et al. Single-centre validation of the EASL-CLIF Consortium definition of acute-on-chronic liver failure and CLIF-SOFA for prediction of mortality incirrhosis. *Liver Int*. 2015;35:16–23.

23. McPhail M, Shawcross D, Ables R, et al. Increased survival for patients with cirrhosis and organ failure in liver intensive care and validation of the Chronic Liver Failure–Sequential Organ Failure Scoring System. *Clin Gastroenterol Hepatol*. 2015;13:1353–60.

24. Ferreira F, Bota D, Bross A, et al. Serial evaluation of the SOFA score to predict outcome in critically ill patients. *JAMA*. 2001;286:1754–8.

25. Maddrey W, Boitnott J, Bedine M, Weber F, Mezey E, White R. Corticosteroid therapy of alcoholic hepatitis. *Gastroenterology*. 1978;75:193–9.

26. Louvet A, Naveau S, Abdelnour M, et al. The Lille model: a new tool for therapeutic strategy in patients with severe alcoholic hepatitis treated with steroids. *Hepatology*. 2007;45:1348–54.

27. O'Shea R, Dasarathy S, McCullough A. Alcoholic liver disease. *Hepatology*. 2010;51:307–28.

28. Gustot T, Maillart E, Bocci M, et al. Invasive aspergillosis in patients with severe alcoholic hepatitis. *J Hepatol*. 2014;60:267–74.

29. O'Grady J, Alexander G, Hayllar K, Williams R. Early indicators of prognosis in fulminant hepatic failure. *Gastroenterology.* 1989;97:439–55.

30. Child C, Turcotte J. Surgery and portal hypertension. In: Child GC (ed) *The Liver and Portal Hypertension.* Philadelphia, PA: Saunders; 1964, pp. 50–64.

31. Malinchoc M, Kamath P, Gordon F, Peine C, Rank J, Borg P. A model to predict poor survival in patients undergoing transjugular intrahepatic portosystemic shunts. *Hepatology.* 2000;31:864–71.

32. Merion R, Schaubel D, Dykstra D, Freeman R, Port F, Wolfe R. The survival benefit of liver transplantation. *Am J Transplant.* 2005;5:307–13.

33. Dunn W, Jamil L, Brown L, et al. MELD accurately predicts mortality in patients with alcoholic hepatitis. *Hepatology.* 2005;41:353–8.

34. Londono M, Cardenas A, Guevara M, et al. MELD score and serum sodium in the prediction of survival of patients with cirrhosis awaiting liver transplantation. *Gut.* 2007;56:1283–90.

35. Kim W, Biggins S, Kremers W, et al. Hyponatremia and mortality among patients on the liver-transplant waiting list. *N Engl J Med.* 2008;359:1018–26.

36. Vincent J, Moreno R, Takala J, et al. The SOFA (Sepsis-related Organ Failure Assessment) score to describe organ dysfunction/failure. *Intensive Care Med.* 1996;22:707–10.

37. Jalan R, Saliba F, Pavesi M, et al. CANONIC study investigators of the EASL-CLIF Consortium. Development and validation of a prognostic score to predict mortality in patients with acute-on-chronic liver failure. *J Hepatol.* 2014;61:1038–47.

38. Levesque E, Hoti E, Azoulay D, et al. Prospective evaluation of the prognostic scores for cirrhotic patients admitted to an intensive care unit. *J Hepatol.* 2012;56:95–102.

39. Saliba F, Ichai P, Levesque E, Samuel D. Cirrhotic patients in the ICU: prognostic markers and outcome. *Curr Opin Crit Care.* 2013;19:154–60.

40. Jalan R, Pavesi M, Saliba F, et al. The CLIF Consortium Acute Decompensation score (CLIF-C ADs) for prognosis of hospitalised cirrhotic patients without acute-on-chronic liver failure. *J Hepatol.* 2015;62:831–40.

41. Edmark C, McPhail M, Bell M, Whitehouse T, Wendon J, Christopher K. LiFe: a liver injury score to predict outcome in critically ill patients. *Intensive Care Med.* 2016;42:361–9.

42. Forrest E, Evans C, Stewart S, et al. Analysis of factors predictive of mortality in alcoholic hepatitis and derivation and validation of the Glasgow alcoholic hepatitis score. *Gut.* 2005;54:1174–9.

43. Forrest E, Morris A, Stewart S, et al. The Glasgow alcoholic hepatitis score identifies patients who may benefit from corticosteroids. *Gut.* 2007;56:1743–6.

44. Vilstrup H, Amodio P, Bajaj J, et al. Hepatic encephalopathy in chronic liver disease: 2014 Practice Guideline by the American Association for the Study of Liver Diseases and the European Association for the study of the Liver. *Hepatology.* 2014;60:715–35.

45. Cordoba J, Ventura-Cots M, Simón-Talero M, et al. Characteristics, risk factors, and mortality of cirrhotic patients hospitalized for hepatic encephalopathy with and without acute-on-chronic liver failure (ACLF). *J Hepatol.* 2014;60:275–81.

46. Córdoba J, Gottstein J, Blei A. Chronic hyponatremia exacerbates ammonia-induced brain edema in rats after portacaval anastomosis. *J Hepatol.* 1998;29:589–94.

47. D'Amico G, Garcia-Tsao G, Pagliaro L. Natural history and prognostic indicators of survival in cirrhosis: a systematic review of 118 studies. *J Hepatol.* 2006;44:217–31.

48. Ferenci P, Lockwood A, Mullen K, et al. Hepatic encephalopathy—Definition, nomenclature, diagnosis, and quantification: Final report of the Working Party at the 11th World Congresses of Gastroenterology, Vienna, 1998. *Hepatology.* 2002;35:716–21.

49. Lockwood A. Blood ammonia levels and hepatic encephalopathy. *Metab Brain Dis.* 2004;19:345–9.

50. Bernal N, Hall C, Karvellas CJ, Auzinger G, Sizer E, Wendon J. Arterial ammonia and clinical risk factors for encephalopathy and intracranial hypertension in acute liver failure. *Hepatology.* 2007;46:1844–52.

51. Bernal W, Wendon J. Acute liver failure. *N Engl J Med.* 2016;370:1170–1.

52. Jalan R, Olde Damink S, Ter Steege J, et al. Acute endotoxemia following transjugular intrahepatic stent-shunt insertion is associated with systemic and cerebral vasodilatation with increased whole body nitric oxide production in critically ill cirrhotic patients. *J Hepatol*. 2011;54:265–71.

53. Jalan R, Dabos K, Redhead D, et al. Elevation of intracranial pressure following transjugular intrahepatic portosystemic stent-shunt for variceal haemorrhage. *J Hepatol*. 1997;27:928–33.

54. Joshi D, O'Grady J, Patel A, et al. Cerebral oedema is rare in acute-on-chronic liver failure patients presenting with high-grade hepatic encephalopathy. *Liver Int*. 2014;34:362–6.

55. Als-Nielsen B, Gluud L, Gluud C. Non absorbable disaccharides for treatment of hepatic encephalopathy: systematic review of randomised trials. *BMJ*. 2004;328:1046–50.

56. Prasad S, Dhiman R, Duseja A, Chawla Y, Sharma A, Agarwal R. Lactulose improves cognitive functions and health-related quality of life in patients with cirrhosis who have minimal hepatic encephalopathy. *Hepatology*. 2007;45:549–59.

57. Bajaj J, Sanyal A, Bell D, Gilles H, Heuman D. Predictors of the recurrence of hepatic encephalopathy in lactulose-treated patients. *Aliment Pharmacol Ther*. 2010;31:1012–17.

58. Bass N, Mullen K, Sanyal A, et al. Rifaximin treatment in hepatic encephalopathy. *N Engl J Med*. 2010;362:1071–81.

59. Jiang Q, Jiang X, Zheng M, Chen Y. L-Ornithine-L-aspartate in the management of hepatic encephalopathy: a meta-analysis. *J Gastroenterol Hepatol*. 2009;24:9–14.

60. Abid S, Jafri W, Mumtaz K, et al. Efficacy of L-ornithine-L-aspartate as an adjuvant therapy in cirrhotic patients with hepatic encephalopathy. *J Coll Physicians Surg Pak*. 2011;21:666–71.

61. Wright G, Noiret L, Olde Damink S, Jalan R. Interorgan ammonia metabolism in liver failure: the basis of current and future therapies. *Liver Int*. 2011;31:163–75.

62. Slack A, Auzinger G, Willars C, et al. Ammonia clearance with haemofiltration in adults with liver disease. *Liver Int*. 2014;34:42–8.

63. Slowinski T, Morgera S, Joannidis M, et al. Safety and efficacy of regional citrate anticoagulation in continuous venovenous hemodialysis in the presence of liver failure: the Liver Citrate Anticoagulation Threshold (L-CAT) observational study. *Critical Care*. 2015;19:349.

64. Cabral C, Burns D. Low protein diets for hepatic encephalopathy debunked: let them eat steak. *Nutr Clin Pract*. 2011;26:155–9.

65. Cordoba J, Lopez-Hellin J, Planas M, et al. Normal protein diet for episodic hepatic encephalopathy: results of a randomized study. *J Hepatol*. 2004;41:38–43.

66. Saliba F. The Molecular Adsorbent Recirculating System (MARS®) in the intensive care unit: a rescue therapy for patients with hepatic failure. *Crit Care*. 2006;10:118.

67. Bañares R, Nevens F, Larsen F, et al. RELIEF study group. Extracorporeal albumin dialysis with the molecular adsorbent recirculating system in acute-on-chronic liver failure: the RELIEF trial. *Hepatology*. 2013;57:1153–62.

68. Thursz M, Richardson P, Allison M, et al. STOPAH trial. Prednisolone or pentoxifylline for alcoholic hepatitis. *N Engl J Med*. 2015;372:1619–28.

69. Mathurin P, O'Grady J, Carithers R, et al. Corticosteroids improve short-term survival in patients with severe alcoholic hepatitis: meta-analysis of individual patient data. *Gut*. 2011;60:255–60.

70. Finkenstedt A, Nachbaur K, Zoller H, et al. Acute-on-chronic liver failure: excellent outcomes after liver transplantation but high mortality on the wait list. *Liver Transpl*. 2013;19:879–86.

71. Larsen FS, Schmidt LE, Bernsmeier C, et al. High-volume plasma exchange in patients with acute liver failure: An open randomised controlled trial. *J Hepatol*. 2016;64:69–78.

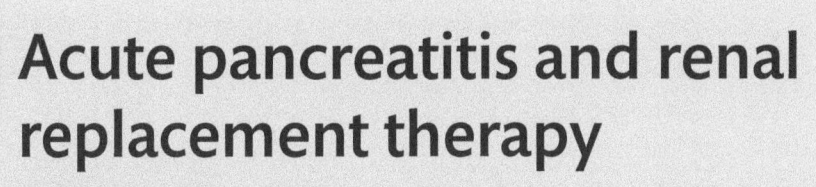

12 Acute pancreatitis and renal replacement therapy

Clinton Lobo

⊕ **Expert Commentary** Kim Gupta and Matt Thomas

Case history

A 51-year-old male patient was admitted under the surgical team with upper abdominal pain following a single alcohol binge. He had no known medical conditions, did not take any medications, had stopped smoking 10 years previously, and exercised regularly. On examination, he was haemodynamically stable and had an arterial blood oxygen saturation (SpO_2) of 96% in air, but had marked tenderness and guarding in the epigastrium. A diagnosis of acute pancreatitis was made following identification of a raised serum amylase value, and he was admitted to the surgical ward.

> ✪ **Learning point** The revised Atlanta classification
>
> The revised Atlanta classification 2012 for the diagnosis of acute pancreatitis [1] requires at least two from:
>
> 1. acute-onset, severe abdominal pain
> 2. raised serum amylase (or lipase) at least three times the upper limit of normal
> 3. characteristic findings on contrast-enhanced computed tomography (CT) scanning, magnetic resonance imaging (MRI), or abdominal ultrasonography.
>
> Serum amylase rises within hours of onset of acute pancreatitis, returning to normal within 3–5 days. Serum lipase remains elevated for 8–14 days, and therefore in late presentation (>48 hours after symptom onset) has better diagnostic sensitivity than amylase (80% vs 30%). The degree of enzyme elevation does not correlate with disease severity.

An initial abdominal ultrasound scan showed a non-dilated, non-obstructed biliary tract, with no evidence of gallstones. The pancreatitis was considered to be secondary to the alcohol binge. A nasogastric tube and urinary catheter were sited, and he was managed conservatively with analgesia and enteral nutrition.

> ✪ **Learning point** Causes of acute pancreatitis
>
> Acute pancreatitis has many causes. Between 75% and 85% of cases are associated with gallstones or excess alcohol, with gallstones being the most common cause in most European and North American studies. Fifteen per cent of cases have no clear cause (idiopathic). In these cases, endoscopic ultrasound examination detects occult bile duct stones or biliary sludge in approximately two-thirds of cases. Rarer causes (<10% of cases) include drugs (e.g. valproate and steroids), trauma, endoscopic retrograde cholangiopancreatography (ERCP), hypertriglyceridaemia, hypercalcaemia, and viral infections (e.g. mumps and cytomegalovirus).

> ⊕ **Clinical tip** Morphine
>
> Although there is a theoretical risk of morphine exacerbating acute pancreatitis through spasm of the sphincter of Oddi, there is little human evidence that this is clinically significant in acute pancreatitis, or that any particular opioid is more likely to cause a problem.

Table 12.1 Blood results and arterial blood gas results 48 hours after admission

Variable	Result	Reference range
Full blood count		
Hb (g/L)	142	130–180
WCC (×10⁹/L)	16.1	4–11
Neut (×10⁹/L)	13.9	2–6.5
Platelets (×10⁹/L)	286	150–400
Urea and electrolytes		
Na (mmol/L)	141	135–145
K (mmol/L)	4.7	3.5–5.0
Urea (mmol/L)	14.1	3–7
Creatinine (µmol/L)	185	<110
Glucose (mmol/L)	7.6	3.5–8.5
CRP (mg/L)	285	<10
Liver function tests		
Bilirubin (µmol/L)	25	3–17
ALT (IU/L)	360	3–35
AST (IU/L)	393	3–35
Alk P (IU/L)	240	30–130
Alb (g/L)	33	35–50
Ca (mmol/L)	2.10	2.12–2.65
Amylase	1240	<100
Arterial blood gas		
pH	7.24	7.35–7.45
PaCO₂ (kPa)	2.9	4.4–6.1
PaO₂ (kPa)	6.8	>10
Base excess (mmol/L)	− 8.9	± 2
Bicarbonate (mmol/L)	14.3	22–26
Lactate (mmol/L)	2.1	<2

Alb, albumin; Alk P, alkaline phosphatase; ALT, ALT, AST, aspartate transaminase; AST, aspartate transaminase; CRP, C-reactive protein; Hb, haemoglobin; K, potassium; Na, sodium; Neut, neutrophils; PaCO₂, partial pressure of carbon dioxide; PaO₂, partial pressure of oxygen; WCC, white cell count.

Over the subsequent 48 hours, his condition deteriorated, and he was referred to the intensive care unit (ICU) with escalating oxygen requirements and development of a metabolic acidosis. His blood tests and arterial blood gas results are shown in Table 12.1. His Ranson score at 48 hours was 4 (scoring for partial pressure of oxygen, urea, aspartate transaminase, and base excess). He was admitted to the ICU for monitoring.

---

⑥ Expert comment

Early recognition of severe disease is important to guide appropriate allocation of ICU resources and treatment. Ranson criteria and the Glasgow (Imrie) criteria, shown in Table 12.2, remain widely used to assess severity, but do not provide a full score until 48 hours after admission [2, 3]. The presence of fewer than three Ranson's criteria reliably represents mild disease and the presence of six or more criteria correlates with necrosis and an increased risk of mortality. However, the presence of three to five Ranson's criteria is very common, but correlates poorly with clinical severity or development of necrosis. Many other validated scoring systems exist, based on physiological variables, biochemical markers, or radiological appearance, but none have shown clear superiority in balancing predictive power with ease of use. Severity scores based on CT imaging (e.g. Balthazar score or CT severity index) have no clear advantage over clinical scoring systems in predicting severe disease or prognosis [4, 5]. Most scoring systems have limited day-to-day value in the clinical management of patients with acute

(continued)

pancreatitis, but detection of organ dysfunction using regular clinical observations summarized into early warning scores has similar accuracy for prediction of severity in acute pancreatitis and is of greater value in detecting clinical deterioration.

Table 12.2 Ranson and Glasgow criteria for assessment of acute pancreatitis severity at 48 hours

Ranson criteria (non-gallstone pancreatitis)	Ranson criteria (gallstone pancreatitis)	Glasgow (Imrie) criteria
[a]Age >55 years	[a]Age >70 years	Age >55 years
[a]Glucose >11.1 mmol/L	[a]Glucose >12.2 mmol/L	Glucose >10.0 mmol/L
[a]WBC >16 × 10^9/L	[a]WBC >18 × 10^9/L	WBC >15 × 10^9/L
[a]Serum AST >250 IU/L	[a]Serum AST >250 IU/L	Serum LDH >600 IU/L
[a]Serum LDH >350 IU/L	[a]Serum LDH >400 IU/L	Serum albumin <32 g/L
Hct fall >10%	Hct fall >10%	BUN >16.1 mmol/L
Fluid sequestration >6 L	Fluid sequestration >4 L	Serum Ca^{2+} <2 mmol/L
Base deficit >4 mEq/L	Base deficit >5 mEq/L	Arterial PO_2 <8 kPa
BUN rise >1.8 mmol/L	BUN rise >0.7 mmol/L	
Serum Ca^{2+} <2 mmol/L	Serum Ca^{2+} <2 mmol/L	
Arterial PO_2 <8 kPa	Arterial PO_2 <8 kPa	

AST, aspartate transaminase; BUN, blood urea nitrogen; Hct, haematocrit; LDH, lactate dehydrogenase; PO_2, partial pressure of oxygen; WBC, white blood cell.
[a] Measurements taken on admission.

Because of rapidly escalating oxygen requirements, the patient was anaesthetized, intubated, and his lungs ventilated. A CT scan of his abdomen and chest demonstrated pancreatic necrosis and signs of early acute respiratory distress syndrome (Figure 12.1). He was discussed by consultant intensivists and surgeons and the consensus was for conservative management of the pancreatic necrosis, with the assumption that this was not infected.

> **✪ Learning point Initial imaging in acute pancreatitis**
> - Ultrasonography should be used within 24 hours of admission to assess for the presence of gallstones and biliary tract obstruction.
> - Contrast-enhanced CT is the gold standard for diagnostic imaging in acute pancreatitis.
> - Optimal timing for the initial CT scan is greater than 96 hours after onset of symptoms.
> - Early CT assessment (<96 hours) should be obtained only for diagnostic uncertainty or to identify other life-threatening disorders or complications.
> - Follow-up CT or MRI in acute pancreatitis is indicated only when there is a lack of clinical improvement, clinical deterioration, or when invasive intervention is considered.

The patient was commenced on noradrenaline to maintain a mean arterial pressure of 65 mmHg, with intravenous fluid therapy, initially clinically guided, and continuation of enteral feeding, but it was decided not to commence antibiotics. His renal function and metabolic acidosis deteriorated and, despite use of a non-invasive cardiac output monitor incorporating pulse contour analysis to optimize fluid balance, this continued. On day 2 he was commenced on renal replacement therapy (RRT) using a continuous venovenous haemofiltration (CVVHF) mode, at a rate of 30 mL/kg/h, to target a neutral fluid balance, and anticoagulated with heparin to target an activated partial thromboplastin time ratio of 1.5.

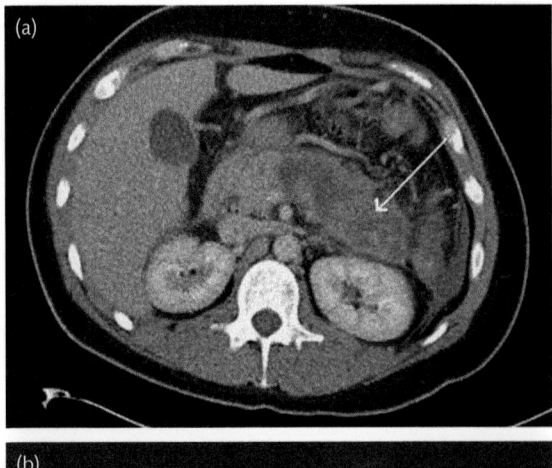

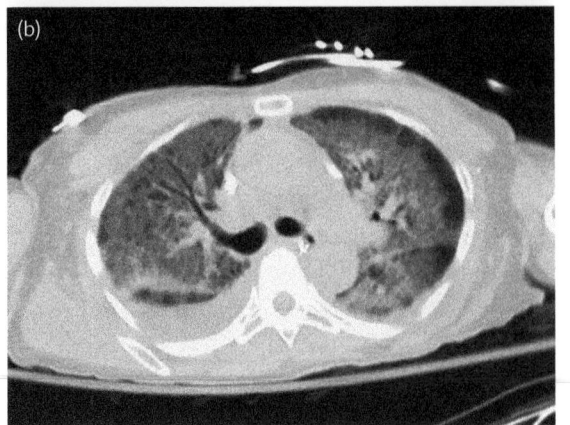

Figure 12.1 CT scans.
(a) Abdomen: pancreatitis with evidence of pancreatic necrosis as demonstrated by the non-enhancing pancreatic body (arrow). (b) Chest: bilateral diffuse ground-glass infiltrates consistent with acute respiratory distress syndrome, a moderate right-sided and small left-sided effusion.

✪ Learning point Types of renal replacement therapy

Peritoneal dialysis

Peritoneal dialysis (PD) involves insertion of a dialysis catheter into the peritoneal cavity, and then filling the cavity with dialysis fluid [6]. It works on the principle that the peritoneum is a semipermeable membrane, enabling transfer of solutes between the dialysis fluid and the blood vessels of the peritoneum. The dialysis fluid is left for 3–4 hours to achieve solute equilibration, and is then drained and replaced with fresh dialysis fluid.

The advantages of PD include no requirement for anticoagulation or expensive machinery, therapy can be continuous, and the patient can mobilize almost normally. The most serious potential risk of PD is infection, either through external contamination or from abdominal viscus translocation, a risk which often precludes its use in critically ill patients [7]. It is contraindicated with most intra-abdominal surgical pathologies (including pancreatitis), and its efficacy is influenced by previous abdominal surgery, duration of use, and constipation. For these reasons, and with the development of continuous RRTs, it is only rarely used in adult critical care. PD is still used in paediatric critical care, where vascular access and extracorporeal circuit management can be very difficult.

Haemodialysis

Haemodialysis (HD) also relies on the principle of solute diffusion across a semipermeable membrane [6]. Vascular access is usually achieved by insertion of a large-bore dual-lumen venous catheter in the short term, or creation of a permanent arteriovenous fistula in the long term. An extracorporeal

(continued)

blood circuit is separated from dialysis fluid by a semipermeable membrane. Solute diffusion rate is determined by the difference in solute concentration between the blood and dialysate. This is augmented in HD by using countercurrent flow of the dialysate to the blood.

HD is very efficient for solute clearance (particularly low-molecular-weight solutes), and is most commonly used outside the ICU as part of an intermittent regimen. Use of rapid intermittent regimens minimizes patient immobility and usually precludes the need for anticoagulation (and the associated potential complications). However, intermittent HD is unsuitable for patients with cardiovascular instability (due to the high blood flow rate) or cerebral injury (due to the associated fluid shifts and the potential for cerebral oedema), which means it is only suitable for critically ill patients who are stable or in the convalescent phase of their illness.

Haemofiltration

Haemofiltration (HF) relies on the principle of convection for the transport of solutes. A pressure is applied across a semipermeable membrane, which results in the transfer of solvent (water) across the membrane. As the solvent crosses the membrane, solutes are carried with it, depending on the pore size of the membrane. This is known as 'solvent drag', and is the main principle behind HF. The transmembrane pressure is the pressure difference between the blood and filtrate compartments, and is directly related to blood flow in the circuit. This pressure difference can also be adjusted by applying a negative pressure to the filtrate side, which often becomes necessary as the membrane degrades. As the transmembrane pressure is directly related to the rate of blood flow, HF is a continuous form of RRT.

During HF, water and solutes are removed from the blood, leading to an increase in oncotic pressure. The fraction of water removed needs to be limited to 25%, otherwise the increased oncotic pressure counteracts the transmembrane pressure. This is achieved by adjusting the blood pump speed according to the ultrafiltration dose. Replacement of plasma water and additional electrolytes is required prior to return of blood to the circulation. This replacement fluid can be administered before or after the filtration process. Post-filtration replacement makes the solute clearance more effective, but pre-filtration replacement increases the life of the haemofilter (by reducing haemoconcentration and so protein build-up on the membrane fibres), and so a combination of pre- and post-filtration replacement is generally used.

Haemodiafiltration

The addition of a transmembrane pressure to the process of HD is called haemodiafiltration, which allows solute transfer to occur by diffusion and convection, and is the most effective method of solute clearance.

> **⊛ Expert comment**
>
> Many of the drugs used in the ICU are cleared by the kidneys. There are often important changes to be made in dose and frequency of these medications. There are several reference books that give advice on changes in medication schedules in the presence of acute kidney injury (AKI). *The Renal Drug Handbook* is frequently used for this and is also available as a database (https://renaldrugdatabase.com).

The metabolic acidaemia was corrected while on CVVHF, and the noradrenaline requirements reduced. However, on day 4 on ICU, the patient's inflammatory markers increased, as did the noradrenaline and oxygen requirements. The patient also had increased respiratory secretions and was commenced on antibiotics (piperacillin/tazobactam) for a suspected ventilator-associated pneumonia. Enteral nutrition was administered at a rate of 10 mL/hour, but despite the introduction of metoclopramide and erythromycin as prokinetic drugs, the patient had high gastric aspirates. It was decided to start post-pyloric feeding and a nasojejunal tube was sited.

> **✪ Learning point Nutrition in acute pancreatitis**
>
> - In mild acute pancreatitis, oral feeding can be started immediately.
> - In severe acute pancreatitis, oral feeding is usually inhibited by nausea.
> - Enteral nutrition is recommended in moderate and severe acute pancreatitis as it may help preserve gut mucosal function and reduce the risk of multiorgan failure and pancreatic infectious complications [8, 9].
>
> (continued)

- Nasogastric and nasojejunal delivery of enteral feed appear comparable in efficacy and safety. Nasogastric tube placement is easier than nasojejunal tube placement, and should be the initial, preferred mode of delivery of enteral nutrition.
- Use parenteral nutrition if the enteral route is unavailable or not tolerated.

On day 6, the patient's platelet count was 73×10^9/L, having decreased from 358×10^9/L over the preceding 2 days. He was deemed to have an intermediate risk of heparin-induced thrombocytopenia and the decision was made to stop his haemofilter heparin anticoagulation, and commence an epoprostenol infusion. Fondaparinux was prescribed for venous thromboembolism prophylaxis.

> ✪ **Learning point** Anticoagulation during extracorporeal renal replacement
>
> RRT activates the clotting cascade because blood is exposed to non-biological surfaces. This usually manifests in clots blocking the haemofilter membrane, and will require replacement with a new filter circuit. Anticoagulation is used to try to prevent this occurring.
>
> The most common modes of anticoagulation for RRT are as follows:
>
> *Unfractionated heparin*—the haemofilter circuit is usually flushed with 2 L of crystalloid with 5000 IU heparin before use. Give a bolus of 2000–5000 IU heparin followed by an infusion starting at a rate of 5–10 IU/kg/hour aiming for an activated partial thromboplastin time ratio of 1.5–2.0 [7]. Occasionally, heparin is used for 'regional anticoagulation' of the haemofilter only. This is achieved by infusing heparin into the blood entering the haemofilter and infusing protamine into the blood returning to the patient.
>
> *Prostacyclin (PGI$_2$)*—often used when there are contraindications to heparin. Prostacyclin inhibits platelet aggregation and is infused at a rate of 2.5–5.0 ng/kg/min. It is short acting and has minimal systemic effects.
>
> *Citrate*—there is growing popularity in the use of citrate as regional anticoagulation to prolong haemofilter use. Citrate chelates calcium, reducing activation of both the clotting cascade and platelet aggregation. It increases haemofilter lifespan compared to using heparin [10]. Citrate is infused into blood entering the haemofilter and calcium is infused into blood leaving the filter so that ionized calcium values are restored in the blood returning to the patient. Much of the citrate is removed in the filtration process, but citrate returning to the patient is metabolized to bicarbonate by the liver.

Between days 8 and 10 in the ICU, the patient developed a fever and raised inflammatory markers. The patient underwent a full line change and septic screen. On day 10, infection of the pancreatic necrosis was suspected as the underlying cause and the patient's antibiotic regimen was escalated (meropenem and vancomycin). A percutaneous tracheostomy was undertaken in anticipation of a prolonged period of ventilation (the patient's platelet count had increased to 121×10^9/L). Two radiologically guided percutaneous drains were inserted into the pancreatic bed, enabling samples to be taken for microbiological analysis. Surgical large-bore drains were then inserted using the percutaneous drains as a guide. One of the large-bore drains was used to infuse warm saline into the pancreatic bed, and the second drain was allowed to freely drain the pancreatic bed.

These washouts continued for 4 days, during which there was a clinical and biochemical improvement in the patient's condition. The washouts were then stopped and the drains left to drain freely for a further 24 hours before being removed. Daily samples of drain fluid were analysed during this time, but did not grow any organisms.

> **ⓕ Expert comment**
>
> Severe acute pancreatitis causes a profound inflammatory response. The associated elevation in inflammatory and infective markers can make the diagnosis of coexisting infection extremely difficult, for example, acute cholangitis on initial presentation, and infected necrosis later in the disease process. A high index of suspicion is required, coupled with focused imaging and targeted microbiological sampling.
>
> Indications for endoscopic or surgical intervention in acute pancreatitis include [8, 9] the following:
>
> - Patients with gallstone pancreatitis with coexisting cholangitis or biliary obstruction should be considered for early ERCP.
> - Routine early ERCP is not needed in most patients with gallstone pancreatitis who lack clinical or biochemical evidence of ongoing biliary obstruction.
> - Patients with mild gallstone pancreatitis should undergo cholecystectomy during their hospital admission. In severe acute pancreatitis, this should be delayed until active inflammation subsides and fluid collections resolve.
> - Asymptomatic pseudocysts and pancreatic or extrapancreatic sterile necrosis do not warrant intervention.
> - Stable patients with infected necrosis which has not responded to antibiotic treatment, should be considered for drainage or resection of infected necrosis.
> - Drainage procedures can be open (via laparotomy) or minimally invasive. In general, minimally invasive techniques approach the necrosis via a retroperitoneal or transgastric route, and laparoscopic, endoscopic, or percutaneous techniques (radiologically guided, with or without lavage) are used to achieve drainage.
> - Comparative studies of different drainage techniques are few, but minimally invasive techniques appear to be associated with lower rates of postoperative complications (e.g. new-onset organ failure, bleeding, visceral perforation) compared to open necrosectomy [11].
> - Drainage procedures should usually be delayed for more than 4 weeks after the onset of the pancreatitis to enable the necrosis to become liquefied, discrete, and walled-off.

Following removal of the pancreatic bed drains, the patient continued to clinically improve, and ventilation weaning was commenced. He started to pass urine while undergoing CVVHF and the decision was made to stop RRT for a trial period. During this trial period, although there was a modest deterioration in his renal function tests, he continued to pass urine, and did not require further RRT. Meropenem and vancomycin were continued for 14 days, during which time there was a marked improvement in his inflammatory markers. At day 27, the patient's tracheostomy was successfully decannulated, and he was discharged to the ward the following day.

Discussion

Acute pancreatitis is a common inflammatory condition, with an incidence of 1–4 cases per 10,000 per year in the UK [12]. Most cases are mild and self-limiting, but approximately 20% of cases are classified as severe, according to the revised Atlanta criteria 2012 [1, 13]. Based on these criteria, this patient had severe acute pancreatitis because he had organ failure lasting more than 48 hours.

Revised Atlanta criteria (2012) for severity grading of pancreatitis
Atlanta symposium—grades of severity of pancreatitis:

Mild acute pancreatitis:

- Absence of organ failure.
- Absence of local complications.

Moderately severe acute pancreatitis:

- Local complications and/or
- Transient organ failure (< 48 hours).

Severe acute pancreatitis:

- Persistent organ failure (> 48 hours).

Acute pancreatitis with pancreatic necrosis has a mortality of approximately 10 % if sterile, but this rises to around 30 % if the necrosis becomes infected. The debate surrounding the use of prophylactic antibiotics to prevent sterile pancreatic necrosis from becoming infected is driven by this stark contrast in mortality. The lack of consensus on this issue is due in part to the lack of consistency in variables in the antibiotic prophylaxis trials. These include choice and duration of antibiotic, the extent of pancreatic necrosis, and the confounding issue of treatment antibiotics in the placebo group. A Cochrane systematic review of available trials in 2010 did not show a significant difference in mortality between use of prophylactic antibiotics and the control group. In this review, only the imipenem prophylaxis subgroup demonstrated a significant reduction in pancreatic infections, albeit without affecting the mortality rate [14].

> ✪ **Learning point** Indication for antimicrobials in acute pancreatitis
>
> - Routine use of antibiotics is not indicated in patients with acute pancreatitis [9].
> - Give antibiotics for coexistent extrapancreatic infections (e.g. acute cholangitis, pneumonia, and urinary tract infection).
> - The use of prophylactic antibiotics to prevent sterile necrosis from becoming infected is not supported by current evidence.
> - Consider a diagnosis of infected pancreatic necrosis in patients with pancreatic or extrapancreatic necrosis who deteriorate or fail to improve after 7–10 days of hospital treatment. In these patients, antibiotic treatment is either guided by culture of the infected pancreatic necrosis (usually obtained by fine-needle aspiration), or given empirically after necessary cultures are obtained.
> - In patients with infected pancreatic necrosis, antibiotics known to penetrate pancreatic necrosis (carbapenems, quinolones, and metronidazole) may be useful in delaying or avoiding intervention.
> - Routine treatment with antifungal drugs along with prophylactic or therapeutic antibiotics is not recommended.

The development of renal injury is common among critically ill patients. There are several classifications of renal injury, although the most commonly used are the Risk, Injury, Failure, Loss, End-stage (RIFLE) criteria and the Acute Kidney Injury Network (AKIN) criteria [15, 16]. More recently, Kidney Disease: Improving Global Outcomes (KDIGO) has created a classification based on both these criteria (Table 12.3) [17].

AKI is usually caused by a combination of several factors, the main ones being:

- hypoperfusion
- sepsis/systemic inflammatory response
- direct nephrotoxicity.

Hypoperfusion is addressed by treating hypovolaemia with fluid resuscitation, and then optimizing renal perfusion with the use of inotropes and vasopressors. There is no evidence for the use of renal vasodilators in the management of AKI [18].

Although the systemic inflammatory response (usually caused by sepsis) is the most common cause of AKI in critically ill patients, the pathophysiology is not fully

Table 12.3 KDIGO classification for acute kidney injury

Stage	Serum creatinine	Urine output
1	1.5–1.9 times baseline Or Increase by ≥0.3 mg/dL or ≥26.5 μmol/L	<0.5 mL/kg/hour for 6–12 hours
2	2.0–2.9 times baseline	<0.5 mL/kg/hour for ≥12 hours
3	≥3.0 times baseline Or Increase to ≥4.0 mg/dL or ≥353.6 μmol/L Or Initiation of renal replacement therapy	<0.3 mL/kg/hour for ≥24 hours Or Anuria for ≥12 hours

understood. It is generally accepted to have a multifactorial pathway, with components including ischaemia–reperfusion injury, direct inflammatory injury, coagulation and endothelial cell dysfunction, and apoptosis [19]. Many treatments used in critical care can be nephrotoxic, including antibiotics, vasoactive drugs, diuretics, and intravenous contrast, the use of which is often unavoidable.

❻ Expert comment

In AKI in critical care facilities, it is important to not forget the basic investigations and treatments. The NCEPOD report 'Adding insult to injury' showed that common tests such as renal tract imaging (ultrasonography or CT) and urinalysis were often omitted. It is important to perform these on the ICU [20]. This report also showed that potentially nephrotoxic drugs are often left prescribed.

Numerous guidelines list indications for the initiation of RRT, including those published by Acute Dialysis Quality Initiative, KDIGO, and the UK Intensive Care Society [17, 21, 22]. These guidelines all vary slightly, and there are no universally accepted biochemical values at which therapy should be started. Several studies have also attempted to determine the optimal timing for initiation of RRT. While there are studies which demonstrate improved outcomes with early versus late initiation of RRT [23–27], other studies have failed to show a difference in outcome [28, 29], and so the timing of initiation is still in question. Although many have attempted to address the issues of indications and timing of RRT, there is very little guidance for stopping this treatment. The KDIGO guidelines recommend discontinuing RRT when it is no longer required, either when renal function has recovered or when it is no longer consistent with the patient's treatment goals [17].

✪ Learning point Indications for renal replacement therapy

UK Intensive Care Society indications for starting RRT [22] are as follows:

Classic 'renal' indications include:

- rapidly rising serum urea and creatinine or the development of uraemic complications
- hyperkalaemia unresponsive to medical management
- severe metabolic acidosis
- diuretic resistant pulmonary oedema
- oliguria or anuria.

'Non-renal' indications include:

- management of fluid balance (e.g. cardiac failure)
- clearing of ingested toxins
- correction of electrolyte abnormalities
- temperature control
- removal of inflammatory mediators in sepsis.

(continued)

Whether a continuous or an intermittent mode of RRT is superior to the other remains controversial. In ICUs in the UK, Western Europe, and Australia, continuous RRT is the predominant mode—approximately 90% of ICUs in the UK use continuous techniques [30]. In the US, a greater proportion of ICUs deliver intermittent RRT, as often this is overseen by renal physicians. Proponents of continuous RRT suggest it offers greater haemodynamic stability, leading to fewer episodes of renal hypoperfusion and earlier renal recovery. Data from the BEST Investigators found that although there was no hospital survival benefit from either mode of therapy, continuous RRT was associated with a higher incidence of renal recovery among survivors [31]. This finding was replicated in a systematic analysis of observational studies in 2013. However, when the analysis was restricted to randomized controlled trials (RCTs), there was no evidence of difference between the two forms of RRT [32].

The optimal dose of RRT is still disputed. Several studies demonstrated an improvement in survival with higher doses of RRT [24, 33]. The authors of a landmark, single-centre RCT observed a reduction in mortality from 59% to 43% when the ultrafiltration dose was increased from 20 to 35 mL/kg/hour [24]. A 2007 survey of adult ICUs found that 49% of units using CVVHF and 67% of units using continuous venovenous haemodiafiltration (CVVHDF) were using a dose of at least 35 mL/kg/hour, which differed from 2003 when 88% of units chose a dose of 14–29 mL/kg/hour [30, 34].

More recent studies have cast doubt over the optimal RRT dose. A large US multicentre RCT found no difference in mortality between low-intensity RRT (CVVHDF 20 mL/kg/hour or intermittent HD three times a week) and high-intensity RRT (CVVHDF 35 mL/kg/hour or intermittent HD six times a week) [35]. A similar large multicentre RCT in Australia and New Zealand found no difference in mortality between high- (40 mL/kg/hour) and low-dose (25 mL/kg/hour) CVVHDF [36].

A final word from the expert

Pancreatitis is a common condition and is associated with considerable morbidity and mortality. The systemic effects from pancreatic inflammation can lead to multiple organ failure, with patients requiring long admissions to the ICU. Decisions about antimicrobial use and timing of surgery are not straightforward. Optimal management involves close working between intensivists, microbiologists, radiologists, and surgeons as well as multidisciplinary team working providing supportive care and long-term rehabilitation.

References

1. Banks PA, Bollen TL, Dervenis C, et al. Classification of acute pancreatitis—2012: revision of the Atlanta classification and definitions by international consensus. *Gut*. 2013;62:102–11.
2. Ranson JH, Rifkind KM, Roses DF, Fink SD, Eng K, Spencer FC. Prognostic signs and the role of operative management in acute pancreatitis. *Surg Gynecol Obstet*. 1974;139:69–81.
3. Blamey SL, Imrie CW, O'Neill J, Gilmore WH, Carter DC. Prognostic factors in acute pancreatitis. *Gut*. 1984;25:1340–6.
4. Balthazar EJ, Ranson JH, Naidich DP, Megibow AJ, Caccavale R, Cooper MM. Acute pancreatitis: prognostic value of CT. *Radiology*. 1985;156:767–72.
5. Balthazar EJ, Robinson DL, Megibow AJ, Ranson JH. Acute pancreatitis: value of CT in establishing prognosis. *Radiology*. 1990;174:331–36.
6. Waldmann C, Soni N, Rhodes A. *Oxford Desk Reference: Critical Care*. Oxford: Oxford University Press; 2008.

7. Hall NA, Fox AJ. Renal replacement therapies in critical care. *Cont Educ Anaesth Crit Care Pain*. 2006;6:197–202.

8. Lankisch PG, Apte M, Banks P. Acute pancreatitis. *Lancet*. 2015;386:85–96.

9. Tenner S, Baillie J, DeWitt J, Vege SS. American College of Gastroenterology guideline: management of acute pancreatitis. *Am J Gast*. 2013;108:1400–15.

10. Oudemans-van Straaten HM, Kellum JA, Bellomo R. Clinical review: anticoagulation for continuous renal replacement therapy—heparin or citrate? *Crit Care*. 2011;15:202.

11. van Santvoort HC, Besselink MG, Bakker OJ, et al. A step-up approach or open necrosectomy for necrotizing pancreatitis (PANTER trial). *N Engl J Med*. 2010;362:1491–502.

12. Young SP, Thompson JP. Severe acute pancreatitis. *Cont Educ Anaesth Crit Care Pain*. 2008;8:125–8.

13. Johnson CD, Besselink MG, Carter R. Acute pancreatitis. *BMJ*. 2014;349:g4859.

14. Villatoro E, Mulla M, Larvin M. Antibiotic therapy for prophylaxis against infection of pancreatic necrosis in acute pancreatitis. *Cochrane Database Syst Rev*. 2010;5:CD002941.

15. Bellomo R, Ronco C, Kellum JA, et al. Acute renal failure—definition, outcome measures, animal models, fluid therapy and information technology needs: the Second International Consensus Conference of the Acute Dialysis Quality Initiative (ADQI) Group. *Critical Care* 2004;8:R204–12.

16. Mehta RL, Kellum JA, Shah SV, et al. Acute Kidney Injury Network: report of an initiative to improve outcomes in acute kidney injury. *Crit Care*. 2007;11:R31.

17. Kidney Disease: Improving Global Outcomes (KDIGO) Acute Kidney Injury Work Group. KDIGO clinical practice guideline for acute kidney injury. *Kidney Int Suppl*. 2012;2:1–138.

18. Belloma R, Chapman M, Finfer S, Hickling K, Myburgh J. Low-dose dopamine in patients with early renal dysfunction: a placebo-controlled randomised trial. Australian and New Zealand Intensive Care Society (ANZICS) Clinical Trials Group. *Lancet*. 2000;356:2139–43.

19. Majumdar A. Sepsis-induced acute kidney injury. *Indian J Crit Care Med*. 2010;14:14–21.

20. National Confidential Enquiry into Patient Outcome and Death (NCEPOD). *Adding Insult to Injury*. London: NCEPOD; 2009. Available from: http://www.ncepod.org.uk/2009report1/Downloads/AKI_report.pdf.

21. Ronco C, Kellum JA, Mehta R. Acute Dialysis Quality Initiative (ADQI). *Nephrol Dial Transplant*. 2001;16:1555–8.

22. Intensive Care Society. *Standards and Recommendations for the Provision of Renal Replacement Therapy on Intensive Care Units in the United Kingdom*. London: Intensive Care Society; 2009. Available from: https://www.ics.ac.uk/ICS/guidelines-and-standards.aspx.

23. Gettings LG, Reynolds HN, Scalea T. Outcome in post-traumatic acute renal failure when continuous therapy is applied early vs late. *Intensive Care Med*. 1999;25:805–13.

24. Ronco C, Bellomo R, Homel P, et al. Effects of different doses in continuous venovenous haemofiltration on outcomes of acute renal failure: a prospective randomised trial. *Lancet*. 2000;356:26–30.

25. Wang C, Lv LS, Huang H, et al. Initiation time of renal replacement therapy on patients with acute kidney injury: a systematic review and meta-analysis of 8179 participants. *Nephrology (Carlton)*. 2016;22:7–18.

26. Zarbock A, Kellum JA, Schmidt C, et al. Effect of early vs delayed initiation of renal replacement therapy on mortality in critically ill patients with acute kidney injury: the ELAIN Randomized Clinical Trial. *JAMA*. 2016;315:2190–9.

27. Park JY, An JN, Jhee JH, et al. Early initiation of continuous renal replacement therapy improves survival of elderly patients with acute kidney injury: a multicenter prospective cohort study. *Crit Care*. 2016;20:260.

28. Xu Y, Gao J, Zheng X, Zhong B, Na Y, Wei J. Timing of initiation of renal replacement therapy for acute kidney injury: a systematic review and meta-analysis of randomized-controlled trials. *Clin Exp Nephrol*. 2017;552–62.

29. Gaudry S, Hajage D, Schortgen F, et al. Initiation strategies for renal-replacement therapy in the intensive care unit. *N Engl J Med*. 2016;375:122–33.

30. Gatward J, Gibbon GJ, Wrathall G, Padkin A. Renal replacement therapy for acute renal failure: a survey of practice in adult intensive care units in the United Kingdom. *Anaesthesia*. 2008;63 959–66.

31. Bell M, Martling C-R. Long-term outcome after intensive care: can we protect the kidney? *Crit Care*. 2007;11:147–9.

32. Schneider AG, Bellomo R, Bagshaw SM, et al. Choice of renal replacement therapy modality and dialysis dependence after acute kidney injury: a systematic review and meta-analysis. *Intensive Care Med*. 2013;39:987–97.

33. Schiffl H, Lang SM, Fischer R. Daily hemodialysis and the outcome of acute renal failure. *N Eng J Med*. 2002;346:305–10.

34. Wright SE, Bodenham A, Short A, Turney JH. The provision and practice of renal replacement therapy on adult intensive care units in the United Kingdom. *Anaesthesia*. 2003;58:1063–9.

35. Pallevsky PM, Zhang JH, O'Connor TZ, et al. The VA/NIH Acute Renal Failure Trial Network. Intensity of renal support in critically ill patients with acute kidney injury. *N Engl J Med*. 2008;359:7–20.

36. Bellomo R, Cass A, Cole L, et al. The RENAL Replacement Therapy Study Investigators. Intensity of continuous renal replacement therapy in critically ill patients. *N Engl J Med*. 2009;361:1627–38.

13 Feeding, access, and thromboprophylaxis

Martin Huntley

❝ Expert Commentary Ramani Moonesinghe

Case history

A 38-year-old man presented to the emergency department with a 3-day history of abdominal pain and vomiting. He had had a poor diet for the past month because of intermittent abdominal cramps and vomiting after eating. He had a history of fistulating Crohn's disease that had been treated with monoclonal antibody therapy in the past. His current medications included mesalazine 2 g once daily, azathioprine 100 mg once daily, lansoprazole 30 mg once daily, ferrous sulphate 200 mg three times daily, and Calcichew D_3 forte 2 tablets once daily. He had a body mass index (BMI) of 15.2 kg/m².

On examination, he was tachycardic, tachypnoeic, and had cool peripheries with a capillary refill time greater than 4 seconds. His abdomen was distended, painful on palpation with generalized guarding, and absent bowel sounds. His initial blood results are presented in Table 13.1.

Table 13.1 Blood results on presentation

Arterial blood gas (FiO₂ 0.35)

pH	7.14	(7.35–7.45)
PaCO₂ (kPa)	2.7	(4.7–6)
PaO₂ (kPa)	18	(>10)
BE (mmol/L)	− 12	(± 2)
Lactate (mmol/L)	5.3	(0.5–2)

Full blood count

Hb (g/L)	82	(130–180)
MCV (fL)	74	(76–96)
Plat (× 10⁹/L)	64	(150–400)
WCC (× 10⁹/L)	3.7	(4–11)

Clotting

INR	1.6	
PT (sec)	19.2	(10.7–13.6)
APTT (sec)	46	(21–34)
Fib (g/L)	0.6	(1.5–4)

Urea and electrolytes

Na (mmol/L)	131	(135–145)
K (mmol/L)	3.0	(3.5–5)
Urea (mmol/L)	16	(2.5–6.7)
Cr (µmol/L)	115	(60–110)
Alb (g/L)	18	(35–50)
CRP (mg/L)	365	(<10)

Alb, albumin; APTT, activated partial thromboplastin time; BE, base excess; Cr, creatinine; CRP, C-reactive protein; Fib, fibrinogen; FiO₂, fraction of inspired oxygen; Hb, haemoglobin; K, potassium; MCV, mean corpuscular volume; Na, sodium; PaCO₂, partial pressure of carbon dioxide; PaO₂, partial pressure of oxygen; Plat, platelets; PT, prothrombin time; WCC, white cell count.

After initial resuscitation with 30 mL/kg of intravenous crystalloid and administration of broad-spectrum antibiotics, he was transferred for an abdominal computed tomography scan. This showed gross small bowel dilatation with mucosal thickening and free air and fluid in the peritoneal cavity. He was transferred urgently to the operating room where he had a right internal jugular central line and radial arterial line inserted and was anaesthetized for an emergency laparotomy. He was found to have multiple small bowel perforations and faecal peritonitis, and underwent extensive adhesiolysis, small bowel resection, and formation of an end ileostomy. He received multiple blood products intraoperatively for an estimated blood loss of 1.3 L.

ⓕ Expert comment

Emergency laparotomy is a high-risk procedure—data from the UK's National Emergency Laparotomy Audit indicate a population mortality of 11%. Although this patient is young, he has several features which place him at very high risk of a poor outcome, including chronic ill health, faecal peritonitis, and the requirement for significant blood and fluid transfusion. The principles of management for these high-risk patients include consultant delivered care, surgery to be conducted as soon as possible, and postoperative critical care admission. Risk stratification at the time of diagnosis and at the end of surgery, using an objective risk score such as P-POSSUM (Portsmouth Physiological and Operative Severity Score for the Enumeration of Mortality and Morbidity) or the Surgical Outcome Risk Tool (SORT; http://www.sortsurgery.com), alongside clinical judgement from senior anaesthetists and surgeons, will also support decision-making and optimal management (see Case 9).

Following surgery, he is transferred to the intensive care unit (ICU) with propofol and fentanyl sedation, mechanical ventilation, and a noradrenaline infusion at 0.45 mcg/kg/min. Overnight he is resuscitated with further crystalloid and blood products and is started on a vasopressin infusion and hydrocortisone 50 mg four times daily for persistent hypotension. On day 1, he is reviewed by the general surgical registrar who enquires about nutritional support for the patient.

✪ Learning point The when, what, and how of feeding in critical illness

The catabolic state associated with critical illness can lead rapidly to a progressive energy deficit that is associated with adverse clinical outcomes, for example, prolonged mechanical ventilation, increased rates of infection, poor wound healing, and loss of gastrointestinal integrity [1, 2]. In view of this, nutritional support in critical care has stimulated substantial interest [3]. The timing, route of delivery, and amount and type of nutrients that are administered has been the focus of research in this area.

The Early Parenteral Nutrition Completing Enteral Nutrition in Adult Critically Ill Patients (EPaNIC) trial, randomized 4640 ICU patients with insufficient enteral nutrition to either additional parenteral nutrition within 48 hours (early) of ICU admission or after at least 7 days (late) [4]. The trial showed no difference in ICU, hospital, or 90-day mortality between groups and a higher rate of infections, duration of mechanical ventilation, hospital length of stay, and total healthcare cost in the early intervention group. An important criticism of this trial was that it consisted of low mortality-risk patients (ICU mortality = 6.2%) and excluded malnourished patients (BMI <17 kg/m^2), which limits the ability to generalize these finding to higher-risk ICU patients.

The initial trophic versus full enteral feeding in patients with acute lung injury (EDEN) trial studied a more specific high-risk group of patients with acute lung injury and found no difference in 60-day

(continued)

mortality, organ failure, or ICU-free days, or incidence of infection between the two groups [5]. Full enteral-fed patients did experience more gastrointestinal intolerances; however, the incidence of this was relatively low and may have been biased by the open-label design of the study.

The Tight Calorie Control Study (TICACOS) also evaluated higher-risk ICU patients, and showed that providing enteral nutrition supported by additional parenteral nutrition significantly reduced in-hospital and 60-day mortality [6]. This suggests that meeting calorie requirements early with additional parenteral nutrition is beneficial and safe.

More recently, the Intensive Care National Audit and Research Centre (ICNARC) conducted a multicentre randomized controlled trial (RCT) of the route of early nutritional support in critically ill patients (CALORIES) [7]. This was a pragmatic trial, which included a heterogeneous ICU patient population who had an unplanned admission and were expected to remain on the ICU for at least 3 days. The trial showed no difference in 30-day mortality or infectious complications between groups receiving enteral or parenteral nutrition. Importantly, more than 60% of patients failed to reach their calorie targets during the trial, which highlights a significant problem with feeding protocols in ICU patients.

Summary points:

1. Patients commonly develop a nutritional deficit during critical illness that increases the probability of adverse outcomes.
2. Patients receiving artificial nutrition on the ICU often fail to reach their daily nutritional targets.
3. Current evidence favours early initiation (i.e. within 24–48 hours) of feeding in critical illness.
4. Assessment of nutritional intake should form part of the daily multidisciplinary review of the ICU patient so that the adequacy and most appropriate route of nutritional support can be determined (Figure 13.1).
5. If patients are unable or unlikely to tolerate enteral nutrition, then the parenteral route can be used safely.

---

⑥ Expert comment

Previous concerns about the safety of enteral nutrition following emergency gastrointestinal surgery, particularly where there has been an intestinal anastomosis, have now been appeased. Principles of enhanced recovery support early return to enteral nutrition. However, in this patient, there are several additional factors which may indicate that enteral nutrition may not be successful, such as multiple organ dysfunction, particularly with the use of vasoactive drugs, and the requirement for sedation including opioid therapy. Therefore, starting parenteral nutrition as opposed to enteral nutrition seems sensible and justified by the evidence.

The ICU team decided to start early parenteral nutrition because of his extensive bowel surgery, pre-existing malnutrition, and likely gastrointestinal dysfunction. A standard formula was ordered from pharmacy and started while awaiting review by the ICU dietician.

---

⑥ Expert comment

In view of his likely chronic malnutrition and his acute critical illness, estimation of this patient's caloric and other dietary requirements is likely to be challenging. Thus, expert review by the dietician is important. Although the Surviving Sepsis Campaign guidelines make a strong recommendation against the use of early parenteral nutrition in sepsis, the trials contributing to this systematic review either excluded or rarely incorporated patients who were malnourished. These patients may represent a particular subgroup where early parenteral nutrition could be considered when enteral nutrition is not feasible.

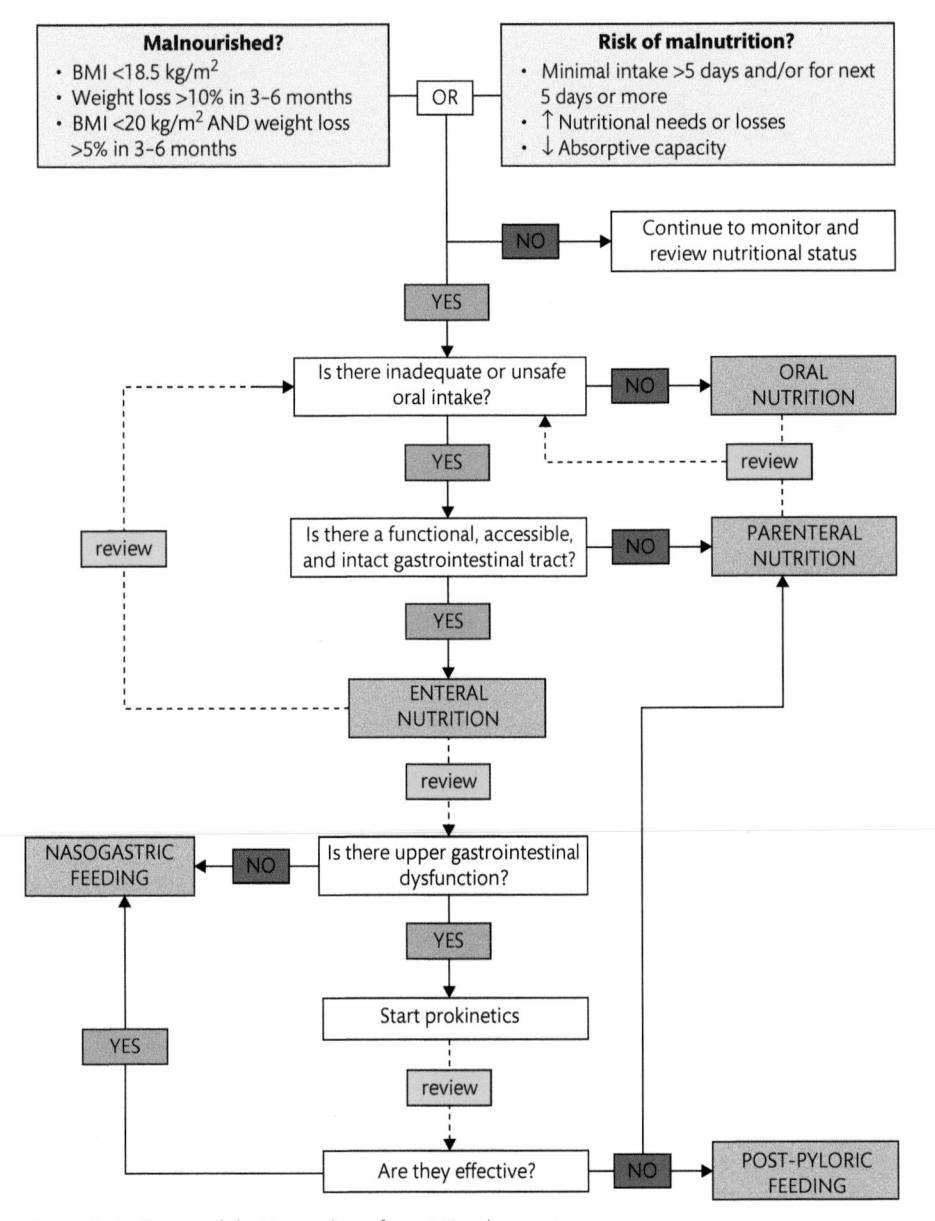

Figure 13.1 Suggested decision pathway for nutritional support.

✪ **Learning point** Predicting caloric requirements in critical illness

Calculating caloric requirements in critical illness is difficult and may involve the use of either predictive formulas (e.g. Oxford, Harris Benedict, or Schofield) or indirect calorimetry [3, 8].

❝ **Expert comment**

Indirect calorimetry measures CO_2 production and O_2 consumption (using a device known as a metabolic cart) to calculate the total energy production. In ventilated patients in critical care, the metabolic cart interacts with the ventilator via the tracheal tube; in spontaneously breathing

(continued)

patients, a face mask, canopy (hood), or Douglas bag (inflatable airtight bag) are used. Both the respiratory quotient and the resting energy expenditure (REE) (which can be used to calculate 24-hour caloric requirements) are provided.

Predictive formulas are simpler to use but they are not as accurate as indirect calorimetry, especially in certain patient groups (e.g. obesity). They are also modelled on afebrile healthy individuals, which may limit their relevance to ICU patients.

Indirect calorimetry calculates caloric requirement by measuring the patient's inspired and expired gases and directly relating the measured oxygen consumption (VO_2) and carbon dioxide production (VCO_2) to the oxidation of substrate fuel. The REE can then be calculated by using the abbreviated Weir equation:

$$REE = (3.94 \times VO_2) + (1.1 \times VCO_2)$$

It is a more accurate and reproducible method that has been shown to increase the amount of nutrition received by ICU patients [6]. However, its use is limited by the technical difficulty of performing it, and consequently most ICU dieticians use predictive formulas and make adjustments for specific patient factors (Table 13.2).

Table 13.2 Calorie adjustments for specific patient factors

Patient factor	Additive calorie adjustment
Fever	↑ by 10% for each 1°C above 37°C (max. 40°C)
Sepsis	↑ by 9%
Surgery or trauma	↑ by 6%
Burns	↑ by 100% for any size >30%

Source: data from Bratanow, S. and Brown, S. Nutrition in the critically ill. *Update in Anaesthesia*. 2012; 28, 79–87. Copyright © 2012 World Federation of Societies of Anesthesiologists.

⊗ **Learning point** How to commence feeding in critical illness

- It is not necessary to correct low plasma electrolyte values before commencing feeding [9].
- Start enteral nutrition or parenteral nutrition at less than 50% of the estimated target energy and protein needs.
- Increase to meet full needs over the first 24–48 hours according to the metabolic and gastrointestinal tolerances.
- Provide the full requirement of fluid, electrolytes, vitamins, and minerals from the outset of feeding.

⊗ **Learning point** What are the components of basic nutritional support?

Macronutrients

These are the main sources of energy and include proteins (4 kcal/g), lipids (9.3 kcal/g), and carbohydrates (3.75 kcal/g) [8]. The suggested total daily calorie requirement is estimated at 25–35 kcal/kg [9]. The contribution made to this by proteins and lipids should be calculated first and the remainder made up by carbohydrates (Table 13.3).

Table 13.3 The daily requirement of macronutrients

Macronutrient	Daily requirement
Protein	0.8–1.5 g/kg
Lipid	40% of total calories
Carbohydrate	3–4 g/kg

Source: data from Bratanow, S. and Brown, S. Nutrition in the critically ill. *Update in Anaesthesia*. 2012; 28, 79–87. Copyright © 2012 World Federation of Societies of Anesthesiologists.

(continued)

Micronutrients

These include trace elements (e.g. zinc, copper, and selenium) and vitamins (e.g. thiamine (B_1), riboflavin (B_2), and vitamin D) [8]. They play vital roles in enzyme function and the metabolic pathways essential to health and recovery from critical illness [10]. Micronutrient deficiencies contribute to reduced antioxidant defence and impaired immune function resulting in increased complication rates (e.g. infection and poor wound healing). Despite their widespread use in ICUs, clinical trials involving several micronutrients (e.g. selenium and vitamin D) have failed to show a significant mortality benefit in ICU patients and they remain a controversial area of nutritional support [11, 12].

Fluid and electrolytes

The daily maintenance requirements for fluid and electrolytes are listed in Table 13.4. Allowances should also be made for pre-existing deficits, extra losses (e.g. drains and fistulae), and extra input (e.g. intravenous drugs).

Table 13.4 Daily maintenance fluid and electrolyte requirement

Fluid	Electrolyte	Daily requirement
Water		30 mL/kg
	Sodium	1–1 mmol/kg
	Potassium	0.7–1 mmol/kg
	Calcium	0.1 mmol/kg
	Magnesium	0.1 mmol/kg
	Chloride	1–2 mmol/kg
	Phosphate	0.4 mmol/kg

Source: data from Bratanow, S. and Brown, S. Nutrition in the critically ill. *Update in Anaesthesia.* 2012; 28, 79–87. Copyright © 2012 World Federation of Societies of Anesthesiologists; and National Institute for Health and Care Excellence (NICE). (2006) *Guidance for nutrition support in adults: oral nutrition support, enteral tube feeding and parenteral nutrition.* Copyright © 2006 NICE.

⭐ **Learning point The changing focus of nutrition**

The concept of nutrition in critical care is progressively changing from a purely 'supportive' to a more 'therapeutic' focus, where the constituents of nutritional formulations can be altered to improve the management of certain disease states [8, 10]. This may be through preventing certain disease-specific complications, reducing oxidative stress and inflammation, enhancing beneficial stress responses, or reducing gastrointestinal dysfunction (Table 13.5).

Table 13.5 Potential formulations for specific disease states

Disease state	Formulation	Effect
Liver failure	↓ Na^+	↓ Ascites and oedema
	Altered amino acids	↓ Encephalopathy
Renal failure	↓ PO_4^{2-} and K^+	↓ Electrolyte excess
	↑ Calorie concentration (2 kcal/mL)	↓ Volume
Respiratory failure	↑ Lipid: carbohydrate ratio	↓ CO_2 and improved weaning
Acute respiratory distress syndrome	↑ Micronutrients	↑ Antioxidant effect
	↑ Fish and borage oil	↑ Anti-inflammatory effect
Surgery, trauma, and burns	↑ Arginine and glutamine	Maintains immune cells and facilitates tissue repair
Intestinal failure	↓ Fibre	↓ Gut transit time
	↑ Hydrolysed proteins and medium-chain triglycerides	↑ Absorption
	↑ Probiotics	↑ Protective bowel flora

Source: data from National Institute for Health and Care Excellence (NICE). (2006) *Guidance for nutrition support in adults: oral nutrition support, enteral tube feeding and parenteral nutrition.* Copyright © 2006 NICE; and Hegazi, R., et al. Clinical review: optimizing enteral nutrition for critically ill patients – a simple data-driven formula. *Critical Care* 2011; 15:234. Copyright © 2006 BioMed Central Ltd.

> **✪ Learning point Summary guidelines for feeding in critical illness**
>
> - Haemodynamically stable patients with a functioning gastrointestinal tract who are not expected to be on a full oral diet within 3 days should receive enteral nutrition within 24 hours of admission.
> - In patients where enteral nutrition is not feasible, there is currently no clear benefit for commencing early parenteral nutrition and consequently intravenous glucose should be initiated with enteral feeds advanced as tolerated. However, malnourished patients may represent a particular subgroup of critically ill patients who benefit from early parenteral nutrition if enteral nutrition is not feasible [13–15].
> - In the absence of indirect calorimetry, patients should receive 25 kcal/kg/day increasing to target over the following 2–3 days.
> - All patients receiving less than their targeted enteral feeding after 2 days should be considered for supplementary parenteral nutrition.
> - All parenteral nutrition prescriptions should include a daily dose of multivitamins and trace elements.
> - The use of gastric residual volume as a marker of intolerance to enteral feeding and for preventing aspiration is controversial and poorly evidence based [16].
> - Traditional practice is to slow or stop enteral nutrition if residual gastric volumes exceed 200 mL every 4 hours. Using a higher threshold for gastric residual volume (>500 mL) improves the provision of enteral nutrition without clearly increasing the risk of ventilator-associated pneumonia [17, 18].
> - Consider intravenous metoclopramide and/or erythromycin in patients with high gastric residual volumes.
> - Position patients receiving enteral nutrition at 30° head elevation to reduce the risk of aspiration and ventilator-associated pneumonia.
> - There is no need to 'rest' patients receiving enteral feeding overnight.
> - Avoiding gastric acid suppression and allowing breaks in enteral feeding to let gastric pH decrease help to prevent bacterial overgrowth.
> - Hyperglycaemia (glucose >10 mmol/L) should be avoided/treated in order to minimize infectious complications.

ⓘ Expert comment

Small intestinal bacterial overgrowth is an over-proliferation of bacteria in this part of the bowel which is usually much less colonized than the large bowel. It can lead to abdominal bloating, pain, nausea, vomiting/poor absorption of feed, and diarrhoea with consequent risks of malnutrition and weight loss. In critically ill patients, therefore, the commonest presentation will be poor absorption. Elemental diets or cyclical antibiotic therapy may be used to treat this.

Use of gastric acid suppression in critically ill patients is generally considered to be unnecessary once full enteral feeding is established, unless there is a particularly high risk of gastrointestinal bleeding. In general hospital settings, three systematic reviews have concluded that proton pump inhibitors (PPIs) are associated with an increased risk of *Clostridium difficile* (toxin) (CDT) infection, and while a causal link has not been established, the use of PPIs has been discouraged in critical care, where H_2 antagonists can be used as an alternative [19–21]. However, a recent meta-analysis specifically of critical care trials found that PPIs were superior to H_2 antagonists in the prevention of significant gastrointestinal bleeding and did not lead to a greater risk of pneumonia or mortality; however, none of the 19 trials reported CDT infection, and therefore the concern about CDT preponderance in critically ill patients has not been addressed [22]. While trials in this area are continuing (e.g. SUP-ICU), it may be preferable to use H_2 antagonists as first-line therapy for gastric protection, unless the patient is on long-term PPIs or there is a reason to consider the patient at high risk for gastrointestinal bleeding. Once enteral feed has been fully established, gastric acid suppression can be stopped, again unless there is an indication to continue it because the patient is at high risk for gastrointestinal bleeding.

The central venous catheter (CVC) that was inserted in the operating theatre did not have any sterile ports and so a peripherally inserted central catheter (PICC) line was inserted into his right cephalic vein. The position was confirmed on chest radiography and the administration of parenteral nutrition was started.

> ✪ **Learning point** European Society of Parenteral and Enteral Nutrition (ESPEN) guidelines for venous access in parenteral nutrition
>
> **Route**
> - A CVC should be used for most patients receiving parenteral nutrition [23].
> - Peripheral access (short cannula or midline catheter) can be used safely for a limited period with solutions that have an osmolarity < 850 mOsm/L.
>
> > ℹ **Expert comment**
> >
> > A midline catheter is a peripherally inserted catheter which is shorter than a PICC and does not lie in a central vein—that is, the tip usually lies in the axillary vein. It is more secure than a short peripheral cannula and is commonly used for prolonged antibiotic courses.
>
> **Device**
> - Short term—peripheral cannula, non-tunnelled CVC, and PICC.
> - Medium term—tunnelled CVC and ports, and PICC.
> - Long term—tunnelled CVC and totally implantable devices.
>
> **Vein**
> - The choice of vein is affected by several factors (i.e. familiarity with technique, body habitus, risk of complications, and presence of thrombus and/or infection).
> - The subclavian vein has the lowest rate of infectious complications, followed by the internal jugular and femoral vein.
> - High approaches to the internal jugular vein restrict nursing access and increase the risk of catheter contamination and infection.

> ✪ **Learning point** Intravascular complications of central venous catheter insertion
>
> In a multicentre trial published in 2015, 3027 adult ICU patients were randomly assigned to have a non-tunnelled CVC inserted in either the subclavian, jugular, or femoral vein [24]. A total of 3471 catheters were inserted and the median duration of catheter use was 5 days.
>
> Catheterization of the subclavian vein, as compared with the jugular or femoral vein, was associated with a significantly lower risk of catheter-related bloodstream infection (0.5% vs 1.4% vs 1.2% respectively) and symptomatic deep vein thrombosis (DVT) (0.5% vs 1.4% vs 1.2% respectively). However, the subclavian vein was associated with a higher risk of mechanical complications (2.1% vs 1.4% vs 0.7% respectively), which was primarily pneumothorax (1.5%). Interestingly, the risk of catheter-related bloodstream infection and symptomatic DVT was similar for jugular and femoral sites.
>
> This trial highlights the significant complication rates associated with CVC insertion, despite the increasing use of ultrasound guidance. This is often an underappreciated problem, which accounted for 14% of all litigation claims associated with intensive care treatment in England between 1995 and 2012 [25].

> ✪ **Learning point** Prevention and management of catheter-related infection
>
> **Interventions to reduce the risk of catheter-related infection**
>
> (For guidance, see references [23,26].)
> - Regular education and competence-based training of staff involved in catheter insertion and/ or care.
>
> *(continued)*

- Appropriate choice of catheter insertion site.
- Use of an all-inclusive catheter insertion kit and a procedural checklist.
- Use of single-lumen catheters whenever possible.
- Use of a chlorhexidine/silver sulfadiazine or antibiotic-impregnated catheter if it is expected to remain in place for longer than 5 days.
- Ultrasound-guided venepuncture.
- Maximal barrier precautions during insertion.
- An appropriate hand-washing policy.
- Use of 2% chlorhexidine on the skin at insertion and for daily washes on ICU.
- Appropriate dressing of the exit site.
- Disinfection of hubs, stopcocks, and needle-free connectors before accessing.
- Regular change of administration sets.
- Daily review of the catheter insertion site.
- Prompt removal of catheters when central access is no longer required.

There is no evidence to suggest that routine, scheduled replacement of catheters reduces the risk of catheter-related infections and therefore the decision to replace a catheter should be based on clinical assessment and culture results [27].

Diagnosis of catheter-related infection

- Quantitative or semi-quantitative culture of the catheter tip (after removal), or
- Paired quantitative blood cultures or paired qualitative blood cultures from a peripheral vein and the catheter.

Treatment of catheter-related sepsis (short-term lines)

- A short-term CVC should be removed if there are:
  o signs of local infection at the exit site
  o clinical signs of sepsis in the absence of other obvious sources
  o positive paired blood cultures.
- Where there is suspicion of infection, the tip should be sent for culture and this may assist in diagnosis of line-associated infection and choice of appropriate antibiotics.
- Appropriate antibiotic therapy should be continued after catheter removal.

Treatment of catheter-related sepsis (long-term lines)

- A long-term CVC should be removed if there is:
  o tunnel infection or port abscess
  o clinical signs of septic shock
  o positive paired blood cultures for fungi or highly virulent bacteria
  o complicated infection (e.g. endocarditis, septic thrombosis).

In patients who have limited or difficult venous access, an attempt to save the device may be tried by 'locking' the line with antibiotic. Vancomycin is commonly used as empirical therapy in view of the prevalence of methicillin-resistant *Staphylococcus aureus* in healthcare settings [28].

On day 4, he became confused, hypotensive, and developed atrial fibrillation. On examination, he had cool peripheries and reduced muscle power. His repeat blood results are shown in Table 13.6.

Table 13.6 Repeat blood results

Urea and electrolytes		
PO_4^{2-} (mmol/L)	**0.2**	(0.8–1.4)
Mg^{2+} (mmol/L)	**0.5**	(0.7–1.0)
K^+ (mmol/L)	**2.7**	(3.5–5.0)
Glucose (mmol/L)	**18.0**	(6–10)

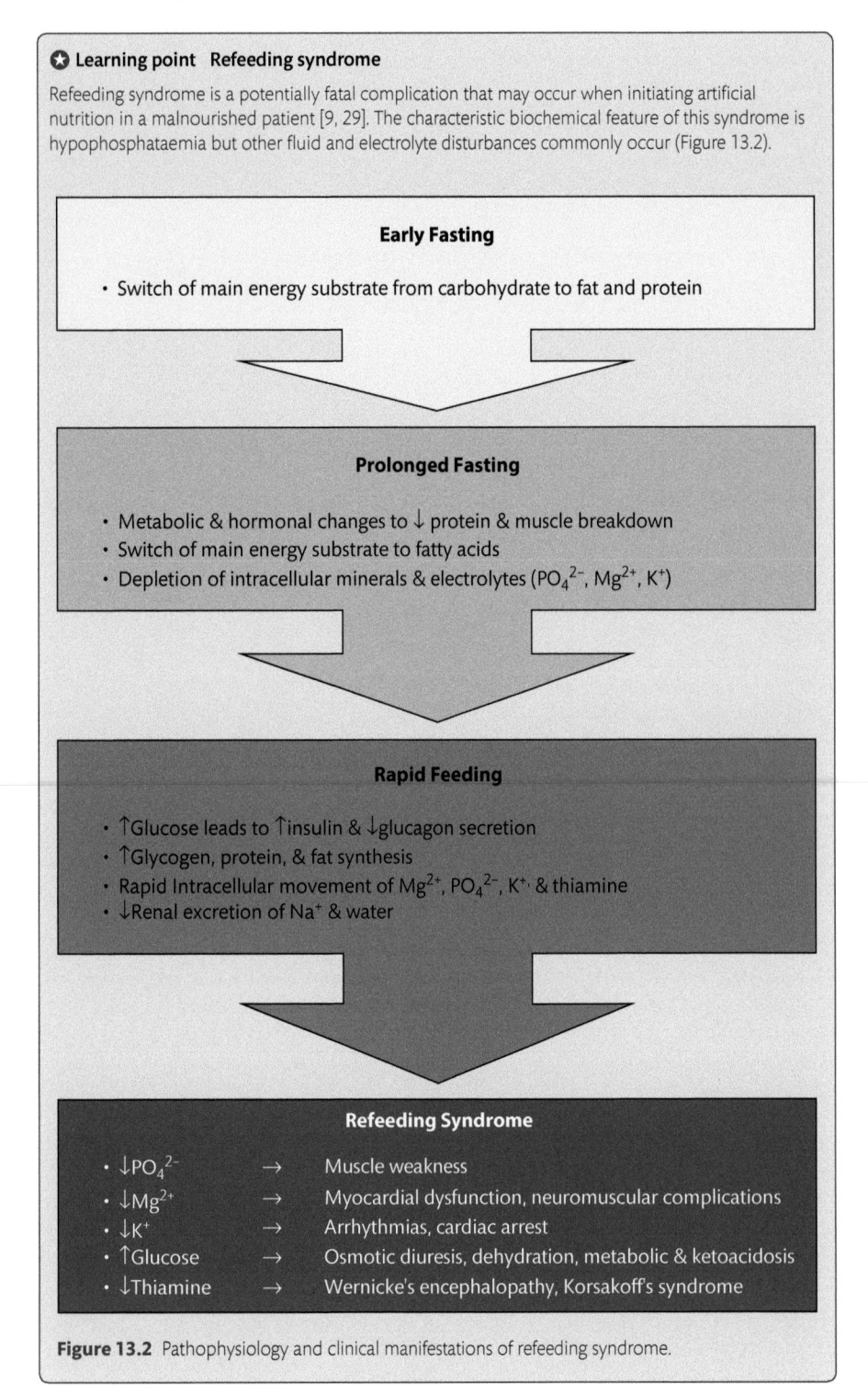

⭐ **Learning point   Refeeding syndrome**

Refeeding syndrome is a potentially fatal complication that may occur when initiating artificial nutrition in a malnourished patient [9, 29]. The characteristic biochemical feature of this syndrome is hypophosphataemia but other fluid and electrolyte disturbances commonly occur (Figure 13.2).

Early Fasting

• Switch of main energy substrate from carbohydrate to fat and protein

Prolonged Fasting

• Metabolic & hormonal changes to ↓ protein & muscle breakdown
• Switch of main energy substrate to fatty acids
• Depletion of intracellular minerals & electrolytes (PO_4^{2-}, Mg^{2+}, K^+)

Rapid Feeding

• ↑Glucose leads to ↑insulin & ↓glucagon secretion
• ↑Glycogen, protein, & fat synthesis
• Rapid Intracellular movement of Mg^{2+}, PO_4^{2-}, K^+, & thiamine
• ↓Renal excretion of Na^+ & water

Refeeding Syndrome

• ↓PO_4^{2-}	→	Muscle weakness
• ↓Mg^{2+}	→	Myocardial dysfunction, neuromuscular complications
• ↓K^+	→	Arrhythmias, cardiac arrest
• ↑Glucose	→	Osmotic diuresis, dehydration, metabolic & ketoacidosis
• ↓Thiamine	→	Wernicke's encephalopathy, Korsakoff's syndrome

Figure 13.2 Pathophysiology and clinical manifestations of refeeding syndrome.

✪ **Learning point** Identifying patients at risk of refeeding syndrome

Patients at high risk of refeeding syndrome should be identified on admission to the ICU. This is to ensure that close monitoring and timely replacement of electrolytes and vitamins occurs, and if necessary, the appropriate clinical specialists are involved in their management at the earliest opportunity (Figure 13.3).

National Institute for Health and Care Excellence criteria for patients at risk of refeeding syndrome

Patient has one or more of the following [9]:

- BMI less than 16 kg/m².
- Unintentional weight loss greater than 15% within the last 3–6 months.
- Little or no nutritional intake for longer than 10 days.
- Low concentrations of potassium, phosphate, or magnesium prior to feeding.

Or patient has two or more of the following [9]:

- BMI less than 18.5kg/m².
- Unintentional weight loss greater than 15% within the last 3–6 months.
- Little or no nutritional intake for longer than 5 days.
- A history of alcohol abuse or drugs including insulin, chemotherapy, antacids, or diuretics.

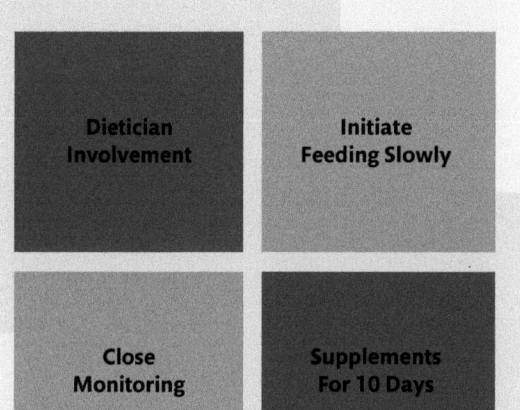

- Expert knowledge and advice
- Max 10 kcal/kg/day
- ↑ Slowly over 4–7 days

Dietician Involvement

Initiate Feeding Slowly

Close Monitoring

Supplements For 10 Days

- Fluid balance
- Electrolytes
- Overall clinical status

- Thiamine & vitamin B
- Multivitamin
- K⁺ 2–4 mmol/kg
- PO_4^{2-} 0.3–0.6 mmol/kg
- Mg^{2+} 0.2–0.4 mmol/kg

Figure 13.3 Managing patients at high risk of refeeding syndrome.
Source: data from National Institute for Health and Care Excellence (NICE) (2006). *Guidance for nutrition support in adults: oral nutrition support, enteral tube feeding and parenteral nutrition.* Copyright © 2006 NICE.

He was given intravenous replacement of phosphate, potassium, and magnesium and commenced on an insulin infusion to control his blood glucose. He was also started on regular intravenous vitamin B replacement (a 7-day course). The parenteral nutrition rate was gradually increased over the next week during which time his electrolytes were monitored closely. On day 9, he suddenly developed a swollen, painful, and warm left arm and the nurse looking after him commented that she was no longer able to aspirate blood from the PICC line. An urgent Doppler ultrasound scan of his left arm showed a DVT involving the left axillary and subclavian veins.

✪ **Learning point** **Prevention of catheter-related central venous thrombosis**

Critically ill patients exhibit several general and ICU acquired risk factors (Table 13.7) for venous thromboembolism and the incidence of DVT in those not treated with thromboprophylaxis can be as high as 81% [30]. In view of this, almost all ICU patients will require pharmacological thromboprophylaxis. This presents several challenges for the intensivist as haemorrhage, coagulopathy, and thrombocytopenia are common in ICU patients. Furthermore, the need for effective thromboprophylaxis often must be balanced carefully with the need for antiplatelet therapy, for example, acute coronary syndromes, invasive procedures and expectant surgery.

CVC insertion in ICU patients is a significant risk factor for venous thromboembolism, with catheter-related thrombosis rates of 10–69% with femoral catheters, 40–56% with internal jugular catheters, and 2–10% with subclavian catheters [31]. The risk of thrombosis increases with the duration of catheter placement, but while the risk of pulmonary embolism (PE) increases fourfold with a lower-limb DVT, there doesn't appear to be an increased risk of PE with an upper-limb DVT.

Several strategies to reduce catheter-related thrombosis have been suggested [26]:

● Use an insertion technique that limits damage to the vein, such as:
  o ultrasound guidance at insertion
  o selection of the smallest calibre compatible with the required infusion therapy
  o positioning the tip of the catheter at or near the atriocaval junction.
● Use of a CVC rather than a PICC. There is a higher reported rate of upper extremity superficial venous thrombosis with PICCs, especially in critically ill and cancer patients [32].
● Use routine thromboprophylaxis in all critically ill patients unless contraindicated.

ICU patients should also be considered routinely for mechanical protection against venous thromboembolism (pneumatic calf pumps and compression stockings) and active early immobilization.

Table 13.7 Risk factors for venous thromboembolism

General	ICU acquired
Increased age	Sepsis
Past history of venous thromboembolism	Vasopressor use
Past history of cancer	Respiratory or cardiac failure
Immobilization	Pharmacological sedation
Obesity	Mechanical ventilation
Pregnancy	Central venous catheter
Trauma, spinal cord injury	End-stage renal failure
Recent surgery	
Stroke	

Source: data from Hegazi, R., et al. Clinical review: optimizing enteral nutrition for critically ill patients – a simple data-driven formula. *Critical Care* 2011; 15:234. Copyright © 2006 BioMed Central Ltd.

> **⊕ Clinical tip Correct positioning of a central venous catheter**
>
> A well-positioned CVC should be ± 2 cm from the carina on the chest radiograph, with the tip not pointing at the wall of the superior vena cava. Other methods for establishing correct positioning include Peres' height formula (height (cm)/10 for the right internal jugular vein (IJV) and (height (cm)/10) + 4 cm for the left IJV) and the use of electrocardiographic guidance. Catheters that are too short may result in drug extravasation from proximal lumens that are not in the vein, an increased risk of DVT because of slow venous flow, and poor drug dissemination. Catheters that are too long or point directly at the vessel wall may result in arrhythmias, damage to the tricuspid valve, or erosion and puncture of the vessel wall (especially when larger diameter catheters are used, e.g. Vascaths).

His parenteral nutrition was discontinued, the PICC line was removed, and he was prescribed treatment dose low-molecular-weight heparin. After discussion with the general surgeons and dietician, the decision was made to commence enteral nutrition at an initial rate of 10 mL/hour. This is increased over the next 4 days; however, he developed abdominal pain, a high stoma output, and steatorrhoea. Because of this, he developed a negative fluid balance and it became difficult to maintain his electrolyte levels.

> **✪ Learning point Short bowel syndrome**
>
> Short bowel syndrome is a rare condition where patients are incapable of maintaining adequate nutrition and hydration through oral intake because of a reduction in functional intestinal area [33]. This may be the consequence of small bowel resection, when less than 200 cm of small bowel

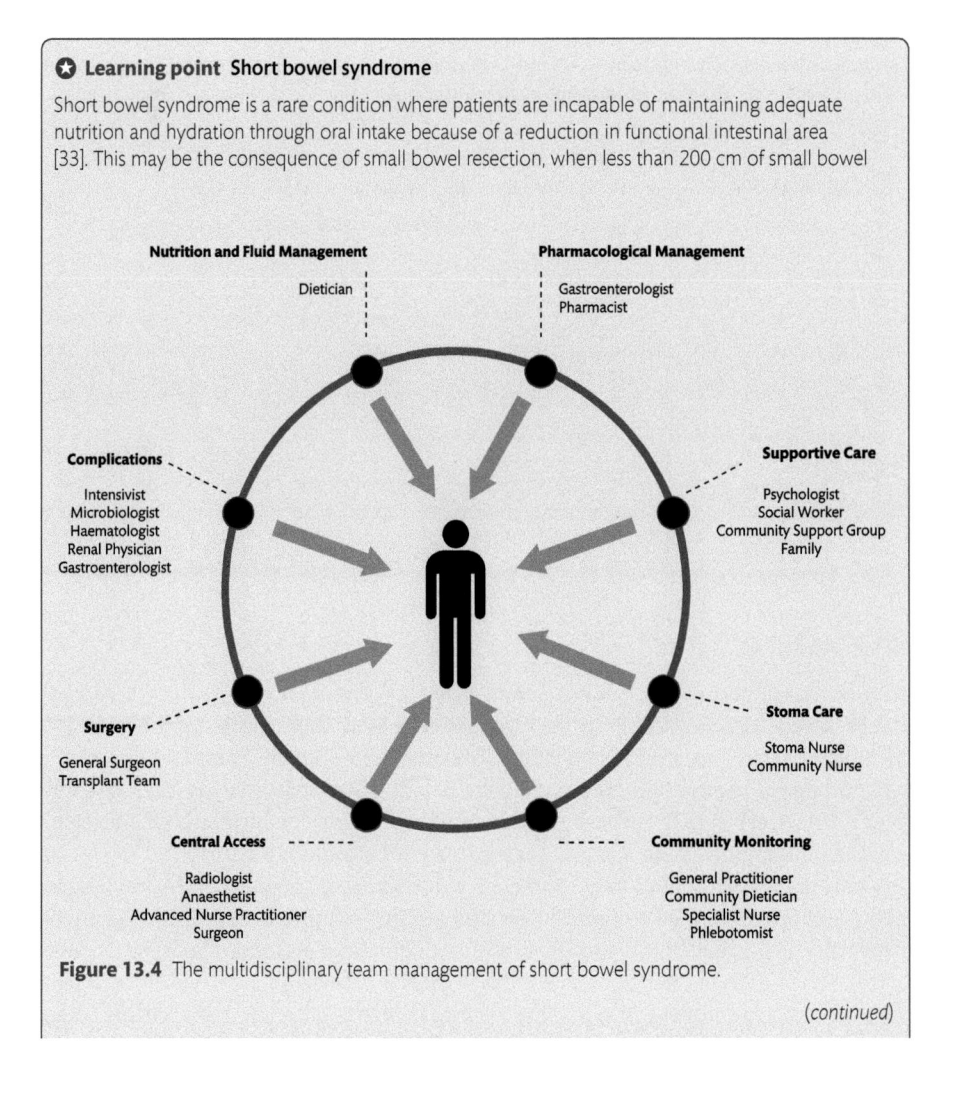

Figure 13.4 The multidisciplinary team management of short bowel syndrome.

(continued)

remains, or diseases that affect the absorptive capacity of the intestines (e.g. radiation enteritis) [34–36]. The characteristic symptoms of short bowel syndrome are:

- abdominal pain
- diarrhoea and steatorrhoea
- fluid and micronutrient depletion (often with high stoma output)
- weight loss and malnutrition
- fatigue.

Short bowel syndrome may be permanent or temporary depending on the ability of the remaining small bowel to increase its absorptive capacity. Most patients with short bowel syndrome develop complex long-term nutritional problems because of intestinal failure and require a coordinated multidisciplinary team approach to manage their disease during the acute ICU admission, on the general ward and on discharge to the community (Figure 13.4) [37].

Over the next few days he was given further micronutrients and fluid replacement intravenously and his enteral nutrition formula was altered to a low-fibre feed with medium-chain triglycerides and hydrolysed proteins. He was prescribed regular probiotic supplements and started on codeine phosphate 30 mg four times daily. A multidisciplinary team meeting was held to discuss his long-term nutritional support and he was subsequently referred to the interventional radiology department for insertion of a tunnelled CVC for supplemental parenteral nutrition.

> ★ **Learning point** Strategies for managing a high output stoma (>1500 mL/day)
>
> 1. Exclude organic causes (e.g. infection, steroid withdrawal, subacute obstruction, and sepsis).
> 2. Restrict oral intake to 500 mL/day.
> 3. Commence loperamide 4 mg four times daily.
> 4. Add codeine phosphate 15–60 mg four times daily.
> 5. Commence omeprazole 40 mg twice daily.
> 6. Consider a trial of antibiotics for bacterial overgrowth.
> 7. Commence St Mark's glucose–electrolyte replacement solution and consider keeping nil by mouth for 24–48 hours.
> 8. Increase loperamide dose to 8 mg four times daily.
> 9. Further increase loperamide dose by 2–4 mg.
> 10. Consider octreotide 200 micrograms three times daily for 3–4 days.

Discussion

Nutritional support is an evolving area of intensive care medicine that has the potential to have a significant impact on mortality and morbidity. Feeding protocols have historically been based on poor-quality observational or single-centre studies, which have produced inconsistent and conflicting results. There has recently been a resurgence of interest in ICU nutrition with investment in larger multicentre RCTs investigating both pragmatic and specific questions about nutritional support [7].

Nutrition is clearly important for recovery from critical illness [38–40]. Deciding on how to optimally provide cost-effective support in this complex heterogeneous group of patients is a real challenge. Critically ill patients often have gastrointestinal dysfunction and have multiple interruptions to feeding regimens because of the need for recurrent surgery, radiological investigations, and dislodgment/complications with feeding tubes or vascular access. This results in a progressive energy deficit and it is now increasingly apparent that most ICU patients regularly fail to reach their nutritional targets [7]. This is compounded by the fact that feeding guidelines have previously favoured enteral nutrition because of concerns about the risks of parenteral nutrition [4, 41]. However, the increased incidence of infective complications, previously associated with parenteral nutrition, is now less evident [6, 7]. This has facilitated a change in practice to earlier initiation of parenteral nutrition in patients failing to tolerate enteral nutrition and will hopefully translate into improved levels of nutrition and patient outcomes in future.

Tailoring nutritional formulas more specifically to patient and clinical characteristics is another area of development [10], and a wider range of feeds, additives, and supplements is now available to support this. It is likely that nutrition will increasingly be considered in terms of a therapeutic option as opposed to just providing generic support. Similarly, improved matching of the type and amount of nutritional support at the various stages of critical illness may help to mitigate the prevalence and effects of under- and overfeeding. This will rely on an improved understanding of the patterns of critical illness and the establishment of more robust mechanisms for determining optimal macro- and micronutrient requirements. Nutrition in critical care is ultimately going through a transition from a 'one-size-fits-all' approach to a more disease- and patient-specific approach to prescribing.

A final word from expert

As with the rest of medicine, critical care nutrition is moving towards a protocolized but personalized approach. Both patient- and disease-related factors will influence the route, volume, and content of nutritional supplementation. Thus, while there is a clear benefit in conducting large-scale RCTs, the need for focused evaluations in specific groups of patients should not be overlooked, and may explain the reason why many large trials are unable to find significant differences between therapeutic approaches. Further, the role of technology advancement and improvements in the prevention of infection associated with intravenous catheterization mean that previous concerns about parenteral nutrition can be overcome with careful attention to detail in high-quality generic patient care. The input of critical care dieticians is important in developing a safe and effective approach to feeding. Gastrointestinal dysfunction can drive both malnutrition and the risk of infectious complications, thus vigilance and maintenance of nutrition via the parenteral route if required are important principles of management. Future advances, including developing approaches to measuring demand (by using indirect calorimetry) so that supply can be more accurately matched to nutritional demand, may present opportunities for quality improvement in this field.

References

1. Alberda C, Gramlich L, Jones N, et al. The relationship between nutritional in- take and clinical outcomes in critically ill patients: results of an international multi-center observational study. *Intensive Care Med.* 2009;35:1728–37.
2. Peuhkuri K, Vapaatalo H, Korpela R. Even low-grade inflammation impacts on small intestinal function. *World J Gastroenterol.* 2010;16:1057–62.

3. Casaer M, Van den Berghe G. Nutrition in the acute phase of critical illness. *N Engl J Med.* 2014;370:1227–36.

4. Casaer M, Mesotten D, Hermans, et al. Early versus late parenteral nutrition in critically ill adults. *N Engl J Med.* 2011;365:506–17.

5. Rice T, Wheeler A, Thompson B, et al. Initial trophic vs full enteral feeding in patients with acute lung injury: the EDEN randomized trial. *JAMA.* 2012;307:795–803.

6. Singer P, Anbar R, Cohen J, et al. The tight calorie control study (TICACOS): a prospective, randomized, controlled pilot study of nutritional support in critically ill patients. *Intensive Care Med.* 2011;37:601–9.

7. Harvey S, Parrott F, Harrison, et al. Trial of the route of early nutritional support in critically ill adults (CALORIES). *N Engl J Med.* 2014;371:1673–84.

8. Bratanow S, Brown S. Nutrition in the critically ill. *Update Anaesth.* 2012;28:79–87.

9. National Institute for Health and Care Excellence (NICE). *Nutrition Support in Adults: Oral Nutrition Support, Enteral Tube Feeding and Parenteral Nutrition.* Clinical guideline [CG32]. London: NICE; 2006. Available from: https://www.nice.org.uk/guidance/cg32.

10. Hegazi R, Wischmeyer P. Clinical review: optimizing enteral nutrition for critically ill patients—a simple data-driven formula. *Crit Care.* 2011;15:234.

11. Angstwurm M, Engelmann L, Zimmermann T, et al. Selenium in intensive Care (SIC): results of a prospective randomized, placebo-controlled, multi-center study in patients with severe systemic inflammatory response syndrome, sepsis, and septic shock. *Crit Care Med.* 2007;35:118–26.

12. Amrein K, Schnedl C, Holl A, et al. Effect of high-dose vitamin D3 on hospital length of stay in critically ill patients with vitamin D deficiency: the VITdAL-ICU randomized clinical trial. *JAMA.* 2014;312:1520–30.

13. Lochs H, Valentini L, Schutz T, et al. ESPEN Guidelines for adult enteral nutrition. *Clin Nutr.* 2006;25:177–360.

14. Cano N, Aparicio M, Brunori G, et al. ESPEN Guidelines for adult parenteral nutrition. *Clin Nutr.* 2009;28:359–479.

15. McClave S, Taylor B, Martindale R, et al. Guidelines for the provision and assessment of nutrition support therapy in the adult critically ill patient. *JPEN J Parenter Enteral Nutr.* 2016;40:159–211.

16. Reignier J, Mercier E, Le Gouge, et al. Effect of not monitoring residual gastric volume on risk of ventilator-associated pneumonia in adults receiving mechanical ventilation and early enteral feeding. *JAMA.* 2013;309:249–56.

17. Pinilla J, Samphire J, Arnold C, et al. Comparison of gastrointestinal tolerance to two enteral feeding protocols in critically ill patients: a prospective, randomized controlled trial. *JPEN J Parenter Enteral Nutr.* 2001;25:81–6.

18. Montejo J, Minambres E, Bordeje L, et al. Gastric residual volume during enteral nutrition in ICU patients: the REGANE study. *Intensive Care Med.* 2010;36:1386–93.

19. Tleyjey I, Bin Abdulhak A, Riaz M, et al. Association between proton pump inhibitor therapy and Clostridium difficile infection: a contemporary systematic review and meta-analysis. *Plos One.* 2012;7:e50836.

20. Kwok C, Arthur A, Anibueze C, et al. Risk of Clostridium difficile infection with acid suppressing drugs and antibiotics: meta-analysis. *Am J Gastroenterol.* 2012;107:1011–19.

21. Janarthanan S, Ditah I, Adler D and Ehrinpresis M. Clostrisium difficile—associated diarrhoea and proton pump inhibitor therapy: a meta-analysis. *Am J Gastroenterol.* 2012;107:1001–10.

22. Alshamsi F, Belley-Cote E, Cook D, et al. Efficacy and safety of proton pump inhibitors for stress ulcer prophylaxis in critically ill patients: a systematic review and meta-analysis of randomized trials. *Crit Care.* 2016;20:120.

23. Pittiruti M, Hamilton H, Biffi R, et al. ESPEN guidelines on parenteral nutrition: central venous catheters (access, care, diagnosis and therapy complications). *Clin Nutr*. 2009;28:365–77.

24. Parienti J-J, Mongardon N, Megarbane B, et al. Intravascular complications of central venous catheterization by insertion site. *N Engl J Med*. 2015;373:1220–9.

25. Pascall E, Trehane S-J, Georgiou A, Cook TM. Litigation associated with intensive care unit treatment in England: an analysis of NHSLA data 1995–2012. *Br J Anaesth*. 2015;115:601–7.

26. Marschall J, Leonard M, Fakih M, et al. Strategies to prevent central line-associated bloodstream infections in acute care hospitals: 2014 update. *Infect Control Hosp Epidemiol*. 2014;35:772–96.

27. McGee D, Gould K. Preventing complications of central venous catheterization. *N Engl J Med*. 2003;348:1123–33.

28. Mermel L, Allon M, Bouza E, et al. Clinical practice guidelines for the diagnosis and management of intravascular catheter-related infection: 2009 update by the Infectious Diseases Society of America. *Clin Infect Dis*. 2009;49:1–45.

29. Mehanna H, Moledina J, Travis J. Refeeding syndrome: what it is, and how to prevent it. *BMJ*. 2008;336:1495–8.

30. Adriance S, Murphy C. Prophylaxis and treatment of venous thromboembolism in the critically ill. *Int J Crit Illn Inj Sci*. 2013;3:143–51.

31. Minet C, Potton L, Bonadona A, et al. Venous thromboembolism in the ICU: main characteristics, diagnosis and thromboprophylaxis. *Crit Care*. 2015;19:287.

32. Smith R, Nolan J. Central venous catheters. *BMJ*. 2013;347:f6570.

33. Storch K. Overview of short bowel syndrome: clinical features, pathophysiology, impact and management. *JPEN J Parenter Enteral Nutr*. 2014;38:5S–7S.

34. Pironi L, Arends J, Baxter J, et al. ESPEN endorsed recommendations. Definition and classification of intestinal failure in adults. *Clin Nutr*. 2015;34:171–80.

35. O'Keefe S, Buchman A, Fishbein T, et al. Short bowel syndrome and intestinal failure: consensus definitions and overview. *Clin Gastroenterol Hepatol*. 2006;4:6–10.

36. Buchman A, Scolapio J, Fryer J. AGA technical review on short bowel syndrome and intestinal transplantation. *Gastroenterology*. 2003;124:1111–34.

37. Matarese L, Jeppesen P, O'Keefe S. Short bowel syndrome in adults: the need for an interdisciplinary approach and coordinated care. *JPEN J Parenter Enteral Nutr*. 2014;38:60S–64S.

38. Sandstrom R, Drott C, Hyltander A, et al. The effect of postoperative intravenous feeding (TPN) on outcome following major surgery evaluated in a randomized study. *Ann Surg*. 1993;217:185–95.

39. Simpson F, Doig GS. Parenteral vs. enteral nutrition in the critically ill patient: a meta-analysis of trials using the intention to treat principle. *Intensive Care Med*. 2005;31:12–23.

40. Giner M, Laviano A, Mequid MM, Gleason JR. In 1995 a correlation between malnutrition and poor outcome in critically ill patients still exists. *Nutrition*. 1996;12:23–9.

41. Gramlich L, Kichian K, Pinilla J, et al. Does enteral nutrition compared to parenteral nutrition result in better outcomes in critically ill adult patients? A systematic review of the literature. *Nutrition*. 2004;20:843–8.

14 Malignancy and critical illness

Nishita Desai

✪ **Expert Commentary** Gary Wares

Case history

A previously fit and well 63-year-old lady presented to her general practitioner with a 1-month history of generalized weakness and fatigue. On examination, she had an enlarged spleen and petechiae on her legs. Her blood tests revealed that she was anaemic, thrombocytopenic, and a blood film revealed blast cells. She was urgently referred to the haematology outpatient clinic and a bone marrow biopsy showed the presence of blast cells at 35%. Subsequently, she was diagnosed with acute myeloid leukaemia. She was admitted to hospital electively and underwent an allogenic haematopoietic stem cell transplantation (HSCT) from a human leucocyte antigen (HLA)-matched unrelated donor with a reduced-intensity myeloablative preconditioning regimen comprising total body irradiation and FMC (fludarabine, melphalan, and alemtuzumab) chemotherapy.

During her pre-engraftment period (defined as a period up to 30 days post HSCT), from day 5 after HSCT she was reviewed regularly by the critical care outreach team because of a high National Early Warning Score (NEWS) of 5 [1]. She had a productive cough and, given the high risk of pneumonia, was commenced on a 7-day course of intravenous Tazocin (piperacillin/tazobactam) and clarithromycin and oral oseltamivir. She was already taking prophylactic co-trimoxazole and fluconazole as part of the post-HSCT regimen. On day 11 after the HSCT, due to persistent pyrexia, tachypnoea, and an additional oxygen requirement of 4 L/min, in consultation with microbiology, her antibiotics were changed to intravenous (IV) meropenem. On day 13 after the HSCT, her clinical condition deteriorated further and she was reviewed urgently by the critical care outreach team because of hypotension, a NEWS score of 7, and a quick Sequential (Sepsis-Related) Organ Failure Assessment (qSOFA) score of 3. At this point, she had a temperature of 38°C, a lactate value of 2.5 mmol/L, and her blood pressure was 78/40 mmHg following an IV infusion of 3 L of Hartmann's solution. Following discussion with the haematology team, the patient, and her family, the decision was made to admit her to the intensive care unit (ICU) for further investigation and management. Within 2 hours, the patient was transferred to the ICU.

⓫ Expert comment

The use of HSCT for curative treatment of malignant and non-malignant disease has increased over the last 10 years. Previously, outcomes for patients who were admitted to ICU following HSCT were poor, partly because 'treatment apathy' provoked suboptimal treatment from the outset. Overall improvements in care through initiatives such as the Surviving Sepsis Campaign [2] have led to an improvement in outcomes in many centres.

(continued)

During HSCT, haemopoietic stems cells are transfused into a recipient from a donor with the intention of repopulating and replacing the haemopoietic system. The donor cells can be the patient's own (autograft) or from another donor (allograft). The cells can be harvested from bone marrow, umbilical cord blood, or peripheral blood.

Autografts are performed using the patient's own cells when their cancer is in remission following chemotherapy and/or radiotherapy. This can be days, weeks, or months following disease control, or even after years where there has been relapse of the primary condition. The patient undergoes a period of intensive preconditioning before infusion of the autograft resulting in a period of profound immunosuppression. Engraftment and return of marrow synthetic function can take up to 25 days after the transplant and patients remain vulnerable to infective complications during this time. During an autograft, the patient acts as their own donor so risks of incompatibility, graft-versus-host disease (GvHD), and the requirement for long-term immunosuppression are negated. There is a low early mortality from autografts, with large-volume centres expecting a mortality of less than 5% and a much lower long-term morbidity profile compared to allograft HSCT. There is a risk of repopulating the patient's marrow with tumour cells and the risk of recurrence in subsequent years.

Allografts involve a more intensive preconditioning regimen with chemotherapy and/or radiotherapy causing early profound immunosuppression to the same extent as autografts; however, the patient's marrow is repopulated with cells that have antigenic properties. Donors and recipients are matched to the same HLA profile. Cytomegalovirus (CMV) status is matched between donor and recipient to ensure that avoidable CMV reactivation with potential for disseminated CMV infection is minimized in the post-transplant period. Immunosuppression is also required to prevent graft rejection and to reduce the incidence of GvHD. Allogenic transplantation has a high morbidity and mortality (20–40% in the early treatment phase) and is usually offered to patients with limited comorbidities who are younger and able to tolerate the more intensive conditioning regimens. Because of the intensive preconditioning, early mortality in allogenic stem cell transplant is in the order of 20%, but is sometimes the only chance of a cure.

Having undergone HSCT, patients present many challenges to the critical care team both during and after their initial period of treatment. They often present diagnostic and therapeutic quandaries for a team that may not be experienced in treating such patients. The immunosuppression required following allograft in the presence of systemic infection may lead to therapeutic indecision and treatment delay. There may be treatment apathy among teams unfamiliar with disease progress and treatment options in such patients with complex multisystem disease. Treatment of HCST patients in high-volume centres is associated with reduced mortality [3] and, where possible, these patients should be transferred to the centre that provided the initial therapy and subsequent transplant.

The patient was admitted into a side room on the ICU and reverse-barrier nursed using protective isolation precautions. Clinical findings and examination were consistent with septic shock [4, 5], with tissue hypoperfusion, hypotension, and a raised serum lactate at 3.0 mmol/L, but she had no clear evidence of organ dysfunction at this time. Blood test results revealed the patient to be pancytopenic (Table 14.1) and following discussion with the haematology team she was commenced on granulocyte-colony stimulating factor (G-CSF). Following discussion with the microbiologist, therapeutic-dose IV co-trimoxazole and anidulafungin was started. The patient was already on IV meropenem, having already completed the course of IV Tazocin and clarythromycin. In view of her deterioration and diagnosis of neutropenic sepsis, antibiotics were escalated to include IV amikacin (requiring drug monitoring with daily trough levels).

Table 14.1 Initial blood results

Blood test	Result	Reference range
Haemoglobin (g/L)	80	115–165
Platelets (× 10⁹/L)	72	140–400
White cell count (× 10⁹/L)	0.8	3.6–11
Neutrophils (× 10⁹/L)	0.1	1.8–7.5
Lymphocytes (× 10⁹/L)	0.5	1.0–4.0
Sodium (mmol/L)	141	135–145
Potassium (mmol/L)	4.7	3.5–5
Urea (mmol/L)	10	1.2–8
Creatinine (µmol/L)	108	70–100
Bilirubin (µmol/L)	10	3–22
ALP (U/L)	115	9–52
GGT (U/L)	66	12–43
AST (U/L)	55	14–36
Albumin (g/L)	18	34–48
CRP (mg/L)	200	<5

ALP, alkaline phosphatase; AST, aspartate transaminase; CRP, C-reactive protein; GGT, gamma glutamyl transferase.

> ✪ **Learning point Management of neutropenic sepsis**
>
> Mortality from neutropenic sepsis is between 45% and 50% among critically ill patients admitted to ICUs [6] and it is therefore considered an acute medical emergency. Neutropenic sepsis as defined by the National Institute for Health and Care Excellence (NICE) is an absolute neutrophil count of 0.5 × 10⁹/L or less (neutropenia) in association with a temperature higher than 38 °C (fever) or other signs and symptoms consistent with clinically significant sepsis [7]. Patients are at risk of severe neutropenia and bacterial infections in the pre-engraftment period (up to 30 days after HSCT). It is important to identify neutropenic fever early and look for signs and symptoms of infection and evidence of systemic inflammation.
>
> Low-risk patients can be discharged home with oral antibiotics and outpatient follow-up. High-risk patients should be given IV broad-spectrum antimicrobials within 60 min of presentation. High-risk patients are those expected to be neutropenic for more than 7 days with active comorbidities or ongoing organ dysfunction. Effort should be made to conduct appropriate microbiological surveillance including two sets of blood cultures and urine cultures before starting antimicrobials. The patient should be isolated and full reverse-barrier precautions should be undertaken by staff and visitors.
>
> The choice of antimicrobial therapy will depend on several factors including the degree of immunosuppression, infection history, previous antimicrobial use, and local patterns of antimicrobial exposure and resistance. There is some debate on whether initial empirical monotherapy or combination therapy should be used. Advantages of combination therapy include broad-spectrum coverage and possible synergistic activity which may reduce resistant strains. However, cost and significant side effects such as ototoxicity and nephrotoxicity are important disadvantages to combination therapy. No randomized controlled trial or meta-analysis has provided evidence that adding an aminoglycoside or quinolone to a beta-lactam is superior to broad-spectrum beta-lactam alone. Meta-analysis has shown that initially, monotherapy with an anti-pseudomonal beta-lactam agent should be considered [8]. In the UK, the current NICE recommendation is piperacillin-tazobactam (Tazocin) as first-line empirical therapy [7]. NICE and the Infectious Diseases Society of America guidelines [9] have specific antibiotic recommendations for high-risk patients with neutropenic sepsis (Figure 14.1). Although most episodes of febrile neutropenia are assumed to be caused by an infection, blood cultures are positive in less than 30% of febrile neutropenic episodes [10]. It is important to maintain antibiotic stewardship and switch from intravenous to oral antibiotics after 48 hours in patients whose risk of developing septic complications has been reassessed to be low.
>
> *(continued)*

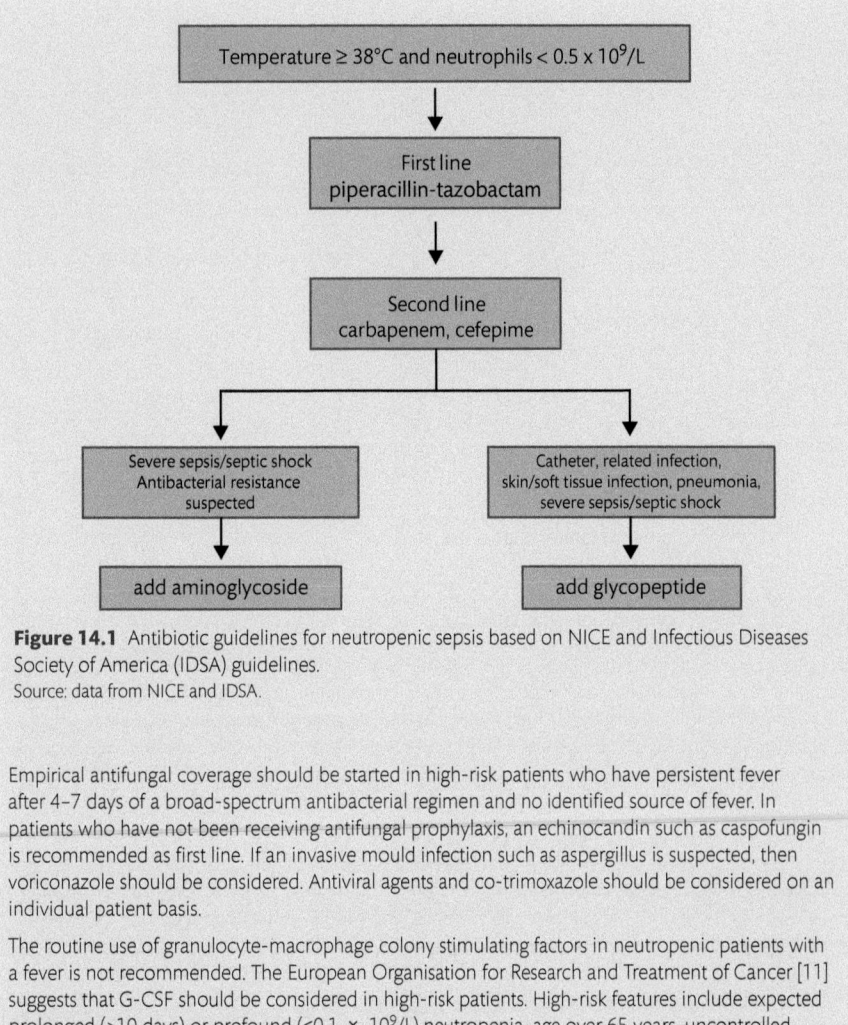

Figure 14.1 Antibiotic guidelines for neutropenic sepsis based on NICE and Infectious Diseases Society of America (IDSA) guidelines.
Source: data from NICE and IDSA.

Empirical antifungal coverage should be started in high-risk patients who have persistent fever after 4–7 days of a broad-spectrum antibacterial regimen and no identified source of fever. In patients who have not been receiving antifungal prophylaxis, an echinocandin such as caspofungin is recommended as first line. If an invasive mould infection such as aspergillus is suspected, then voriconazole should be considered. Antiviral agents and co-trimoxazole should be considered on an individual patient basis.

The routine use of granulocyte-macrophage colony stimulating factors in neutropenic patients with a fever is not recommended. The European Organisation for Research and Treatment of Cancer [11] suggests that G-CSF should be considered in high-risk patients. High-risk features include expected prolonged (>10 days) or profound ($\leq$0.1 $\times$ 10^9/L) neutropenia, age over 65 years, uncontrolled primary disease, pneumonia, hypotension, and multiorgan dysfunction, invasive fungal infection, or being hospitalized at the time of the developing fever.

⊗ **Learning point Fungal infections**

The incidence of fungal infections is 10–20% after HSCT. Allogenic HSCT transplant recipients and patients with severe GvHD are at the highest risk of serious invasive fungal infections from yeasts and moulds. Other risk factors include previous azole exposure, prior colonization, prolonged antibiotic use, duration and severity of neutropenia, use of corticosteroids, and gastrointestinal damage caused by total body irradiation or chemotherapy with high-dose cytosine arabinoside [12]. Fifty per cent of individuals are colonized with *Candida albicans* and this is the most common fungal infection in the pre-engraftment period (Figure 14.2), due to breakdown of the gastrointestinal mucosa caused by chemotherapy or GvHD. Azoles, such as fluconazole, are the most common prophylactic antifungal: they reduce the number of invasive fungal infections and decrease all-cause mortality [13]. Although mould-active prophylaxis (e.g. voriconazole or amphotericin), compared with fluconazole prophylaxis, significantly reduces fungal infection-related

(continued)

mortality in cancer patients receiving chemotherapy or HSCT, it also increases adverse effects and does not reduce all-cause mortality [14].

The engraftment period is usually from 3 weeks to 3 months. During the immediate and late post-engraftment period, during which the T-cells begin to recover, infection with *Aspergillus* spp. is the most common. The use of prophylactic fluconazole has reduced invasive *C. albicans* infection, but has led to an increase in invasive mould infections, particularly with *Aspergillus* spp., *Pneumocystis jirovecii* pneumonia (PJP) occurs late after transplant and is discussed in detail later.

Concerns over antimicrobial resistance, toxicity, drug interactions, over-treatment, and cost have limited routine antifungal prophylaxis. Anti-candida prophylaxis with fluconazole is recommended in selected high risk solid-organ transplant recipients, patients with chemotherapy-induced neutropenia, HSCT recipients with neutropenia, and those receiving allogenic HSCT. Posaconazole, caspofungin, and itraconazole are alternatives. Treatment with echinocandins such as caspofungin, micafungin, and anidulafungin is recommended for candidaemia in neutropenic patients. For patients who are less critically ill with no previous exposure to azoles, fluconazole is a reasonable alternative. Recommended duration of treatment is 14 days after resolution of attributable signs and symptoms, clearance of the bloodstream of *Candida* spp. and recovery of neutropenia. Removal of indwelling catheters is recommended if practical.

In patients who are at high risk of invasive aspergillosis (e.g. HSCT recipients requiring high-dose steroids for GvHD or those with a history of invasive aspergillosis), prophylaxis with a mould-active extended spectrum azole (voriconazole or posaconazole) is recommended. For the treatment of invasive aspergillosis, voriconazole is recommended as first line. Liposomal amphotericin B, caspofungin, micafungin, and posaconazole are all second line.

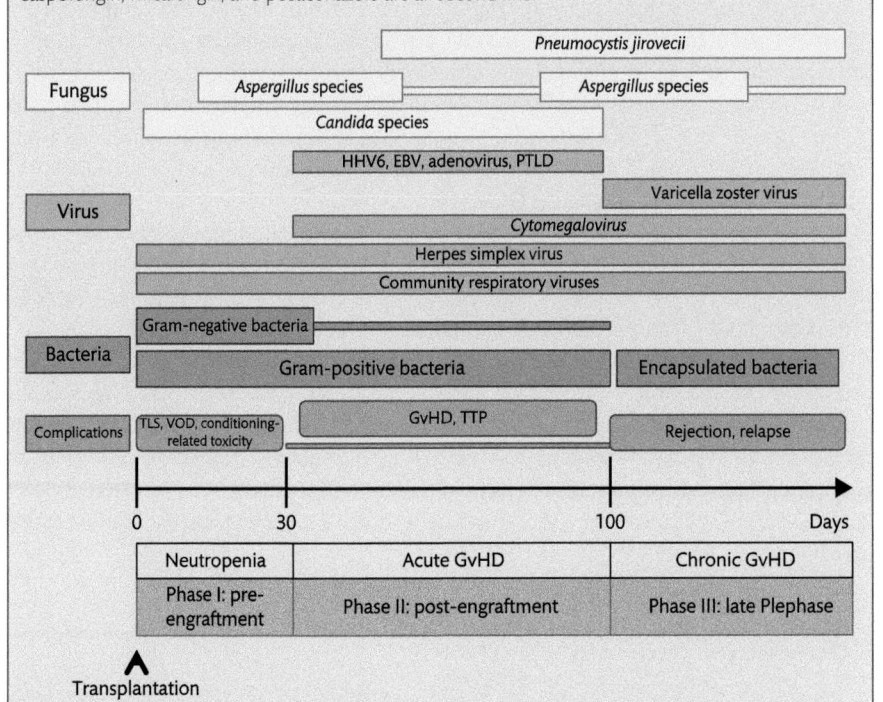

Figure 14.2 Phases of opportunistic infections and complications in allogenic HSCT recipients. EBV, Epstein–Barr virus; HHV6, human herpes virus 6; PTLD, post-transplant lymphoproliferative disorder; TLS, tumour lysis syndrome; TTP, thrombotic thrombocytopenia purpura; VOD, hepatic veno-occlusive disease.

Source: data from Kedia, S. et al. Infectious Complications of Hematopoietic Stem Cell Transplantation. *Journal of Stem Cell Research & Therapy.* 2013; S3: 2. Copyright © 2013 OMICS International—Open Access Publisher.

On admission to the ICU, an internal jugular central venous catheter (CVC) and a radial arterial line were inserted. Following ongoing fluid resuscitation guided by dynamic cardiac output monitoring with a LiDCO (Lithium Dilution Cardiac Output) monitor, she was started on 0.1 mcg/kg/min of noradrenaline to maintain her mean arterial blood pressure (MAP) above 65 mmHg. During the first day in the ICU, her arterial blood gases indicated worsening hypoxaemia (partial pressure of arterial oxygen (PaO_2) 7.0 kPa on 0.6 fraction of inspired oxygen (FiO_2) via facemask). Nasal high-flow oxygen was started. Alongside the initial blood tests (Table 14.1), a full septic screen was sent to microbiology including blood, urine and sputum cultures, and a respiratory viral screen. A chest X-ray showed bilateral interstitial shadowing, worse bi-basally, suggestive of severe bilateral pneumonia.

By day 3 on the ICU she had deteriorated further, now requiring an FiO_2 of 0.9 with flows of 50 L/min cmH_2O. She was visibly tiring, with use of accessory muscles. Following discussion with the patient, her family, and the haematology team, the decision was made to intubate her trachea for airway protection, bronchial toileting, and ventilation.

She was preoxygenated with FiO_2 1.0 on continuous positive airway pressure of 10 cmH_2O, induced with a rapid sequence induction. An 8 mm internal diameter tracheal tube with a subglottic suction port was inserted. Mechanical ventilation was started with tidal volumes of 6 mL/kg ideal body weight and positive end-expiratory pressure of 12 cm H_2O. She was maintained with deep sedation and an atracurium infusion was started to eliminate respiratory effort. After a period of assessment, as she remained hypoxaemic despite an FiO_2 of 1.0 she was turned prone. She was maintained prone for 16 hours daily and lung protective ventilation was maintained with permissive hypercapnia and a target peripheral capillary oxygen saturation of 88–92% [15]. This is discussed further in Case 3.

On day 5 of admission, when she was more stable, she underwent a chest computed tomography scan. This did not show evidence of pulmonary embolism but there were lung parenchymal changes with ground-glass change within the lungs bilaterally. The differential diagnosis included an infection or a drug reaction (Figure 14.3).

There were no positive microbiological cultures to date. Influenza A and B polymerase chain reaction (PCR) assays were negative, so oseltamivir was discontinued. Serum beta-d-glucan assay was positive at 200 pg/mL (> 80 pg/mL positive) and galactomannan serum antigen was negative (< 0.5 index). Collectively these results suggested that an invasive aspergillus infection was unlikely but indicated the possibility of a *P. jirovecii* infection. Treatment-dose IV co-trimoxazole, anidulafungin, meropenem, and amikacin were continued.

> ✚ **Clinical tip** Bronchoalveolar lavage
>
> Often microbiological cultures are negative. Consider bronchoalveolar lavage early, if safe to do so, so that samples for PCR and microscopy and culture can be obtained.

> ✪ **Learning point** Biomarkers for fungal infection
>
> Invasive fungal infections can be difficult to diagnose, particularly invasive *Aspergillus* spp. Inhalation of *Aspergillus* spp. is common, so culture isolation from the airway does not necessarily indicate disease: conversely, many patients with invasive *Aspergillus* are culture negative. The gold standard for diagnosis is a tissue biopsy with microscopic visualization of the organism but biopsy is frequently not feasible, is associated with significant risks, and microscopic examination and culture can be insensitive. While PCR has been used for the diagnosis of *P. jirovecii, Candida* spp., and *Cryptococcus* infections, it has shown mixed results for aspergillosis. Imaging can be useful but again is non-specific. Serum biomarkers may therefore provide a non-invasive approach to establishing invasive fungal infection.
>
> *(continued)*

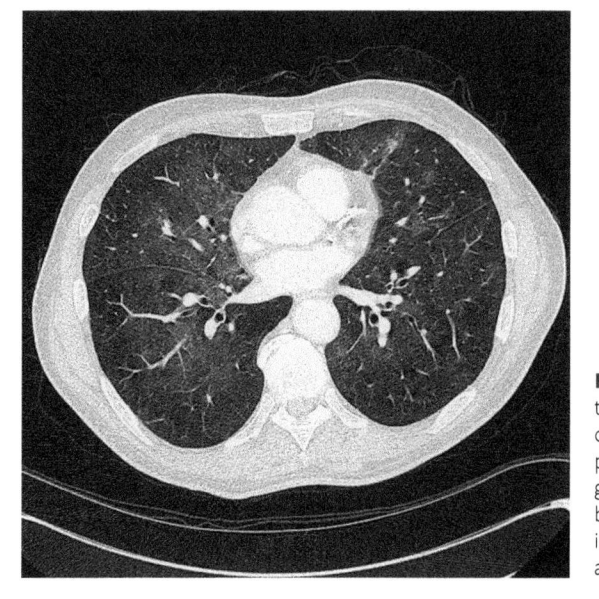

Figure 14.3 Chest computed tomography scan on day 5 of admission, showing lung parenchymal changes with ground-glass change within the lungs bilaterally. The differential diagnosis in this case included an infection or a drug reaction.

Beta-d-glucan is a cell wall component of many fungi including *Candida* spp. and *P. jirovecii*, which makes it useful for diagnosing invasive fungal infection with these organisms but not for invasive aspergillosis. It has a high negative predictive value, making it useful in excluding fungal infection, and it can also be useful when invasive fungal infection is suspected [16]. It is sensitive for *P. jirovecii* and may be used as a screening tool [17].

Galactomannan is a polysaccharide found in fungal cell walls and is a major constituent of the *Aspergillus* cell wall. Galactomannan antigen detection via enzyme immunoassay in serum or bronchoalveolar lavage fluid is relatively specific for invasive *Aspergillus* [18]. Serum screening can be used once or twice weekly to detect invasive fungal infection before clinical signs and symptoms develop, but it has a greater predictive value when there is a high clinical suspicion of infection. False positives can occur in patients who are taking certain beta-lactam antibiotics, with other organisms such as *Penicillium* spp., *Cryptococcus neoformans*, and *Histoplasma* spp. which share the cross-reacting antigens, in patients who may get translocation from reduced mucosal integrity, and by contamination from ingestion of certain foods (pasta, rice).

Maintain a high index of suspicion for the diagnosis of invasive fungal infection and evaluate the clinical risk. The diagnostic accuracy is improved by combining assessment of clinical risk with other diagnostic approaches such as imaging, serial measurements of galactomannan antigen, targeted beta-d-glucan, and serial PCRs.

✪ Learning point   *Pneumocystis jirovecii* pneumonia (PJP)

P. jirovecii is a specific species of pneumocystis affecting human lungs. It was previously called *P. carinii*, an organism that also infects rats, but after determining that the organism infecting humans is genetically and functionally distinct it was renamed *P. jirovecii*. It was also previously thought to be a protozoan, until 1988 when DNA analysis showed it was a fungus, albeit an unusual one lacking in ergosterol and very difficult to grow in culture [19].

PJP presents classically as gradually progressive dyspnoea, with a non-productive cough and a low-grade fever. It is commonly associated with HIV-seropositive individuals, specifically those with a low

(continued)

CD4 count or acquired immunodeficiency syndrome (AIDS). Other risk factors include haematological malignancies (particularly acute lymphoblastic leukaemia), HSCT (specifically allogenic), immunosuppressive chemotherapy, and prolonged high-dose corticosteroids. The ICU mortality of haematological patients with PJP is approximately 30%.

Diagnosis can be made by quantitative PCR, although this should be interpreted alongside clinical and radiological features [20]. Chest X-rays may show bilateral proximal interstitial infiltrates (bat's wing) and CT shows bilateral ground-glass changes with apical predominance and peripheral sparing. Infection beyond the lungs is rare.

Antimicrobial prophylaxis is highly successful in preventing PJP in immunocompromised patients at moderate to high risk. While most antifungal drugs are ineffective against *P. jirovecii*, there is some evidence that echinocandins particularly micafungin may be effective. Co-trimoxazole (trimethoprim–sulfamethoxazole) is first line for prophylaxis and treatment [21]. Second line drugs include dapsone, pentamidine, clindamycin–primaquine, and atovaquone.

High-dose steroid therapy is an effective adjunct during treatment of AIDS-related PJP, because it blunts the inflammatory response and is associated with reduced mortality [22]. In non-HIV-related PJP, there are few studies exploring the use and efficacy of corticosteroids and results are conflicting. Many patients with haematological malignancies who develop PJP are already taking steroids but if not, they can be given to those who develop moderate/severe PJP.

ⓕ Expert comment

Maintain a high index of suspicion for infective complications in these patients and start broad-spectrum cover early based on the local knowledge base of sensitivity patterns. The impact of *P. jirovecii* has changed dramatically over the last 10 years and infections are becoming rarer because of the use of prophylactic co-trimoxazole. A beta-d-glucan assay can help to direct therapy towards PJP, although full investigations include a bronchoalveolar lavage and PCR analysis of the lavage fluid for PJP as well as other bacterial cultures and viral PCR studies. High-resolution CT is useful in the investigation of invasive pulmonary fungal disease.

Broad-spectrum antibacterial, antifungal, and, where appropriate, antiviral therapy is started as soon as cultures have been taken; in practice, these are often started before a full infective screen has been completed.

Consider the CMV status of the patient and start an antiviral agent such as ganciclovir if clinical suspicion for CMV reactivation is high. As ganciclovir is immunosuppressive, it may have to be changed to an alternative agent if there is bone marrow suppression. Diagnosis is confirmed by PCR for viral antigens or CMV DNA polymerase.

On day 7 of ICU admission, oxygenation and ventilation improved. However, hypotension, which was poorly fluid responsive, persisted and she was vasodilated and oligoanuric. A procalcitonin (PCT) assay was higher than 10 ng/mL, which suggested an ongoing bacterial infection. Her CVC was changed (and cultured) and a dialysis catheter was inserted in preparation for renal replacement therapy. Antibiotics were changed empirically on microbiological advice to IV vancomycin, teicoplanin, and voriconazole. Amikacin and co-trimoxazole were continued. Meropenem was stopped.

Renal replacement therapy was started with a 35 mL/kg/hour exchange rate for a severe metabolic acidosis and acute kidney injury (see Case 12). A transthoracic echocardiogram showed a hyperdynamic left ventricle, pulmonary hypertension (systolic pulmonary arterial pressure 70 mmHg), with moderate tricuspid regurgitation and moderate right ventricular failure. The patient had developed acute right ventricular failure secondary to her severe acute respiratory distress syndrome.

On day 10 of the ICU admission, the patient developed diarrhoea, stopped absorbing her nasogastric feeds, and the plasma bilirubin increased to 150 µmol/L and gamma glutamyl transferase to 40 U/L. In view of progressive multiorgan failure (respiratory, cardiovascular, renal, and now gut) there was a suspicion of GvHD. Stools samples were negative for *Clostridium difficile* antigen and toxin. After seeking haematological advice, high-dose methylprednisolone was started.

✚ Clinical tip Central venous catheter-related bloodstream infections

It is often difficult to confirm that a CVC is the source of infection in bacteraemia or fungaemia. There may be no evidence of infection at the insertion site, and the organisms involved are frequently part of the normal skin flora and are common contaminants of blood cultures. A differential quantitative blood culture using time to positivity can be considered: blood cultures taken from the CVC will have a higher bacterial load than those taken peripherally, and therefore a shorter time to positivity. If central blood cultures become positive at least 120 min before peripheral blood cultures taken simultaneously, the CVC is the more likely source of infection [23], though not all studies confirm this result. In the UK, recommendations from Public Heath England [24] are that diagnosis of catheter-related bacteraemia be based on isolation of the same organism from the blood and purulent CVC insertion site or CVC tip. Alternately, catheter-related bloodstream infection can be diagnosed if there is clinical sepsis that is unresponsive to antimicrobial therapy and that resolves on catheter removal. Routine remove of central venous access devices as part of the initial empiric management of suspected neutropenic sepsis is not recommended and should be considered only if there is confirmed infection with *Staphylococcus aureus*, *Pseudomonas aeruginosa*, or *Candida* spp. [10].

✪ Learning point Procalcitonin (PCT)

The management of patients with malignancy (particularly haematological malignancy) and fever can be challenging. It can be difficult to determine whether the fever is related to infection or other causes; including blood transfusions, disease burden, medications, or other disease processes such a GvHD. Conventional markers of sepsis such as C-reactive protein (CRP) and white cell counts can be challenging to interpret in patients who are immunosuppressed and these markers lack sensitivity for bacterial infections. This can lead to unnecessary, prolonged antimicrobial treatment which risks or perpetuates antibiotic resistance. PCT is a useful biomarker for detection of bacteraemia in febrile neutropenia and has a better diagnostic value than CRP [25].

PCT is a peptide precursor of calcitonin, a hormone synthetized by the thyroid parafollicular C cells and involved in calcium homeostasis. It is also produced and released as an acute phase protein by the neuroendocrine cells of the lung and intestine in response to endotoxin and inflammatory cytokines released in response to bacterial infections. For this reason, PCT has been considered as a marker for the diagnosis of bacterial infection and to aid antibiotic stewardship, by enabling earlier cessation of treatment [26]. Serum PCT release in response to viral infections and non-infectious inflammatory stimuli (e.g. autoimmune disease and chronic inflammatory processes) is much less pronounced and rarely exceeds 0.5 ng/mL. It is not metabolized and has a half-life of 30 hours. A PCT-based algorithm for antibiotic discontinuation has been shown to be a cost-effective way of reducing antibiotic exposure [27, 28]. In patients with sepsis, higher PCT values are associated with a greater risk of progression to severe sepsis/septic shock and values fall with successful treatment. Persistent or recurrent PCT elevation may indicate secondary infection. False-positive elevated PCT levels can be caused by massive cell death, such as burns and other microbial infections. False negatives can be seen in early infection or localized infection such as an abscess. PCT can therefore be a useful aid for the diagnosis and risk stratification of bacterial sepsis, choice and timing of the initiation of antibiotic treatment, and in deciding when to discontinue antibiotics. Its routine use remains controversial and further research is required before its use is adopted widely.

> ✪ **Learning point** Graft-versus-host disease
>
> GvHD is a multisystem disorder and a common complication of allogenic HSCT, which classically develops in the early post-transplant period (<100 days). It is a T-cell-mediated disease, whereby the donor graft cells recognize the recipient host cells as foreign. The main antigenic target of the T-cells of the graft is the host major or minor histocompatibility complex molecules. The risk is greater with HLA and sex disparity between recipient and donor. Acute GvHD commonly presents with a classic maculopapular rash, persistent nausea and/or emesis, abdominal cramps with diarrhoea, and a rising serum conjugated bilirubin concentration [29]. The main organs affected are the skin, gastrointestinal tract, and liver. It is usually a diagnosis of exclusion. The differential diagnosis is wide especially in a critically ill patient and includes hepatic veno-occlusive disease (VOD) (see the learning point on 'Hepatic veno-occlusive disease'). Diagnosis can be made by taking a biopsy of the tissue involved. Treatment involves optimizing immunosuppression (usually calcineurin inhibitors such as ciclosporin or tacrolimus), high-dose methylprednisolone 2 mg/kg/day, optimizing nutrition, and use of octreotide which may reduce the diarrhoea. Patients who are refractory to steroids face a poor prognosis as second-line agents, including mycophenolate mofetil and etanercept, are less effective.

> 🕓 **Expert comment**
>
> GvHD is unique to allogenic HSCT and typically presents with one or more of a collection of problems related to eye, skin, intestine, liver, or lungs. Patients often have intractable diarrhoea with ileus, nausea, vomiting, and abdominal pain. This often results in the use of parenteral nutrition to maintain calorific requirements. Diagnosis is via a skin (where the patient has a maculopapular rash) or rectal biopsy. This will distinguish between GvHD and *Clostridium difficile* diarrhoea. As a last resort, a liver biopsy can be used to make the diagnosis. Management of acute GvHD is aimed at immunosuppression: ciclosporin, methotrexate, mycophenolate, and methylprednisolone have all been used with variable effect.

The patient deteriorated rapidly on day 11, bilirubin and gamma glutamyl transferase increased to 236 µmol/L and 300 U/L, respectively. She displayed right upper quadrant abdominal tenderness during a sedation hold. Clinically, she was grossly oedematous and her plasma albumin concentration was 10 g/L. An ultrasound examination of the liver showed no evidence of hepatomegaly or ascites. A blood film showed red cell crenation and occasional red cell fragments. There was a suspicion of hepatic VOD: defibrotide was considered but due to concerns over GvHD and poor gut absorption, it was not started. Bone marrow trephine showed an empty marrow with no haematopoiesis, and no engraftment indicating graft failure.

> ✪ **Learning point** Hepatic veno-occlusive disease
>
> Hepatic sinusoidal obstruction syndrome or hepatic VOD is a complication of allogenic and autologous HSCT. It is a life-threatening condition that usually occurs within the first 30 days after HSCT and is thought to be caused by the high-dose conditioning chemotherapy regimens that precede HSCT. The mean prevalence of VOD is 14% (range 0–60%) [30] and it causes significant morbidity and mortality with severe VOD associated with a mortality of 67–90% in the first 100 days after transplant [31]. The differential diagnosis of deranged liver function following HSCT includes GvHD, infection, drug toxicity, and VOD.
>
> VOD is characterized by damage to sinusoidal and small hepatic vein endothelium, microthrombosis, sinusoidal fibrosis, and hepatocellular necrosis. This can lead to portal hypertension, coagulopathy, fulminant acute liver failure, hepatic encephalopathy, and hepatorenal syndrome, eventually leading to multiorgan failure and death. Risk factors include pre-existing liver disease, allogenic transplant, second transplant, and lower age. The diagnosis is usually made clinically, based on the presence of hepatomegaly, ascites, raised bilirubin, and weight gain. Liver biopsy is often considered too high risk in these patients. Ultrasonography is useful to rule out other causes.
>
> *(continued)*

Treatment is largely supportive, through diuresis, renal replacement therapy, and analgesia. Recent studies using defibrotide are promising, with a complete response rate of 36–42% [31] and it has been approved by the European Medicines Agency for this indication. Defibrotide is an oligonucleotide that acts as a polydeoxyribonucleotide adenosine receptor and it has antithrombotic, anti-inflammatory, and anti-ischaemic properties. It has a protective effect against endothelial cell injury, may stimulate revascularization and has a protective effect against GvHD. Defibrotide has minimal side effects and no known toxicity. Despite reducing procoagulant activity, increasing fibrinolysis, and modulating platelet activity, its use has not been associated with an increased risk of systemic bleeding. Recent guidelines recommend the use of defibrotide in the treatment of VOD at a dose of 25 mg/kg/day [32]. Other treatments include methylprednisolone, careful fluid balance, and, in some cases, consideration of transjugular intrahepatic portosystemic shunt or hepatic transplantation.

In view of her continued deterioration with multiorgan failure (respiratory, cardiovascular, gut, and renal) despite maximal medical management, and with evidence of graft failure, her condition and progress was discussed between the clinical teams and senior nursing staff involved in her care. Her condition was judged to be unsurvivable. A family discussion took place which included the haematology team, the ICU team, and the palliative care team. After this, the decision was made to change the direction of her care from restorative to palliative care. End of life care and comfort measures were started and unnecessary life-sustaining treatment was withdrawn. She died within 12 hours with her family present.

> **✪ Learning point** Outcomes in patients with haematological and solid organ tumours admitted to the ICU in high-volume centres
>
> Outcomes of critically ill cancer patients have improved over the last decade. An increasing number of patients with solid and haematological malignancies will benefit from ICU support and this is associated with a decreased mortality. Intensivists are increasingly willing to admit patients with advanced cancer to the ICU [33]. Advances in cancer diagnosis, improvements in chemotherapy regimens, better patient selection, and improved ICU care have all contributed to better outcomes in these patients. However, prognostication remains challenging and the prognostic significance of certain risk factors has changed over time. Classic predictors of mortality in this group of patients may no longer be relevant and even those that are associated with increased mortality are often unreliable [33, 34]. Performance status and number of organ dysfunctions appear to be important in prognostication.
>
> Mortality on the ICU, although improved, remains high, with cancer patients admitted to ICU having a 25–45% mortality, which is comparable to many other diseases. Over the last decade, some units have reported a 15.7% reduction in hospital mortality of critically ill cancer patients with neutropenic sepsis [35]. Patients with haematological malignancy have the highest ICU mortality at 61% for allograft patients and 39% for autograft patients [36], though treatment in high-volume centres is associated with improved survival [3].
>
> Delayed admission to ICU of cancer patients with acute respiratory failure is associated with increased mortality [37]. A 60% mortality rate was reported in ventilated cancer patients who survived to day 5 on an ICU [38]. Cancer patients with acute respiratory distress syndrome have a 55% mortality compared to 25% in those without cancer. Longer-term outcomes following ICU admission have yet to be evaluated but more than half of cancer patients staying longer than 16 days in an ICU survive for at least 1 year [39].
>
> With poor prognostic certainty in many cases and ever improving outcomes, the focus should be on early multidisciplinary decision making and timely ICU admission when indicated, supported by good ongoing communication between clinical teams and families, and early diagnosis of the condition precipitating admission.

Discussion

This case illustrates the diagnostic and therapeutic challenges in critically ill cancer patients, focusing on high-risk patients following allogenic HSCT for haematological malignancy. It highlights some of the complexities of managing such patients, who are clearly at risk of multiorgan failure with complex pathophysiological states.

Cancer Research UK reports that more than 300,000 people are newly diagnosed with cancer every year in the UK. Overall mortality is improving; however, there is an ageing population and the incidence of cancer is increasing in the elderly and more are dying of cancer. Treatment of cancer is changing with a move towards more targeted therapy and immunotherapy with novel drugs. Over time, an improved understanding of the pathophysiology and toxicity of the novel chemotherapy drugs will facilitate better ICU management.

With improving outcomes and rising expectations, more cancer patients are admitted to ICU. Studies from high-volume specialist ICUs have shown reduced mortality and improved outcomes. Early identification of these patients, early critical care input, understanding patient expectations, and advanced care planning are all key components to high-quality care.

The approach to the management of these complex patients must be multidisciplinary. Despite optimal treatment, some of these patients will require end of life care on the ICU; this should be planned and delivered in a systematic, dignified, and compassionate way.

> **❻ Expert comment**
>
> Selecting which patient with cancer may benefit from ICU care is notoriously difficult, particularly without reliable scoring systems or clear predictors of survival. Cancer diagnosis is often associated with clinical pessimism and ICU management in this population requires considerable resource use, availability of which may vary between smaller hospitals and specialist centres. Intensivists tend to be overly pessimistic and the oncologists similarly overly optimistic. Therefore, a multidisciplinary approach needs to be adopted, requiring excellent communication between the clinical teams involved, not only at admission but also during the time spent on an ICU. Increasingly recognized is the importance of identifying patient expectations and wishes. These require careful exploration, consideration, and management. Equally important, all clinicians and the patient need to understand the goals of the cancer treatment, which may include cure or prolongation of life without cure.
>
> Traditional markers of cancer severity such as stage, disease burden, spread of disease, cycle of chemotherapy, and characteristics of the cancer are inconsistent at predicting mortality. Similarly, patient characteristics such as age and neutropenia are no longer reliable for assessing the potential benefits of ICU care and are not as relevant as previously thought. Hospital mortality is likely to be better determined by performance status, number of organ dysfunctions at admission, and the presence of haematological malignancy. Further research is required into the triage criteria for ICU referral, the survival rates after full ICU management, and the survival rates after a trial of ICU.

> **✪ Learning point** End of life decision-making and prognostication
>
> Advanced care planning before ICU admission should be instigated as early as possible—ideally before critical illness occurs—to ensure that planned care is appropriate and in accordance with the patient's values and preferences. All parties must understand the goals of ICU care and early involvement of palliative care clinicians may be important components of multidisciplinary approach to care.
>
> *(continued)*

Advanced care planning interventions may increase the frequency of out-of-hospital and out-of-ICU care and increase compliance with patients' end of life wishes. Trials of ICU care lasting 1 to 4 days may be sufficient in patients with poor-prognosis solid tumours, whereas patients with haematological malignant neoplasms or less severe illness seem to benefit from longer trials of ICU care.

Reappraise aggressive ICU management after a few days of full support. Sepsis is a frequent complication of critically ill patients with cancer: sepsis, septic shock, and the need for vasopressor use are all independent predictors of ICU mortality in patients with haematological malignancies. The multidisciplinary teams (intensivist, oncologist/haematologist, palliative care) should regularly assess treatment goals, degree of success, and suitability and where indicated, aid in changing the goals from restorative to palliative care. Postponing end of life decisions increases the physical and emotional burden on patients and relatives and such care should be timely, multidisciplinary, and focused on the patient's autonomy, dignity, and expectations.

Often 'do not attempt cardiopulmonary resuscitation' orders are completed within the first 48 hours of admission to ICU; at this time, patients are often too unwell to participate in such discussions. Such decisions should involve patients where possible, family if this is not possible, and should be reviewed regularly.

Future therapeutic and research considerations for the critically unwell cancer patient should include early palliative care involvement, advanced care planning, and better prognostication.

A final word from the expert

Improvements in outcomes for many cancer patients, particularly for those with complications of cancer treatments, mean that these patients may often benefit from ICU admission if physiological deterioration occurs. Prognostication is complex and imperfect so patients require advance planning and multidisciplinary input to determine the best management. Trials of ICU care may be appropriate in many patients for whom it would not have been appropriate 10 years ago. Included in the group of cancer patients in whom outcomes have improved and in whom ICU care is often appropriate are patients with haematological malignancies. HSCT has transformed the outcomes from haematological malignancy, but the risks and benefits must be considered when offering such therapy, especially to the patient with multiple comorbidities. Because of their complexity, these patents should ideally be managed in high-volume centres with close multidisciplinary working practices to ensure the best outcomes.

References

1. Royal College of Physicians (RCP). *National Early Warning Score (NEWS): Standardising the Assessment of Acute-Illness Severity in the NHS. Report of a Working Party.* London: RCP; 2012.
2. Rhodes A, Evans L, Aihazzani W, et al. Surviving sepsis campaign: international guidelines for management of sepsis and septic shock: 2016. *Intensive Care Med.* 2017;43:304–77.
3. Intensive Care National Audit and Research Centre. Annual quality report 2015/16 for adult critical care [Internet]. 2016. Available from: https://onlinereports.icnarc.org/Reports/2016/12/annual-quality-report-201516-for-adult-critical-care (accessed 3 July 2017).

4. Bone RC, Balk RA, Cerra FB, et al. Definitions for sepsis and organ failure and guidelines for the use of innovative therapies in sepsis. The ACCP/SCCM Consensus Conference Committee. American College of Chest Physicians/Society of Critical Care Medicine. *Chest*. 1992;101:1644–55.

5. Shankar-Hari M, Phillips GS, Levy ML, et al. Developing a new definition and assessing new clinical criteria for septic shock: for the third international consensus definitions for sepsis and septic shock (Sepsis-3). *JAMA*. 2016;315:775–87.

6. Mokart D, Darmon M, Resche-Rigon M, et al. Prognosis of neutropenic patients admitted to the intensive care unit. *Intensive Care Med*. 2015;41:296–303.

7. National Institute for Health and Care Excellence (NICE). *Neutropenic Sepsis: Prevention and Management in People with Cancer*. Clinical guideline [CG151]. London: NICE, 2012. Available from: https://www.nice.org.uk/guidance/cg151.

8. Paul M, Dickstein Y, Schlesinger A, et al. Beta-lactam versus beta-lactam-aminoglycoside combination therapy in cancer patients with neutropenia. *Cochrane Database Syst Rev*. 2013;6:CD003038.

9. Infectious Diseases Society of America (IDSA). Neutropenic sepsis guidelines [Internet]. http://www.idsociety.org/IDSA_Practice_Guidelines (accessed 12 December 2016).

10. Feld R. Bloodstream infections in cancer patients with febrile neutropenia. *Int J Antimicrob Agents*. 2008;32:S30–3.

11. Aapro MS, Bohlius J, Cameron DA, et al. 2010 update of EORTC guidelines for the use of granulocyte-colony stimulating factor to reduce the incidence of chemotherapy-induced febrile neutropenia in adult patients with lymphoproliferative disorders and solid tumours. European Organisation for Research and Treatment of Cancer. *Eur J Cancer*. 2011;47:8–332.

12. Prentice HG, Kibbler CC, Prentice AG. Towards a targeted, risk-based, antifungal strategy in neutropenic patients. *Br J Haematol*. 2000;110:273–84.

13. Robenshtok E, Gafter-Gvili A, Goldberg E, et al. Antifungal prophylaxis in cancer patients after chemotherapy or hematopoietic stem-cell transplantation: systematic review and meta-analysis. *J Clin Oncol*. 2007;25:5471–89.

14. Ethier MC, Science M, Beyene J, Briel M, Lehrnbecher T, Sung L. Mould-active compared with fluconazole prophylaxis to prevent invasive fungal diseases in cancer patients re-ceiving chemotherapy or haematopoietic stem-cell transplantation: a systematic review and meta-analysis of randomised controlled trials. *Br J Cancer*. 2012;106:1626–37.

15. Guérin C, Reignier M, Richard JC, et al. Prone positioning in severe acute respiratory dis-tress syndrome. *N Engl J Med*. 2013;368:2159–68.

16. Odabasi Z, Mattiuzzi G, Estey E, et al. Beta-D-glucan as a diagnostic adjunct for invasive fungal infections: validation, cutoff development, and performance in patients with acute myelogenous leukemia and myelodysplastic syndrome. *Clin Infect Dis*. 2004;39:199–205.

17. Onishi A, Sugiyama D, Kogata Y, et al. Diagnostic accuracy of serum 1,3-β-D-glucan for pneumocystis jiroveci pneumonia, invasive candidiasis, and invasive aspergillosis: system-atic review and meta-analysis. *J Clin Microbiol*. 2012;50:7–15.

18. Zou M, Tang L, Zhao S, et al. Systematic review and meta-analysis of detecting galactomannan in bronchoalveolar lavage fluid for diagnosing invasive aspergillosis. *PLoS One*. 2012;7:e43347.

19. Edman JC, Kovacs JA, Masur H, Santi DV, Elwood HJ, Sogin ML. Ribosomal RNA sequence shows Pneumocystis carinii to be a member of the fungi. *Nature*. 1988;334:519–22.

20. Teh BW, Azzato FA, Lingaratnam SM, Thursky KA, Slavin MA, Worth LJ. Molecular diag-nosis of Pneumocystis jirovecii in patients with malignancy: clinical significance of quanti-tative polymerase chain reaction. *Med Mycol*. 2014;52:427–32.

21. Cooley L, Dendle C, Wolf J, et al. Consensus guidelines for diagnosis, prophylaxis and man-agement of Pneumocystis jirovecii pneumonia in patients with haematological and solid malignancies, 2014. *Intern Med J*. 2014;44:1350–63.

22. Castro JG, Morrison-Bryant M. Management of Pneumocystis jirovecii pneumonia in HIV infected patients: current options, challenges and future directions. *HIV AIDS (Auckl)*. 2010;2:123–34.

23. Garcia X, Sabatier C, Ferrer R, et al. Differential time to positivity of blood cultures: a valid method for diagnosing catheter-related bloodstream infections in the intensive care unit. *Med Intensiva*. 2012;36:169–76.

24. UK Standards for Microbiology Investigations. Issued by the Standards Unit, Public Health England. *Bacteriology*. 2014;37:1–51.

25. Kim DY, Lee YS, Ahn S, Chun YH, Lim KS. The usefulness of procalcitonin and C-reactive protein as early diagnostic markers of bacteremia in cancer patients with febrile neutropenia. *Cancer Res Treat*. 2011;43:176–80.

26. Schuetz P, Albrich W, Mueller B. Procalcitonin for diagnosis of infection and guide to antibiotic decisions: past, present and future. *BMC Med*. 2011;9:107–16.

27. Kip MMA, Kusters R, IJzerman MJ, Steuten LM. A PCT algorithm for discontinuation of antibiotic therapy is a cost effective way to reduce antibiotic exposure in adult intensive care patients with sepsis. *J Med Econ*. 2015;18:944–53

28. Bouadma L, Luyt CE, Tubach F, et al. Use of procalcitonin to reduce patients' exposure to antibiotics in intensive care units (PRORATA trial): a multi-centre randomised controlled trial. *Lancet*. 2000;375:463–74.

29. Dignan FL, Clark A, Amrolia P, et al. Diagnosis and management of acute graft-versus-host disease. *Br J Haematol*. 2012;158:30–45.

30. Carreras E, Bertz H, Arcese W, et al. Incidence and outcome of hepatic veno-occlusive disease after blood or marrow transplantation: a prospective cohort study of the European Group for Blood and Marrow Transplantation. European Group for Blood and Marrow Transplantation Chronic Leukemia Working Party. *Blood*. 1998;92:3599–604.

31. Richardson PG, Ho VT, Giralt S, et al. Safety and efficacy of defibrotide for the treatment of severe hepatic veno-occlusive disease. *Ther Adv Hematol*. 2012;3:253–65.

32. Dignan FL, Wynn RF, Hadzic N, et al. British Society for Blood and Marrow Transplantation. BCSH/BSBMT guideline: diagnosis and management of veno-occlusive disease (sinusoidal obstruction syndrome) following haematopoietic stem cell transplantation. *Br J Haematol*. 2013;163:444–57.

33. Azoulay E, Soares M, Darmon M, Benoit D, Pastores S, Afessa B. Intensive care of the cancer patient: recent achievements and remaining challenges. *Ann Intensive Care*. 2011;1:5.

34. Bird GT, Farquhar-Smith P, Wigmore T, Potter M, Gruber PC. Outcomes and prognostic factors in patients with haematological malignancy admitted to a specialist cancer intensive care unit: a 5 yr study. *Br J Anaesth*. 2012;108:452–9.

35. Legrand M, Max A, Peigne V, et al. Survival in neutropenic patients with severe sepsis or septic shock. *Crit Care Med*. 2012;40:43–9.

36. Schellongowski P, Staudinger T, Kundi M, et al. Prognostic factors for intensive care unit admission, intensive care outcome, and post-intensive care survival inpatients with *de novo* acute myeloid leukemia: a single center experience. *Haematologica*. 2011;96:231–7.

37. Mokart D, Lambert J, Schnell D, et al. Delayed intensive care unit admission is associated with increased mortality in patients with cancer with acute respiratory failure. *Leuk Lymphoma*. 2013;54:1724–9.

38. Lecuyer L, Chevret S, Thiery G, Darmon M, Schlemmer B, Azoulay E. The ICU trial: a new admission policy for cancer patients requiring mechanical ventilation. *Crit Care Med*. 2007;35:808–14.

39. Gruber PC, Achilleos A, Speed D, Wigmore TJ. Long-stay patients with cancer on the intensive care unit: characteristics, risk factors, and clinical outcomes. *Br J Anaesth*. 2013;111:1026–7.

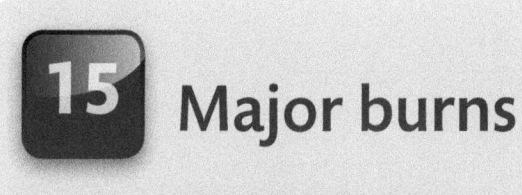

15 Major burns

Sian Alys Moxham

ⓘ **Expert Commentary** Amber E. Young

Case history

An 18-month-old girl weighing 11.5 kg was brought into the regional major trauma centre after becoming trapped in a house fire for 40 minutes. The child was found unconscious with burns. Assessment of her conscious level showed a Paediatric Glasgow Coma Scale score of 6 (E1, M4, V1). She was initially managed by the prehospital team who intubated her on scene with a size 4.0 uncuffed, uncut tracheal tube using ketamine and fentanyl. She received two boluses of 20 mL/kg warmed 0.9% saline before hospital admission.

> ✖ **Learning point** Upper airway injury and intubation
>
> Upper airway injury is typically caused by direct thermal injury with associated oedema that may potentially lead to tracheal obstruction [1]. Early intubation is advised if there are signs of potential upper airway injury, such as singed facial/nasal hairs, carbonaceous sputum, stridor, hoarse voice, drooling, or dysphagia [2]. A child's trachea has a small cross-sectional area and any swelling will cause a disproportionate increase in resistance and risk of airway obstruction.
>
> Continuing facial swelling due to facial burns and fluid administration may displace a tracheal tube, which therefore should be left uncut. Tube fixation is important—attach the tracheal tube to a bony surface or to the teeth as soon as possible after arrival at the burn service.

On arrival at the emergency department a primary survey was completed. She was covered with soot and there were burns on her face, the entire circumference of her thorax, and part of her abdomen.

Her arterial oxygen saturation by pulse oximetry (SpO_2) was 87% despite a fractional inspired oxygen concentration (FiO_2) of 0.8. Arterial blood gas (ABG) analysis showed a partial pressure of oxygen of 7.5 kPa and partial pressure of carbon dioxide of 6.7 kPa. Her lungs were difficult to ventilate; tidal volumes were small and the peak airway pressure was 45 cmH_2O. She was sedated with morphine and midazolam, and given atracurium to facilitate ventilation. Urgent thoracic escharotomy was undertaken which restored her peak airway pressure to normal values. Her oxygenation and carbon dioxide clearance subsequently improved. Sedation was maintained with a combination of weight-adjusted midazolam and morphine infusions.

> **⑥ Expert comment**
>
> Burned skin leads to interstitial oedema that compresses underlying soft tissues. Circumferential burns can cause extremity ischaemia, elevated intra-abdominal pressures, tracheal and jugular venous compression when the neck is involved, and respiratory compromise when the chest and upper abdomen are involved—especially in children [3, 4]. Circumferential chest burns will restrict chest wall movement, leading to decreased tidal volumes and carbon dioxide retention. Escharotomies should be undertaken aseptically in the operating room under general anaesthesia and with blood available. They rarely need to be undertaken outside an operating environment or before burn service admission, unless there are predicted delays of several hours. The exception to this is when circumferential burns impact patient ventilation [5, 6].

The patient had a heart rate of 145 beats per minute. Her blood pressure was 81/ 43 mmHg, capillary refill was 4 seconds, and she had cold peripheries.

Laboratory admission bloods were unremarkable. Her admission ABG, however, revealed a carboxyhaemoglobin (COHb) value of 36%, a lactate concentration of 3.0 mmol/L, and a base deficit of −6 mmol/L—consistent with carbon monoxide (CO) poisoning.

> **✪ Learning point** **Pathology of inhalational injury**
>
> Inhalational injury can occur in isolation or in combination with a cutaneous burn. The presence of inhalational injury is an independent risk factor for death after burn injury [7–9]. Consider inhalational injury in anyone exposed to a fire within an enclosed area [10].
>
> *Pulmonary parenchymal injury*: toxins typically cause local inflammation and hypersecretion which can obstruct the airways causing alveolar collapse and hypoxaemia [11]. The gold standard for diagnosis of inhalational injury is fibreoptic bronchoscopy, although there is no classification system for severity [12–14]. Clinical differentiation between direct chemical irritation of the lungs and the systemic inflammatory response (SIR) to the cutaneous injury may also be difficult [11]. Pulmonary parenchymal injury after inhalation is often delayed and should be anticipated [15]. Treatment is supportive and involves a lung protective ventilation strategy, regular pulmonary toilet, respiratory physiotherapy, humidified oxygen, nebulized *N*-acetylcysteine (a powerful mucolytic), and nebulized heparin to decrease fibrin casts [16–19].
>
> Carbon monoxide (CO) and cyanide are two toxic chemicals that cause severe systemic toxicity and metabolic derangement.
>
> CO causes tissue hypoxia by reducing oxyhaemoglobin and competitively inhibiting cytochrome oxidase enzymes thereby interfering with normal cellular oxygen handling [20]. Carboxyhaemoglobin (COHb) can be directly measured by a blood gas analyser that incorporates co-oximetry. Significant CO poisoning may exist despite normal pulse oximetry. Peak COHb levels may be underestimated on initial co-oximetry because of supplemental oxygen given before hospital admission [21]. Symptoms are non-specific and may not correlate with measured COHb values, but duration of exposure is an important factor in prognosis (Table 15.1). Values of more than 10% may be significant. The
>
> **Table 15.1** Symptoms and signs associated with ranges of carboxyhaemoglobin values
>
> | COHb % | Symptoms/signs |
> |---|---|
> | 10–20 | Asymptomatic, headache |
> | 20–40 | Visual disturbance, tiredness, disorientation |
> | 40–60 | Marked confusion, aggression, seizures, coma, cardiovascular collapse |
>
> *(continued)*

mainstay of treatment is high-concentration oxygen, as the half-life of CO is 250 minutes in air and only 40–60 minutes when breathing 100% oxygen [21]. Evidence is conflicting for the use of hyperbaric oxygen in the treatment of CO poisoning [22]. Practical issues also limit the applicability of this treatment [23].

Cyanide uncouples the mitochondrial respiratory chain (primarily by inhibiting cytochrome C oxidase) causing histotoxic hypoxia. Diagnosis of cyanide poisoning may be difficult, but ST elevation on the electrocardiograph may be suggestive along with an increased anion gap, unexplained lactic acidosis, or raised mixed venous saturation. A high index of suspicion is key. Treatment is with hydroxocobalamin, sodium thiosulphate, sodium nitrate or dicobalt edetate. Hydroxocobalamin is the preferred antidote in the UK as it is relatively safe, easy to give, does not compromise oxygen-carrying capacity, and does not produce hypotension, unlike sodium thiosulphate and sodium nitrate [24–26].

> **🅖 Expert comment**
>
> Early detection of bronchopulmonary injury with bronchoscopy is important to enable appropriate treatment to be undertaken. Inhalation injury substantially increases mortality and often requires tracheal intubation [16–18]. However, as intubation and ventilation will increase the incidence of nosocomial pneumonia, patients with inhalation injury should not be prophylactically intubated, nor should they receive prophylactic antibiotics [9].

The patient had sustained 55% total burn surface area (TBSA) deep partial/full-thickness burns covering her head, neck, chest, parts of her abdomen, and upper limbs.

> **✪ Learning point Pathology of a burn**
>
> Heat denatures proteins and damages plasma membrane integrity resulting in cell necrosis. The temperature and duration of the heat source are synergistic contributors to injury. Necrosis is worst at the centre of the burn, resulting in three zones of injury classically described by Jackson [27]:
>
> 1. Zone of coagulation: no viable cells.
> 2. Zone of stasis: viable and non-viable cells. This is an at-risk area that may convert to full necrosis with hypoperfusion, oedema, and infection. In the elderly and those with significant comorbidities, such as diabetes and chronic illness, this zone is at higher risk of conversion to cell death [28].
> 3. Zone of hyperaemia: viable cells which usually recover completely.
>
> Protection of the zone of stasis involves adequate fluid resuscitation, avoidance of vasoconstrictor drugs, prevention of infection, and excision of non-viable tissue [29–32].

> **✪ Learning point Burns assessment and management**
>
> Modern management of a burn relies on accurate assessment of the size and depth of burn injury. This depends upon clinical expertise and experience.
>
> **Burn assessment involves**
>
> 1. *Determination of the size of the burn (%TBSA) to guide fluid resuscitation and future management.* This is most commonly undertaken either using the 'rule of nines' in adults or more accurately, especially in children, Lund and Browder charts [33] (Figures 15.1 and 15.2). The Mersey Burns App is a free clinical tool which helps calculate burn percentages and fluid regimens [34]. This has been recommended by the National Institute for Health and Care Excellence (NICE) for speed of assessment compared to paper- or calculator-based methods [35].
> 2. *Determining the burn wound depth to guide surgical management.* Wounds that are not predicted to heal within 2–3 weeks (deep partial thickness and full-thickness depth) will require surgical excision and covering with autograft or other means to close the wound.
>
> *(continued)*

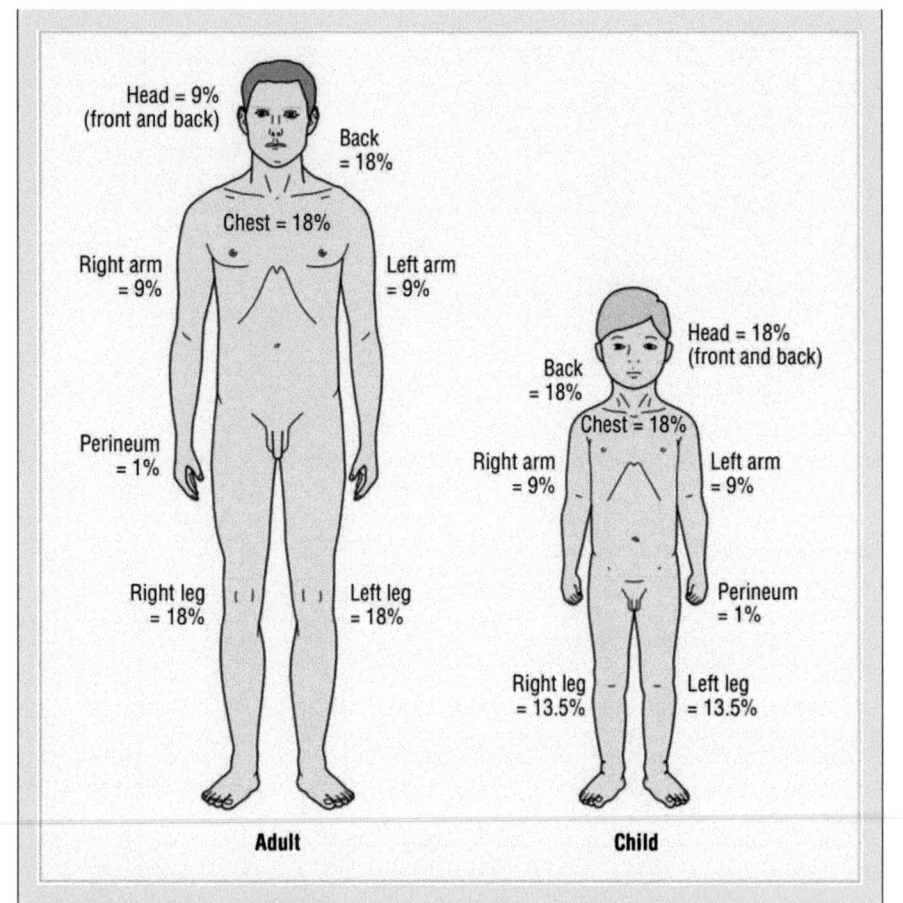

Figure 15.1 Wallace rule of nines.
Reproduced with permission from Shehan Hettiaratchy, S., and Papin, R. ABC of burns—Initial management of a major burn: II—assessment and resuscitation. *British Medical Journal*. 329(7457): 101–103. Copyright © 2004, BMJ Publishing Group Ltd.

> **✎ Expert comment**
>
> Assessing burn depth accurately is key to future management and prognosis. Clinical assessment of burn depth is unreliable and has been shown to be effective only 60-75% of the time [36]. Most burns are mixed-depth partial-thickness burns. Delayed or incorrect diagnosis can lead to unnecessary surgical procedures, or delayed surgery with the development of complications. Laser Doppler imaging is an alternative technique, but uses surrogate markers of burn depth and is limited by the time frame of use, as it cannot be used until 48 hours after injury. In 2011, NICE supported adoption of laser Doppler imaging for guiding treatment decisions where there is uncertainty about the depth and healing potential of burn wounds that have been assessed by experienced clinicians [37].

Superficial burns are erythematous, painful, and non-blistering. Superficial partial-thickness burns form blisters. Once the blister is removed, the wound is red, moist, blanches with pressure, and is hypersensitive [38]. Superficial burns and superficial partial-thickness depth burns typically heal within 2–3 weeks without scarring and with no impact on cosmesis or function.

Deep partial-thickness burns blister and appear mottled pink and white immediately after injury. Full-thickness burns can be recognized by pallor, and a leathery, firm feel. They are insensate and

(continued)

non-blanching [38]. Deeper burns typically take more than 3 weeks to heal. Burns that have longer healing times have an increased risk of scarring, with associated contractures, and impact cosmesis and psychological function. See Table 15.2 for a summary of the clinical features.

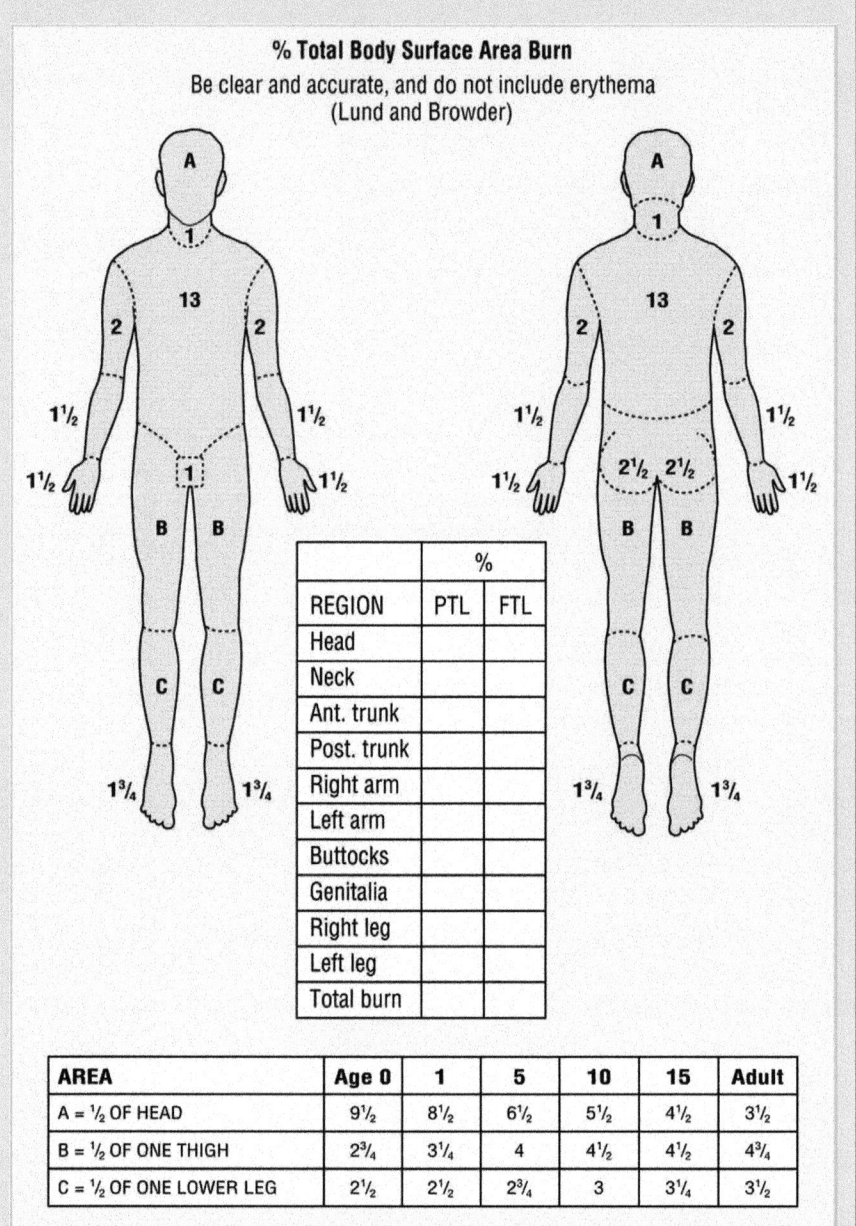

% Total Body Surface Area Burn
Be clear and accurate, and do not include erythema
(Lund and Browder)

REGION	%	
	PTL	FTL
Head		
Neck		
Ant. trunk		
Post. trunk		
Right arm		
Left arm		
Buttocks		
Genitalia		
Right leg		
Left leg		
Total burn		

AREA	Age 0	1	5	10	15	Adult
A = ½ OF HEAD	9½	8½	6½	5½	4½	3½
B = ½ OF ONE THIGH	2¾	3¼	4	4½	4½	4¾
C = ½ OF ONE LOWER LEG	2½	2½	2¾	3	3¼	3½

Figure 15.2 Lund and Browder chart.
Reproduced with permission from Shehan Hettiaratchy, S., and Papini, R. ABC of burns—Initial management of a major burn: II—assessment and resuscitation. *British Medical Journal*. 329(7457): 101–103. Copyright © 2004, BMJ Publishing Group Ltd.

(continued)

Table 15.2 Burn type and clinical features

Burn type	Tissue burnt	Clinical features			
		Appearance	Pain	Capillary refill time	Blisters
Superficial	Epidermis	Red, glistening	Painful	Brisk	No
Partial–superficial	Epidermis, upper dermis	After blistering: red, moist	Painful	Brisk	Yes
Partial–deep	Epidermis, upper and deep dermis	Dry, mottled pink and white	Dull ache	Absent	Yes
Full thickness	Epidermis, upper and deep dermis, subcutaneous tissue	Dry, pale, and leathery	Absent	Absent	No

Burns of more than 20% TBSA will trigger a systemic inflammatory response (SIR). Early surgical excision of the eschar with immediate or delayed skin grafting improves outcomes in terms of organ function, sepsis, and survival by reducing this SIR [32, 38, 40].

Achieving vascular access for the patient was difficult, so an intraosseous device was placed in her proximal tibia. She was commenced on an intravenous infusion of warmed crystalloid fluid (PlasmaLyte 148). The rate and volume was calculated according to the Parkland formula at 4 mL/kg/%TBSA along with maintenance fluid requirement.

The patient received a total of 3816 mL of crystalloid during the first 24 hours. This was calculated from a combination of the resuscitation fluid according to the Parkland formula, two 20 mL/kg fluid boluses given prehospital and 80% maintenance fluid.

Calculation:

Parkland: 4 mL × 11.5 kg × 55% TBSA = 2530 mL over 24 hours with 50% within 8 hours.

Bolus doses: 230 + 230 mL = 460 mL.

Maintenance fluid: (4 mL × 10 kg = 40 mL) + (1.5 kg × 2 mL) = 43 mL/hour × 80% = 826 mL over 24 hours.

A nasogastric tube was sited, and position confirmed, with the expectation that the maintenance fluid would be converted to enteral feed within the first 24–48 hours.

> **⊕ Clinical tip Giving less than 100% calculated fluid**
>
> Children who are critically unwell, or have undergone surgery, do not receive 100% of the traditional maintenance fluid calculation. This is due to increased antidiuretic hormone (ADH) production, resulting in fluid retention, and a less than perfect fluid calculation. Most paediatric intensive care units (PICUs) give between 50% and 80% of maintenance fluid.

> **✪ Learning point Fluid management**
>
> Until the 1950s, patients with major burns died from hypovolaemic shock within a few days. Resuscitation has considerably increased survival [10].
>
> Current recommendations are that intravenous fluid replacement should be started after a 10% TBSA burn in children and 15% TBSA burn in adults. Hypovolaemia associated with burn injury is secondary to evaporative fluid loss and fluid leak from capillaries [41]. Ventricular dysfunction seen after major burn injury can contribute to hypotension and is caused by high concentrations of circulating cytokines [42].
>
> The hypovolaemia caused by burns is biphasic. In the first hour, there is rapid oedema formation within the burned tissue, followed over the next 24 hours, by a more gradual fluid extravasation into whole-body non-burned tissue [43]. Release of inflammatory mediators (stimulated by the burn
>
> (continued)

injury), including histamine, bradykinin, nitric oxide, oxygen free radicals, tumour necrosis factor, interleukins, and arachidonic acid metabolites, increase capillary permeability, which causes fluid extravasation [42]. Normal blood volume is not restored until 24–36 hours post injury, even with appropriate fluid resuscitation [44].

The Parkland formula reflects the biphasic response:

Total crystalloid fluid (a balanced electrolyte solution) volume = 2–4 mL/kg × %TBSA burn [45].

Half of this total volume is given during the first 8 hours after burn injury and the other half infused over the following 16 hours. Fluid resuscitation formulae are only guidelines and under- or over-resuscitation is common. Children have low circulating blood volumes and those with major burns require swift commencement of fluid replacement as delayed fluid resuscitation will worsen outcomes [46–48].

Adequate resuscitation has been traditionally indicated by correction of clinical condition, base deficit, lactate, and pH and achieving a urine output of 0.5 mL/kg/hour in adults, 1 mL/kg/hour in children, and 2 mL/kg/hour in infants [10]. However, normalizing urine output is difficult to achieve with high levels of ADH following burn injury.

Complications of under-resuscitation include acute kidney injury, multiorgan failure, and death [10]. However, in modern practice, complications are more commonly associated with fluid over-resuscitation [10] and include:

- compartment syndromes:
  - abdominal compartment syndrome
  - extremity compartment syndrome
  - thoracic circumferential constriction
- wound-related complications:
  - conversion of viable tissue to non-viable tissue within the burn injury
  - graft failure
- vital organ oedema:
  - pulmonary oedema
  - cerebral oedema
- electrolyte imbalance:
  - hyponatraemia.

⨁ Expert comment

Fluid overload (and associated complications) is common in the early few days after burn injury. This is associated with rigid adherence to guidelines for fluid administration in patients with burns, difficulties with estimating fluid balance, fluid creep, and high levels of ADH [49]. This hypervolaemic state is often associated with hyponatraemia. It commonly manifests as an increased oxygen requirement in those patients with no lung pathology, or increased ventilator requirements in those requiring ventilation. Fluid overload should be anticipated and managed early with fluid restriction and/or diuretics as required.

In the example case described here, it is likely that this child was over-resuscitated because of the use of the Parkland formula at 4 mL/kg/%TBSA, resulting in respiratory dysfunction and difficulty with positive pressure ventilation. Current research suggests that over-resuscitation of patients with burn injuries causes significant harm with respect to respiratory function, other organ function, depth of burn, and mortality [48, 50]. Recent work suggests that using a more restrictive approach to burn resuscitation (permissive hypovolaemia) with appropriate clinical end points produces better outcomes [51, 52]. A challenge in achieving optimal fluid resuscitation for burn patients is that the gold standard is still urine output. However, this is unlikely to reflect hydration status accurately because of the high ADH concentrations associated with significant burn injury (especially in children). Aiming to achieve a 'normal' urine output, will almost always result in fluid overload. Using a collection of clinical end points measured every few hours during the resuscitation period including clinical condition, ABG indices, and serum urea and sodium as well as urine output will ensure the best monitor of fluid status [53, 54].

As the regional major trauma centre was distant to the burns centre, a referral and transfer to the burn service was required. Referral was required because of the size of the burn and the presence of an inhalational injury with associated CO poisoning. The patient was transferred to the regional burn centre, where she was immediately taken to the operating room for:

- reassessment of burn size and depth
- wound cleaning and excision
- early grafting of her deep dermal and full-thickness burns.

> ✪ **Learning point** Referral criteria
>
> Systems for treating severe burns will vary from country to country. The UK is an example of a country with a dedicated network of burn centres offering specialized care. In the UK, the Burn Operational Delivery Networks (burn ODN) comprises a group of geographically related hospitals; a burn centre having the capacity to treat the most severe burn from injury to rehabilitation, along with a constellation of burn units providing care for less complex burns. Uncomplicated small burns may be treated in burn facilities (designated plastic surgery services). The network provides appropriate expertise and resources for the burned patient. There are four burn ODNs within England and Wales [55]. However, not all burn centres are co-located with major trauma centres. If the patient is multiply injured and requires other specialist care the best location for that patient will need to be agreed. If the burn is the predominant injury, care within a burn service is essential.
>
> To guide referral decisions, five criteria are considered—burn size, depth, location, mechanism, and other factors [55]. Criteria are different for adults and children. See Tables 15.3 and 15.4.
>
> **Table 15.3 Paediatric referral criteria**
>
> | Paediatric | Burn unit | Burn centre |
> |---|---|---|
> | TBSA % | >5% | >30%
>15% if <1 year |
> | Depth | >2% full thickness
>1% full thickness if <6 months | >20% full thickness |
> | Site | Any burn to special areas[a]
Any circumferential burn | As for burn unit |
> | Mechanism of Injury | Chemical
Electrical
Friction
Cold injury
Inhalational injury | As for burn unit |
> | Other factors | Any burn not healed within 2 weeks
Physiological instability secondary to burn injury
Suspicion of non-accidental injury | As for burn unit |
>
> [a] Special areas include hands, feet, face, perineum, genitalia.
> Source: data from National Network for Burn Care (NNBC) (2012). *British Burn Association National Burn Care Referral Guidance: Version* 1, 2012. Copyright © 2012 NNBC. Available at www.britishburnsassociation.org.uk.
>
> **Table 15.4 Adult referral criteria**
>
> | Adult | Burn unit | Burn centre |
> |---|---|---|
> | TBSA % | 10–40%
10–25% with associated inhalational injury | >40%
>25% with associated inhalational injury or age >65 years or significant comorbidities |
> | Depth | ≥5% | As for burn unit |
>
> *(continued)*

Table 15.4 Continued

Adult	Burn unit	Burn centre
Site	Any burn to special areas[a] ˙ Any non-blanching circumferential burn	As for burn unit
Mechanism	Chemical Electrical Friction Cold injury	As for burn unit
Other factors	Any burn not healed in 2 weeks Physiological instability secondary to burn injury Suspicion of non-accidental injury Pregnancy	As for burn unit

[a] Special areas include hands, feet, face, perineum, genitalia.
Source: data from National Network for Burn Care (NNBC) (2012). *British Burn Association National Burn Care Referral Guidance: Version 1*, 2012. Copyright © 2012 NNBC. Available at www.britishburnsassociation.org.uk.

ⓖ Expert comment

Early debridement of large area, deep partial-thickness or full-thickness burns improves survival and decreases hospital stay, blood loss, and healthcare costs [56–60]. However, the definition of 'early' still requires clarification. In most burn services in the UK, as full a debridement as possible of the burn eschar occurs when the patient is stable and within the first 48–72 hours.

Definitive wound cover should occur early after debridement as there is a risk of infection until the wound is closed. However, it is the presence of dead tissue that worsens outcomes and therefore the urgency for debridement is more than that for wound coverage. Choice of wound coverage depends upon the size and site of the burn. The ideal cover is the patient's own skin (autograft); however, this will not be possible if the burns are of more than 40–50% TBSA. In these cases, cadaver skin or biosynthetic dressings can be used to temporize, until a further autograft is available or until alternative dermal cover is provided using products such as Matriderm or Integra [49].

After surgery, the patient was nursed in a thermally controlled ICU isolation room with an ambient temperature of 30°C and 60% relative humidity.

The patient became progressively more oedematous over the following few days. It became more difficult to ventilate her lungs, with the FiO_2 increasing to 0.9 and peak inspiratory pressures greater than 30 cmH$_2$O. A positive end-expiratory pressure of 14 cmH$_2$O was required to maintain adequate oxygenation. A chest X-ray showed bilateral diffuse infiltrates consistent with acute respiratory distress syndrome caused by inhalational injury, SIR, and exacerbated by fluid overload. Her serum sodium concentration decreased to 130 mmol/L.

✪ Learning point Mechanical ventilation in the burn patient

Indications for mechanical ventilation in the patient with burns include:

- management of direct airway injury
- nosocomial pulmonary infection
- acute respiratory distress syndrome secondary to inhalational injury, pulmonary infection, iatrogenic pulmonary oedema, or the SIR to severe burns
- abdominal compartment syndrome
- neurological sequelae of CO or cyanide poisoning.

> **ⓕ Expert comment**
>
> Current evidence suggests that mechanical ventilation of patients with burns, but without inhalational injury, is independently associated with poorer outcomes [61]. This may be due to the need to provide more intravenous fluid purely to maintain acceptable clinical end points in patients who are sedated and ventilated [62]. Patients with facial burns, upper airway thermal trauma, or a large burn area should be intubated and ventilated, if required, for transfer to definitive care at the burn service. However, *extubation should then occur as early as possible* [62, 63] and should not be postponed because of a need for daily or alternate day surgery. This management requires careful monitoring of ventilator requirements and airway signs in a high-care area. If extubation is not possible, consider an early tracheostomy and weaning from sedative drugs and positive pressure ventilation.

Over the next day, the patient's temperature increased to 39°C and she became increasingly tachycardic. Propranolol was started to ameliorate the systemic inflammatory response to the burn. Despite earlier placement of a nasogastric tube and early enteral nutrition, absorption of feed was inconsistent. A nasojejunal tube replaced her nasogastric tube and oxandrolone was started once she was fully absorbing her enteral feed.

> **✪ Learning point** Hypermetabolic response
>
> Burn injuries of more than 20% TBSA cause a hypermetabolic response, characterized by a hyperdynamic circulation, increased body temperature, catabolism, and inefficient energy substrate cycling. This is mediated by acute phase response cytokines and increased secretion of catecholamines, glucocorticoids, and glucagon. Protein is preferentially used as the main body substrate. Without treatment, the patient will have muscle wastage, delayed mobilization, impaired rehabilitation, and immunocompromise, increasing the risk of sepsis [10]. Cardiac output and heart rate can often increase by 150–200%, which can last well into the rehabilitative stage [10]. The patient will also typically develop a hyperglycaemic insulin-resistant state and may require insulin supplementation, especially during episodes of sepsis.
>
> Management of the hypermetabolic response includes pharmacological and non-pharmacological methods [64].
>
> Non-pharmacological methods include:
>
> - early wound excision and closure (as described earlier)
> - early enteral nutritional support
> - environmental support: high ambient temperature and humidity to prevent heat loss.
>
> Early enteral feeding is essential to maintain calorific input and to protect the integrity of the bowel mucosa [65]. Repeated operative procedures interrupt feeding regimens and early consideration of a nasojejunal tube is important. Excessively high-calorie feeding is associated with increased mortality. Conversely, failure to meet nutritional requirements impairs wound healing and increases infection risk [66]. Many formulae have been developed but most overestimate calorie requirement. A nutritionist/dietician is a key member of the burn care multidisciplinary team [10].
>
> In patients with burns, an increase in 'normal' central body temperature to 38°C is linked to the hypermetabolic response. Maintaining a warm, humid ambient environment (30–33°C and 60% humidity respectively) prevents heat loss and ameliorates the hypermetabolic response by decreasing resting energy expenditure by up to 20% [64].
>
> Pharmacological treatment includes beta blockers and anabolic agents. Propranolol, starting at 1 mg/kg, is titrated to decrease heart rate by 20%. Propranolol reduces cardiac work, decreases hepatic steatosis, and reduces skeletal muscle catabolism [10]. Oxandrolone, a non-virilizing anabolic steroid, improves efficiency of protein synthesis and healing of the burn wound, and is started when enteral feeding is established [67]. At a dose of 0.1 mg/kg twice daily, lean body mass is maintained and hospital length of stay decreased [68]. Liver function tests should be monitored. Propranolol and oxandrolone should be maintained for at least 1 year after major burn injury [10].

ⓒ Expert comment

Burns of more than 20% TBSA cause stress and inflammatory and hypermetabolic responses which can last up to 3 years. An ebb phase starts immediately after injury with low cardiac output, decreased metabolic rate, and impaired glucose tolerance and may present as shock. The flow or hyperdynamic phase occurs after 3–5 days and comprises increased heart rate, blood pressure, temperature and hypermetabolism, and is associated with protein catabolism [69].

Research supports the safety and effectiveness of drugs such as propranolol and oxandrolone in ameliorating this hypermetabolic response. Propranolol is a non-selective beta blocker, and has undergone significant testing in patients with major burns. It has been shown to decrease heart rate, cardiac work, muscle catabolism, and resting energy expenditure in children with severe burns [70]. A more recent systematic review of ten clinical trials concluded that propranolol was effective and safe for reduction of metabolic rate in patients with burns [49, 71, 72].

Results of smaller studies support a role of the testosterone analogue oxandrolone in reducing muscle loss and hypermetabolism and increasing bone mineral density and promoting growth in children recovering from burns [49, 71].

✪ Learning point General issues for the burned patient

Airway management

A tracheostomy should be considered in the presence of facial burns, and to aid early weaning from ventilation if extubation is otherwise impossible.

Vascular access

The risk of sepsis from vascular access is a constant consideration. Avoid central venous lines if possible; but if deemed essential, site observation is paramount and consider replacement immediately if there are any signs of infection.

Coagulation

The burn patient is at risk of unrecognized blood loss from burn wound ooze. However, burn patients are more commonly in a hypercoagulable state with an increased risk of deep vein thrombosis and other thromboembolic events. Chemical thromboprophylaxis should be initiated as soon as bleeding risk has passed, that is, when surgery resulting in major blood loss is unlikely.

Gastroprotection

Gastrointestinal ulcer formation is common in patients with burns who are not fed enterally. Consider chemoprophylaxis for ulcer prevention when enteral feeding cannot be established or fails at any point.

Hypothermia

Anaesthetic and sedative drugs ablate normal thermoregulation and the patient may need to be fully exposed to enable assessment and surgical management. The burned patient is at high risk of hypothermia and this may exacerbate blood loss from worsening coagulopathy. Ventricular arrhythmias are more likely and the left shift of the oxyhaemoglobin dissociation curve reduces peripheral oxygen delivery, risking burn injury extension and graft failure. During anaesthesia and sedation, core temperatures of higher than 36°C should be maintained.

Altered drug handling

The hypermetabolic state, hypoproteinaemia from capillary protein leak, and catabolism lead to altered drug handling. Free drug concentrations are increased for those drugs that are predominantly protein bound.

Muscle relaxants

Do not use depolarizing neuromuscular blocking drugs (i.e. suxamethonium) from 24 hours after injury to 2 years after burn injury because of an increase in extrajunctional nicotinic acetylcholine receptors. Stimulation of these extrajunctional receptors leads to excessive potassium release with the risk of arrhythmias and cardiac arrest. Burn patients are also relatively insensitive to non-depolarizing neuromuscular blocking drugs.

(continued)

> **Pain**
>
> High doses of opioids are commonly used for long periods leading to tolerance and subsequent withdrawal unless managed carefully. Consider multimodal analgesia including gabapentinoids. Early involvement of an age-appropriate acute pain service is crucial.

After a week in ICU, the patient was extubated. On one dressing change, the surgeon noticed a green discharge from a burn site and skin graft on her torso. Her dressing change was more painful than usual, necessitating ketamine along with Entonox. Her white cell count decreased and C-reactive protein (CRP) increased. Her temperature increased to 40.1°C. She was taken back to the operating room for wound debridement of a likely infected wound site. Broad-spectrum antibiotics were started. After the results of wound swabs and blood cultures were available, the antibiotic spectrum was narrowed to treat identified pathogens.

> ✪ **Learning point Infection**
>
> Burn patients are susceptible to infection because of:
>
> 1. loss of skin integrity
> 2. cellular and humoral immunosuppression due to the SIR
> 3. a requirement for central vascular access and urinary catheters
> 4. prolonged hospital stay and invasive procedures.
>
> Bacterial infections are a consequence of endogenous flora and environmental contaminants including airborne microorganisms [10]. Burned patients commonly acquire multidrug-resistant microbes or fungal infection due to long hospitalization, high carer/patient contact load, and frequent antibiotic therapy. Because of the high incidence of septic episodes and risk of bacterial resistance, prophylactic antibiotics should not be used.
>
> Preventative measures include [10]:
>
> 1. patient isolation
> 2. hand washing
> 3. disposable waterproof full gowns, gloves, and masks
> 4. regular cleaning of isolation rooms with antibacterial solutions
> 5. regular wound, urinary catheter, and venous line inspection plus wound and blood cultures if indicated.
>
> Diagnosis of invasive burn wound infection can be difficult as the standard criteria for sepsis is mimicked by the hypermetabolic response in the non-infected burn patient. Although prophylactic antimicrobial treatment is not appropriate in burn patients, there needs to be scrupulous screening for infection and prompt treatment when there is evidence of active infection.
>
> The American Burn Association developed consensus guidelines to aid diagnosis of sepsis in the burn patient. The trigger for diagnosis of sepsis includes at least three of the following features as detailed in Table 15.5 as well as 'documented infection' (defined in Table 15.5).
>
> Treatment involves source control (usually aggressive surgical debridement of infected wounds) and targeted antimicrobial therapy.
>
> Wound infection leading to systemic sepsis is potentially catastrophic for the burn patient because it may lead to multiorgan failure, haematogenous spread to distant sites, and/or graft failure. A high index of suspicion is key. Organisms cultured during pneumonia often reflect the flora of the burn wound [10].
>
> *(continued)*

Table 15.5 Features of sepsis in the burn patient

	Children	Adults
Temperature	>39°C or <36.5°C	
Progressive tachycardia	>2 SD above age-specific norms	>110 bpm
Progressive tachypnoea	>2 SD above age-specific norms	a. >25 breaths per minute if not ventilated. b. Minute volume >12 L/min if ventilated
Thrombocytopenia	<2 SD below age-specific norms	<100 × 10⁹/L
Hyperglycaemia	a. Blood sugar >20 mmol/L, if untreated b. >7 insulin IU/hour or >25% increase in insulin requirement in a 24-hour period, if supplementation used	
Gastrointestinal stasis	a. Abdominal distension b. Uncontrolled diarrhoea c. Enteral feed intolerance >24 hour: aspirates >150 mL/hour	c. Enteral feed intolerance
Documented infection	a. Culture positive b. Pathological tissue source c. Clinical response to antimicrobials	

bpm, beats per minute; SD, standard deviation.

⊕ Expert comment

Diagnosis of burn wound infection and/or sepsis is difficult in the patient with burns during the acute period after burn injury. The signs of sepsis are identical to those of systemic inflammation except for the presence of blood-borne bacteria. Diagnosis relies on a high index of suspicion. The presence of pyrexia, changes in white blood cell count, and CRP alone, may indicate either state. Intolerance of enteral feed is more helpful, as is glucose instability. Evidence for the use of procalcitonin as a biomarker of sepsis in patients with burns is inconclusive.

If there are signs of sepsis in patients with burns, blood cultures, wound swabs, and urgent assessment of the burn wound are essential. Broad-spectrum antibiotics are started until cultures give definitive results.

Toxic shock syndrome (TSS), usually secondary to the TSST1 toxin of *Staphylococcus aureus*, should always be considered in the child with signs of sepsis after burn injury. Specific management requires anti-staphylococcal antibiotic treatment and wound cleaning. However, management *must* also include anti-toxin treatment with intravenous immunoglobulin (IVIG) or fresh frozen plasma (FFP). FFP is obtained from adults and contains the anti-TSST1 toxin antibody which is low in children of less than 4 years of age compared to older children and adults. FFP is more commonly used than IVIG in the treatment of TSS, although the evidence supporting this use is limited.

The patient was discharged from ICU after 2 weeks. Her total hospital stay was 130 days because she required ongoing dressing changes and further rehabilitation. National benchmarks for length of stay (healing) are related to the size of the burn and are set at 2 days/%TBSA. Following discharge, she will require regular reconstructive surgery for contractures as she continues to grow during childhood and puberty.

> ⚙ **Learning point** Psychosocial aspects
>
> There is increasing interest in the impact of major burn injury on a patient's psychosocial function [10]. Most patients now survive the burn injury, because of improved burn and critical care management. The resultant psychosocial impact has become increasingly apparent. Communication and social interaction may be affected by altered skin and disfigurement, with a resultant impact on social identity (particularly in the adult population). Depressive symptoms, anxiety, hopelessness, and emotional lability (and regressive behavioural patterns in the paediatric patient) are normal reactions to the burn injury during the recovery phase [10].
>
> Some patients develop acute stress disorder (ASD) and post-traumatic stress disorder (PTSD) from the initial burn injury and from multiple medical interventions. The incidence of ASD is 19%, typically occurring immediately following the trauma, and lasting up to 4 weeks. ASD is a predictor of PTSD, but PTSD is the most common psychiatric disorder seen in burn survivors, occurring in approximately 45%. Age-appropriate psychologists are key members of the burns multidisciplinary team.
>
> Burns cases can be complicated by the suspicion of non-accidental injury (NAI) which is not uncommon in children with burns. Burns account for 6–8% of all paediatric abuse cases annually and abuse-associated burns have worse clinical outcomes including higher mortality. The vulnerable adult may also be at risk of NAI. The wider family should be considered, for example, any other siblings who may need emergency social care during any NAI investigation. Clinical notes should be detailed, factual, and objective, and the appropriate safeguarding team involved at an early stage.

Discussion

Death from burn injury has reduced during the twentieth and the early part of the twenty-first century. In the 1940s, a child with 50% TBSA burns had an expected mortality of over 50%. Currently, the same child, has an expected mortality of 16% and survival in children with burns of greater than 80% is now possible [54]. However, this improvement in survival is not reflected in the elderly population; the mortality rate for a 50% TBSA burn is 68% in those older than 60 years. This is most likely because of comorbidities [10]. The difficulty with achieving meaningful estimates for mortality includes varying burn care management, standardizing the burn type, presence of inhalation injury, comorbidity, and agreeing the mortality calculation. Sepsis and multiorgan failure remain the leading causes of death after burn injury [54].

The most important advance in the surgical care of patients with large area burns is early excision of the burn eschar with subsequent wound coverage. This should ideally be from autografting or dermal replacement in larger area burns. This removes the stimulus for the systemic inflammatory and hypermetabolic responses, decreases the incidence of sepsis, and improves survival along with cosmetic and functional outcome [32].

Improved critical care including early and appropriate fluid resuscitation (with a trend towards limiting fluid replacement to 'just enough'), amelioration of the hypermetabolic response, and strict prevention and treatment (but not prophylaxis) of infection have also reduced mortality. Positive pressure ventilation should be used with caution and only when essential. Early extubation of all patients with burns (including those with facial burns) is key to good outcomes.

Incidence and management of inhalational injury remains a major determinant of burn survival. Diagnosis is still a challenge. The aims of critical care management in inhalational injury are early diagnosis, a protective ventilation strategy, conservative fluid management, and pharmacological treatment/prevention of complications.

A final word from the expert

Burn care is improving with advances in surgery, critical care, microbiology, and psychological care. Good outcomes are now possible despite the most severe injuries, although these improvements in outcome have been limited in the elderly. Quality evidence is improving, although multicentre randomized controlled trials with consistent outcome reporting are still limited, with associated difficulties in evidence synthesis.

Areas of research include wound coverage for large area burns (dermal preservation and replacement), improvement of wound healing, early detection of infection with new point-of-care technology, limitation and accuracy of fluid replacement with a clear understanding of clinical end points, the role of ventilation in burn-injured patients, and standardization of care to enable audit of care pathways across services.

The importance of physical and psychological rehabilitation starting early after injury for burns of all sizes is now clear. An understanding of the importance of expert, experienced multidisciplinary teamwork is also clear, as is the need to provide the best outcomes by centralizing care into a few specialized centres for the rare major burns in both adults and children.

References

1. Moritz A, Henriques F, McLean R. The effects of inhaled heat on the air passages and lungs: an experimental investigation. *Am J Pathol*. 1945;21:311–31.
2. Madnani D, Steele N, de Vries E. Factors that predict the need for intubation in patients with smoke inhalation injury. *Ear Nose Throat J*. 2006;85:278–80.
3. Hobson K, Young K, Ciraulo A, et al. Release of abdominal compartment syndrome improves survival in patients with burn injury. *J Trauma*. 2002;53:1129–34.
4. Tsoutsos D, Rodopoulou S, Keramidas E, et al. Early escharotomy as a measure to reduce intraabdominal hypertension in full-thickness burns of the thoracic and abdominal area. *World J Surg*. 2003;27:1323–8.
5. Asch M, Flemma R, Pruitt B Jr. Ischemic necrosis of tibialis anterior muscle in burns patients: report of three cases. *Surgery*. 1969;66:846–69.
6. Hettiaratchy S, Papini R. Initial management of a major burn: II—assessment and resuscitation. *BMJ*. 2004;329:101–3.
7. Palmieri T. Inhalation injury: research progress and needs. *J Burn Care Res*. 2007;28:549–54.
8. Shirani K, Pruitt B Jr, Mason A Jr. The influence of inhalation injury and pneumonia on burn mortality. *Ann Surg* 1987;205:82–7.
9. Jeschke M, Herndon D. Burns in children: standard and new treatments. *Lancet*. 2014;383:1168–78.
10. Herndon D. *Total Burn Care*, 4th edn. Amsterdam: Elsevier Health Sciences; 2012.
11. Demling R. Smoke inhalation lung injury: an update. *Eplasty* 2008;8:e27.
12. Hunt J, Agee R, Pruitt B Jr. Fiberoptic bronchoscopy in acute inhalation injury. *J Trauma*. 1975;15:641–9.
13. Muehlberger T, Kumar D, Munster A et al. Efficacy of fiberoptic laryngoscopy in the diagnosis of inhalation injuries. *Arch Otolaryngol Head Neck Surg*. 1998;124:1003–7.
14. Cancio L. Airway management and smoke inhalation injury in the burn patient. *Clin Plast Surg*. 2009;36:555–67.
15. Woodson L. Diagnosis and grading of inhalation injury. *J Burn Care Res*. 2009;30:143–5.

16. Fu Z, Yang Z, Liu L, et al. The influence of N-acetyl-L-cysteine on pulmonary injury and oxygen stress after smoke inhalation injury. *Zhonghua Shao Shang Za Zhi*. 2002;18:152–4.

17. Desai M, Micak R, Richardson J, et al. Reduction in mortality in paediatric patients with inhalation injury with aerosolized heparin/N-acetlycystine [correction of acetylcystine] therapy. *J Burn Care Rehabil* 1998;19:210–12.

18. Miller A, Elamin E, Suffredini A. Inhaled anticoagulation regimens for the treatment of smoke inhalation-associated acute lung injury: a systematic review. *Crit Care Med*. 2014;42:413–19.

19. Walker P, Buehner M, Wood L, et al. Diagnosis and management of inhalation injury: an updated review. *Crit Care*. 2015;19:351.

20. Kealey G. Carbon monoxide toxicity. *J Burn Care Res*. 2009;30:146–7.

21. Dries D, Endorf F. Inhalation injury: epidemiology, pathology, treatment strategies. *Scand J Trauma Resusc Emerg Med*. 2013;21:31.

22. Buckley N, Juurlink D, Isbister G, et al. Hyperbaric oxygen for carbon monoxide poisoning. *Cochrane Database Syst Rev*. 2011;4:CD002041.

23. Villanueva E, Bennett M, Wasiak J, et al. Hyperbaric oxygen therapy for thermal burns. *Cochrane Database Syst Rev*. 2004;3:CD004727.

24. Murray L, Little M, Pascu O, et al. *Toxicology Handbook*, 3rd edn. Sydney: Elsevier Australia: 2015.

25. Borron S, Baud F, Mégarbane B, et al. Hydroxocobalamin for severe acute cyanide poisoning by ingestion or inhalation. *Am J Emerg Med*. 2007;25:551–8.

26. Fortin J, Giocanti J, Ruttimann M, et al. Prehospital administration of hydroxocobalamin for smoke inhalation associated cyanide poisoning: 8 years of experience in the Paris Fire Brigade. *Clin Toxicol (Phila)*. 2006;44:37–44.

27. Jackson D. The diagnosis of the depth of burning. *Br J Surg*. 1953;40:588–96.

28. Zawacki B. Reversal of capillary stasis and prevention of necrosis in burns. *Ann Surg*. 1974;180:98–102.

29. Shupp J, Nasabzadeh T, Rosenthal D, et al. A review of the local pathophysiologic bases of burn wound progression. *J Burn Care Res*. 2010;31:849–73.

30. Knabl J, Bauer W, Andel H, et al. Progression of burn wound depth by systemical application of a vasoconstrictor: an experimental study with a new rabbit model. *Burns* 1999;25:715–21.

31. Rico R, Ripamonit R, Burns A, et al. The effect of sepsis on wound healing. *J Surg Res*. 2002;102:193–7.

32. Cope O, Langohr J, Moore F, et al. Expeditious care of full-thickness burn wounds by surgical excision and grafting. *Ann Surg*. 1947;125:1–22.

33. Hettiaratchy S, Papini R. ABC of burns: initial management of a major burn: II – assessment and resuscitation. *Br Med J*. 2004;329:101–3.

34. St Helens and Knowsley Teaching Hospitals NHS Trust. Mersey Burns App [Internet]. 2013. Available from: https://www.merseyburns.com (accessed 11 April 2017).

35. National Institute for Health and Care Excellence (NICE). *Mersey Burns for Calculating Fluid Resuscitation Volume when Managing Burns*. NICE Medtech Innovation Briefing [MIB58]. London: NICE; 2016. Available from: https://www.nice.org.uk/advice/mib58/chapter/Introduction.

36. Heimbach D, Afromowitz M, Engrav L, et al. Burn depth estimation—man or machine. *J Trauma*. 1984;24:373–8.

37. National Institute for Health and Care Excellence (NICE). *MoorLDI2-BI: A Laser Doppler Blood Flow Imager for Burn Wound Assessment*. NICE Medical Technologies Guidance [MTG2]. London: NICE; 2011. Available from: https://www.nice.org.uk/guidance/MTG2/chapter/1-Recommendations.

38. Waldmann C, Soni N, Rhodes A. *Oxford Desk Reference: Critical Care*. Oxford: Oxford University Press; 2008.

39. Tompkins R, Remensnyder J, Burke J, et al. Significant reductions in mortality for children with burn injuries through the use of prompt eschar excision. *Ann Surg.* 1988;208:577–85.

40. Herndon D, Barrow R, Rutan R, et al. A comparison of conservative versus early excision. Therapies in severely burned patients. *Ann Surg.* 1989;209:547–53.

41. Cope O, Moore F. The redistribution of body water and fluid therapy of the burned patient. *Ann Surg.* 1947;126:101–45.

42. Youn Y, LaLonde C, Demling R. The role of mediators in the response to thermal injury. *World J Surg.* 1992;16:30–6.

43. Demling R, Mazess R, Witt R, et al. The study of burn wound edema using dichromatic absorptiometry. *J Trauma.* 1978;18:124–8.

44. Cioffi W Jr, Vaughan G, Heironimus J, et al. Dissociation of blood volume and flow in regulation of salt and water balance in burns patients. *Ann Surg.* 1991;214:213–18.

45. Baxter C. Fluid volume and electrolyte changes in the early postburn period. *Clin Plast Surg.* 1974;1:693–703.

46. Wolf S, Rose J, Desai M, et al. Mortality determinants in massive pediatric burns: an analysis of 103 children with > or = 80% TBSA burns (> or = 70% full thickness). *Ann Surg.* 1997;225:554–69.

47. Barrow R, Jeschke M, Herndon D. Early fluid resuscitation improves outcomes in severely burned children. *Resuscitation.* 2000;45:91–6.

48. Klein M, Hayden D, Elson C, et al. The association between fluid administration and outcome following major burn: a multicenter study. *Ann Surg.* 2007;245:622–8.

49. Porter C, Tompkins R, Finnerty C, et al. The metabolic stress response to burn trauma: current understanding and therapies. *Lancet.* 2016;388:1417–26.

50. Saffle J. The phenomenon of "fluid creep" in acute burn resuscitation. *J Burn Care Res.* 2010;28:382–95.

51. Arlati S, Storti E, Pradella V, et al. Decreased fluid volume to reduce organ damage: a new approach to burn shock resuscitation? A preliminary study. *Resuscitation.* 2007;72:371–8.

52. Walker T, Rodriguez D, Coy K, et al. Impact of reduced resuscitation fluid on outcomes of children with 10–20% body surface area scalds. *Burns.* 2014;40:1581–6.

53. Paratz J, Stockton K, Paratz E, et al. Burn resuscitation—hourly urine output versus alternative endpoints: a systematic review. *Shock.* 2014;42:295–306.

54. Henschke A, Lee R, Delaney A. Burns management in ICU: quality of the evidence: a systematic review. *Burns.* 2016;42:1173–82.

55. National Network for Burn Care (NNBC). National Burn Care Referral Guidance: Version 1 [Internet]. 2012. Available from: http://www.britishburnsassociation.org.uk (accessed 11 April 2017).

56. Pietsch J, Netscher D, Nagaraj H, et al. Early excision of major burns in children: effect on morbidity and mortality. *J Pediatr Surg.* 1985;20:754–7.

57. Hernson D, Parks D. Comparison of serial debridement and autografting and early massive excision with cadaver skin overlay in the treatment of large burns in children. *J Trauma.* 1986;26:149–52.

58. Muller M, Herndon D. The challenge of burns. *Lancet.* 1994;343:216–20.

59. Tompkins R, Remensnyder J, Burke J, et al. Significant reductions in mortality for children with burn injuries through the use of prompt eschar excision. *Ann Surg.* 1988;208:577–85.

60. Desai M, Hernson D, Broemeling L, et al. Early burn wound excision significantly reduces blood loss. *Ann Surg.* 1990;211:753–9.

61. Galeiras R, Lorente J, Pértega S, et al. A model for predicting mortality among critically ill burn victims. *Burns.* 2009;35:201–9.

62. Mackie D. Inhalation injury or mechanical ventilation: which is the true killer in burn patients? *Burns.* 2013;39:1329–30.

63. Holst J, Sauaia A, Ivashchenko A, et al. Indications for intubation of the patient with thermal and inhalational burns. *Am J Respir Crit Care Med.* 2015;191:A1619.

64. Williams F, Jeschke M, Chinkes D, et al. Modulation of the hypermetabolic response to trauma: temperature, nutrition, and drugs. *J Am Coll Surg.* 2009;208:489–502.

65. McDonald W, Sharp C Jr, Deitch E. Immediate enteral feeding in burn patients is safe and effective. *Ann Surg.* 1991;213:177–83.

66. Lee J, Benjamin D, Herndon D. Nutrition support strategies for severely burned patients. *Nutr Clin Pract.* 2005;20:325–30.

67. Demling R, Orgill D. The anticatabolic and wound healing effects of the testosterone analog oxandrolone after severe burn injury. *J Crit Care.* 2000;15:12–17.

68. Jeschke M, Finnerty C, Suman O, et al. The effect of oxandrolone on the endocrinologic, inflammatory, and hypermetabolic responses during the acute phase post burn. *Ann Surg.* 2007;246:351–60.

69. Henig O, Avni T, Herndon D et al. Beta adrenergic antagonists for hospitalized burned patients. *Cochrane Database Syst Rev.* 2015;6:CD011713.

70. Herndon D, Hart D, Wolf S, et al. Reversal of catabolism by beta-blockade after severe burns. *N Engl J Med.* 2001;345:1223–9.

71. Porter C, Tompkins R, Finnerty C, et al. The metabolic stress response to burn trauma: current understanding and therapies. *Lancet.* 2016;388:1417–26.

72. Flores O, Stockton K, Roberts J, et al. The efficacy and safety of adrenergic blockade after burn injury: a systematic review and meta-analysis. *J Trauma Acute Care Surg.* 2016;80:146–55.

16 Prolonged mechanical ventilation and delayed weaning

Patrick B. Murphy

ⓘ **Expert Commentary** Nicholas Hart

Case history

A 67-year-old retired lecturer was referred from his local intensive care unit (ICU) to a specialist weaning, rehabilitation, and home mechanical ventilation service. The patient had contracted poliomyelitis when 5 years old and had required respiratory support with 'iron lung tank ventilation' for 4 months during his acute illness. Following this, he made a full respiratory recovery, with no need for ongoing ventilatory support. He did, however, have limited recovery of lower limb strength and the development, despite a spinal brace, of a significant scoliosis. He regained only limited walking with callipers and required a wheelchair for mobility. He worked as a lecturer but noticed progression of his weakness from the age of around 50, which was consistent with post-polio syndrome. Despite this progression, he lived with his wife in an adapted flat with a comprehensive care package and was first reviewed by the home mechanical ventilation and 'post-polio' service aged 57, 10 years before this referral. He had no symptoms of sleep-disordered breathing, normal overnight oximetry, and a vital capacity of 1.9 L (Figure 16.1).

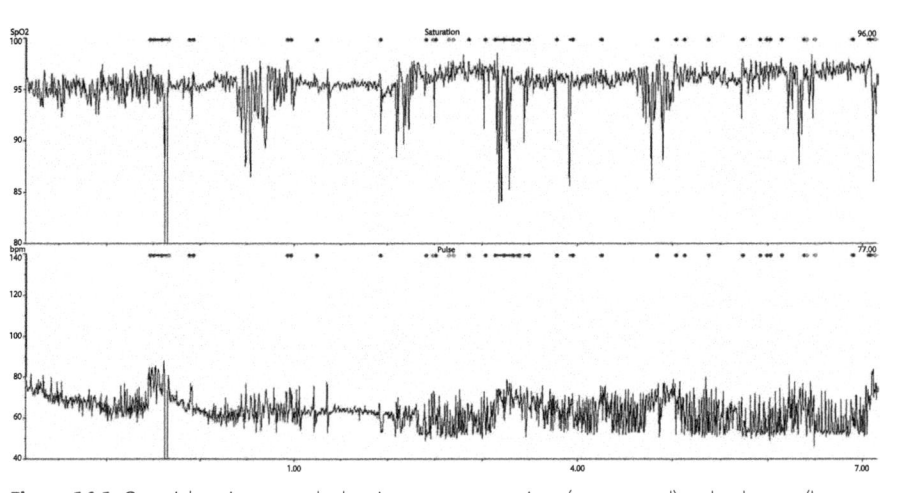

Figure 16.1 Overnight oximetry study showing oxygen saturations (upper panel) and pulse rate (lower panel). Periods of limited desaturations occurring intermittently throughout the night coincide with rapid eye movement sleep or supine position. The study shows no evidence of rapid repetitive desaturation and resaturation consistent with upper airways obstruction and obstructive sleep apnoea or significant prolonged desaturations to suggest clinically significant hypoventilation.

> ❂ **Learning point** Indication for overnight non-invasive ventilation in neuromuscular disease and chest wall deformity: monitoring respiratory function and screening for sleep-disordered breathing
>
> Progressive neuromuscular disease (NMD) may lead to respiratory muscle weakness. Respiratory muscle weakness and chest wall deformity can result in a restrictive ventilatory deficit and chronic respiratory failure, which can often be overlooked. Evidence supports the use of long-term non-invasive ventilation (NIV) to improve mortality in patients with NMD or chest wall deformity [1, 2]. Assessments of respiratory impairment secondary to NMD and chest wall disease can encompass a simple assessment of breathlessness, through to sitting and supine spirometry, to direct measurement of respiratory muscle strength using inspiratory and expiratory mouth pressures as well as sniff nasal pressures [3].
>
> While established chronic respiratory failure is an obvious indicator of the need for ventilatory support, it is ideal to pre-empt this event and initiate NIV prior to the occurrence of diurnal respiratory failure, but not so early as to burden the patient unnecessarily. Assessment of ventilation during sleep offers an ideal opportunity to detect patients at risk of decompensation, in the near future or in the event of a respiratory infection, as the normal physiological changes during sleep [4] stress the respiratory system and identify the need for domiciliary NIV [5, 6]. Such at-risk patients should therefore be closely assessed at presentation with acute illness for features of respiratory muscle weakness and sleep-disordered breathing that places them at risk of sleep hypoventilation and thus subsequent decompensation.

He was admitted to his local hospital with a 10-day history of a productive cough and worsening breathlessness, despite a course of broad-spectrum antibiotics in the community. On admission, he was febrile with right basal crackles. A chest X-ray showed right lower lobe consolidation and sputum culture isolated a sensitive *Klebsiella* species. Despite Tazocin 4.5 g three times daily started on admission he developed acute respiratory failure within 48 hours, which was managed initially with NIV. Over the next 24 hours, his lower airways secretion load increased and hypoxaemia worsened, requiring emergency tracheal intubation for invasive ventilation, oxygenation, and regular bronchial toileting.

> ❂ **Learning point** Predicting failure of non-invasive ventilation/selection for non-invasive ventilation
>
> NIV is increasingly used in acute decompensated hypercapnic respiratory failure within the critical care unit and on the general medical wards. The indications for NIV have expanded over the past 20 years and it is considered first-line therapy in many clinical situations [7]. However, while there is robust evidence supporting its use in patients with acute respiratory acidosis secondary to exacerbations of chronic obstructive pulmonary disease (COPD) [8, 9], the data supporting its use in other situations are less compelling. There have been no randomized controlled trials demonstrating superiority of NIV to invasive ventilation in obesity-related acute hypercapnic respiratory failure, but there is observational evidence to support its use [10]. However, as NIV failure is associated with a poor prognosis in numerous clinical contexts [11–14], it is essential to use NIV appropriately, targeting the patients who will benefit most, such as those with pre-existing chronic respiratory disease and considering carefully which patients should be managed within critical care to facilitate rapid escalation to intubation when appropriate (Table 16.1).
>
> *(continued)*

Table 16.1 Factors associated with non-invasive ventilation failure

Patient factors	Poor nutrition
	Confusion with agitation
	High upper and lower airways secretion load
	Lobar consolidation on the chest radiograph
Intervention factors	Poor patient–ventilator synchrony
	Excessive mask leak
	Insufficient ventilator pressures
Outcome factors	Failure to improve respiratory rate or acidosis within 1 hour of initiating NIV

An experienced multidisciplinary team is vital to the success of acute NIV. Despite the widespread use of NIV including on the ward, its use requires education and training [15]. Regular clinical exposure is important in maintaining skills and use of NIV in multiple clinical settings can lead to dilution of expertise with subsequent erosion of skills whereas consolidation of NIV skills in a single setting, such as a respiratory intermediate care unit, can be both clinically and cost-effective [16].

Over the following 7 days, and despite numerous attempts with differing strategies, he was unable to be weaned from invasive ventilation. After discussion with the respiratory unit which had been undertaking his long-term monitoring, he was transferred to an ICU with an attached weaning, rehabilitation, and home mechanical ventilation centre. This was to facilitate direct input from specialist clinicians to manage his complex neuromuscular condition and likely requirement for prolonged mechanical ventilation.

⊗ Learning point Simple weaning from mechanical ventilation

The process of weaning from mechanical ventilation can only occur when patients have sufficient physiological reserve to respond to the increase in work of breathing that will occur on reduction and withdrawal of ventilator support. 'Readiness to wean' is the term used to describe assessment of a patient's suitability for a trial of weaning. Weaning in this context may involve either a spontaneous breathing trial (SBT) or reduction in pressure support. Criteria for readiness testing are:

- improving clinical picture
- adequate oxygenation (e.g. partial pressure of oxygen (PaO_2) ≥8 kPa breathing a fraction of inspired oxygen (FiO_2) ≤0.4 and positive end-expiratory pressure (PEEP) ≤10 cmH_2O)
- cardiovascular stability (e.g. heart rate ≤120 beats/min (bpm), stable blood pressure, and minimal or no vasopressors)
- afebrile
- no significant respiratory acidosis
- adequate haemoglobin (e.g. haemoglobin concentration ≥70 g/L)
- adequate mentation (e.g. Glasgow Coma Scale score ≥12)
- adequate cough function to allow secretion clearance
- stable metabolic state.

The rapid shallow breathing index (RSBI) has been used as a weaning predictor in patients who are deemed ready to wean [17]. The RSBI is performed in spontaneously breathing, awake patients with

(continued)

minimal respiratory support. This involves monitoring respiratory parameters during a short period (2 min) of self-ventilation using a T-piece. The second minute of the test is used to calculate the RSBI which is the respiratory frequency divided by the average tidal volume. The use of a T-piece most accurately reflects post-extubation work of breathing, with the use of PEEP or pressure support reducing the discriminatory value of the test. A value of greater than 100 breaths/min/L indicates a high risk of extubation failure (95%) with a value less than 100 breaths/min/L indicating an 80% chance of extubation success [17].

Although it has sensitivity to predict weaning failure, it has poor specificity and its routine use has not been shown to improve outcomes [18]. Other weaning predictors have been used including oxygenation, minute ventilation, occlusion pressure, and work of breathing [19–22]. However, and not surprisingly, each of these single predictors has insufficient power to discriminate between weaning success and failure in daily clinical practice. Although integrated measures have been suggested, they have also failed to be translated into a useful clinical tool [23], highlighting that weaning from mechanical ventilation is a complex task. Patients deemed ready to wean but at high risk of extubation failure can be supported after extubation with NIV. The use of NIV in these high-risk patients can reduce the risk of reintubation and improve hospital survival [24]. More recent data suggest that high-flow, humidified nasal oxygen therapy demonstrates equivalent benefits to NIV in the high-risk post-extubation simple weaning group, although interestingly the NIV arm had significant rates of therapy failure (approximately 50%), emphasizing the importance of skill and experience in applying this intervention [25].

✪ Learning point Predicting failure to wean and prolonged mechanical ventilation

Prolonged mechanical ventilation, incorporating weaning failure, is defined as the provision of ventilator support for greater than 21 days, although there are subtle differences between the UK and other international consensus definitions [26, 27]. The UK definition is based on days of invasive ventilation, whereas international consensus incorporates days of invasive ventilation and the number of failed SBTs.

International consensus categorization of weaning

- Simple: progression from weaning to successful extubation at first attempt.
- Difficult: up to three SBTs or 7 days from first SBT prior to extubation.
- Prolonged: failure to extubate after at least three SBTs or more than 7 days following first SBT.

Early identification of patients who are likely to undergo prolonged mechanical ventilation and weaning failure will enhance decision-making and care planning. Factors associated with an increased risk of prolonged mechanical ventilation include admission with pneumonia, acute respiratory distress syndrome, COPD, restrictive lung disease, NMD, poor nutritional state, and severe acute physiological derangement at presentation to ICU [28]. Patients with chronic respiratory failure due to COPD, NMD (pre-morbid or ICU acquired), or obesity are at high risk of prolonged mechanical ventilation and weaning failure and often will require transition to NIV [29]. Generalized skeletal muscle weakness can be assessed by the Medical Research Council (MRC) sum score; this is a manual technique and involves a clinician using opposing force to rate the strength of a patient's peripheral muscle groups. The sum score is calculated by the cumulative score provided by testing the power of three upper and three lower limb groups each rated from 0 to 5 (maximum 60). The MRC sum score has been used to identify potential respiratory muscle weakness and thus risk for extended ventilation, but the test is poorly repeatable in the clinical setting and thus unreliable [30, 31]. Furthermore, the individual predictive power of any of these clinical factors is low and so prognostic assessments are unreliable [28]. Patients who undergo prolonged mechanical ventilation have a high mortality with around half of patients not surviving to 12 months—deaths occur both during and after weaning [32, 33]. Many survivors will have impairment to physical, cognitive, and psychosocial aspects of quality of life [34]. However, the severity of these impairments will be most related to the number of comorbidities and presence of chronic disease, rather than duration of mechanical ventilation [34].

Following transfer, as the patient exhibited agitated delirium, he was sedated with propofol at 100 mg/hour. A size 8.0 mm internal diameter tracheal tube was in place. The ventilatory mode was changed to bi-level pressure control with an inspiratory pressure of 22 cmH$_2$O and an expiratory pressure of 7 cmH$_2$O, a back-up rate of 12 breaths/min, inspiratory time (Ti) of 1.4 seconds with a FiO$_2$ of 0.50. Arterial blood gas (ABG) analysis showed pH 7.53, partial pressure of carbon dioxide (PaCO$_2$) 5.9 kPa, PaO$_2$ 16.9 kPa, base excess 13 mmol/L, and standard bicarbonate (sHCO$_3^-$) 35.6 mmol/L. His heart rate was 57 bpm in sinus rhythm and blood pressure was 97/57 mmHg. He had extensive pitting oedema to the knees bilaterally and was being fed via a nasogastric tube and had a urinary catheter *in situ*. A chest X-ray showed resolution of the original consolidation which was replaced by widespread alveolar shadowing, and with the reduction in inflammatory markers indicated fluid overload and pulmonary oedema rather than a recurrent or persistent respiratory infection (Figure 16.2). The patient was agitated and biting the tube.

🄲 Expert comment

Patients with chronic respiratory failure have elevated serum bicarbonate levels to metabolically compensate for the respiratory acidosis caused by the elevated PaCO$_2$. If aggressive ventilation is pursued in such patients with a view to achieving normocapnia, then the inevitable result is a metabolic alkalosis. This acts to blunt the respiratory centre's response to carbon dioxide and may leave the patient prone to central apnoeas and respiratory centre instability resulting in periodic breathing. The target carbon dioxide values in patients with chronic respiratory failure should be based on the admission bicarbonate values or, if available, the pre-admission PaCO$_2$.

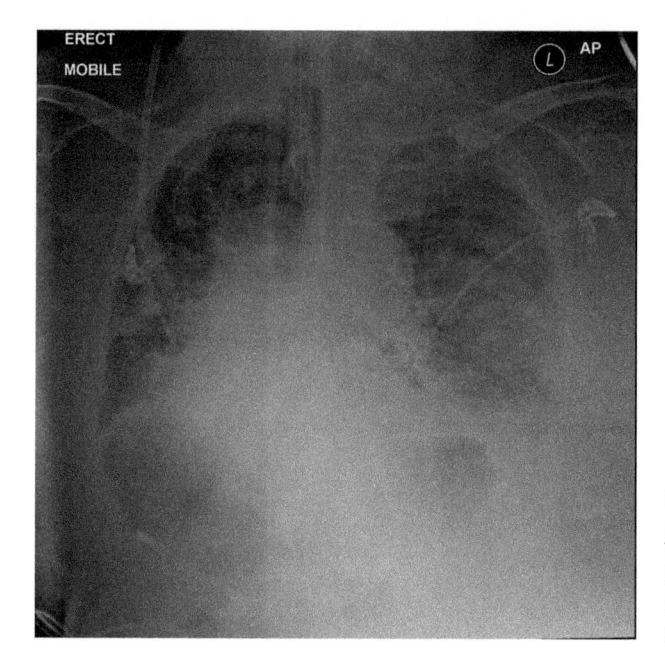

Figure 16.2 Chest radiograph performed following transfer. The image shows extensive bilateral perihilar airspace shadowing consistent with pulmonary oedema.

✪ Learning point Identify causes of prolonged ventilation

Patients who meet the criteria for prolonged mechanical ventilation and weaning failure should have a careful review by an experienced critical care physician to identify potential barriers to weaning. Assuming the initial reversible cause of ventilatory failure has resolved, then further causes can be considered that contribute to failure to wean by causing an imbalance in the load–capacity–drive relationship of the respiratory system.

Increased respiratory load

- Airways disease, such as COPD, results in expiratory flow limitation and increased threshold load (dynamic lung hyperinflation) and elastic load (bronchospasm and secretion load) of the respiratory system. Ventilator setting must accommodate a prolonged expiratory time to prevent hyperinflation.
- Obesity contributes to decreased pulmonary compliance and increased threshold load due to intrinsic PEEP and also contributes to increased elastic load [35]. High intra-abdominal pressure reduces lung volume placing the patient on an inefficient part of the respiratory pressure–volume curve [36]. Obesity also confers a significant increase in work of breathing, placing further demands on the respiratory muscles [37].
- Chest wall deformity, such as scoliosis and kyphosis, can often be overlooked as a cause of increased work of breathing and may contribute to chronic respiratory failure.

Reduced respiratory muscle capacity

- Chronic respiratory muscle weakness secondary to established NMD (e.g. myotonic dystrophy and Duchene muscular dystrophy) is likely to be diagnosed before admission. However, adults may present *de novo* to critical care with an acute decompensation complicating progressive respiratory muscle-predominant neurological diseases such as motor neuron disease or late-onset Pompe's disease. Features of NMD should therefore be assessed on all slowly weaning subjects with attention paid to generalized muscle and tongue fasciculation, loss of muscle bulk, evidence of diaphragmatic weakness or history prior to admission of bulbar dysfunction, features of respiratory muscle weakness, gait abnormalities, or falls.
- Prolonged critical illness can be associated with critical illness polymyoneuropathy which can lead to significant general and respiratory muscle weakness contributing to weaning delays.
- Metabolic derangements and malnutrition are corrected to ensure optimal respiratory muscle function. Magnesium supplementation may augment diaphragmatic function, although whether this is clinically beneficial in the critical care population is unproven [38].

Reduced neural respiratory drive

- Patients presenting with acute ascending radiculopathies, such as Guillain–Barré syndrome and its variants, will have profound generalized and respiratory muscle weakness. While acute treatment with steroids or intravenous immunoglobulin and plasmapheresis may lead to rapid improvement in some, many patients require prolonged weaning because of a profound reduction in respiratory drive and respiratory muscle capacity. The duration of recovery may be many months and is best coordinated across the multidisciplinary team with clear rehabilitation as well as respiratory targets.
- Obesity-related chronic respiratory failure is increasingly common within ICUs, yet it is often undiagnosed [39]. In addition to increased work of breathing, compared to their counterparts with 'simple obesity' these patients also have a marked reduction in ventilatory drive with further suppression in response to an increased FiO_2 [40]. Evidence of chronic respiratory failure, such as elevated base excess and bicarbonate on admission, assists in setting appropriate physiological targets.
- Less commonly, disorders of the neuromuscular junction, such as myasthenia gravis or botulinum toxin poisoning, can impair the ability to transmit respiratory drive from the cortex to the respiratory muscles contributing to weaning failure and, as potentially reversible causes, should be considered, investigated, and when present treated.

In addition to impediments to weaning caused by imbalance in the respiratory muscle load–capacity–drive relationship, non-respiratory factors may inhibit weaning. Severe cardiac dysfunction whether in isolation or comorbid to congenital muscular dystrophies may prevent weaning [41–43]. Left ventricular failure and subsequent pulmonary oedema can contribute to increased work of breathing and the beneficial cardiac effects of positive airway pressure may render patients ventilator dependent. A cardiology review is recommended in these patients.

(continued)

Optimal fluid management along with treatment of any reversible ischaemia and residual heart failure is required to progress weaning. Patients with established cardiac disease have negative physiological consequences of weaning ventilator pressures with one study showing an increase in pulmonary wedge pressure during weaning trials and subsequent improvement of weaning success following diuresis [41]. In some patients, weaning may be facilitated by coronary revascularization [44]. More radical approaches such as the use of cardiac resynchronization devices or long-term inotropes, such as levosimendan, may offer potential salvage therapy for patients with few alternative avenues for liberation from mechanical ventilation. There is experimental evidence that levosimendan, a calcium-sensitizing agent, may have a direct beneficial effect on diaphragm function in these patients [45]. However, recent data in patients with septic shock demonstrated no advantage of levosimendan on sequential organ dysfunction score (the study primary outcome) and interestingly demonstrated delayed weaning in the treatment compared to placebo group [46]. It must be realized when interpreting these data that the patient group were not weaning failure patients and that chronic cardiac dysfunction, despite optimization of other therapy, was not a prerequisite for trial entry. However, these data suggest the indiscriminate use of levosimendan cannot be supported, and it should be reserved for carefully evaluated patients with weaning failure and evidence of cardiac dysfunction.

❝ Expert comment

Patients with profound cardiac dysfunction but without comorbid chronic respiratory disease or NMD may be unable to be liberated from mechanical ventilation. These patients may often be normocapnic with the ability to achieve spontaneous ventilation on modest continuous positive airway pressure (CPAP) support but will rapidly decompensate following its withdrawal. This can be demonstrated by removal of positive pressure at the bedside with a clinical evidence of a fall in cardiac output such as cooling of the peripheries and associated respiratory distress.

A comprehensive case review was undertaken, the issues contributing to delayed weaning were considered in full, and a weaning strategy was developed. A major contributor to the patient's failure to wean was ongoing delirium, exacerbated by poorly controlled musculoskeletal pain, sleep deprivation, and poor positioning in bed because of his significant skeletal deformity. Fentanyl analgesia was added with the aim of reducing the propofol infusion. The goal was a Richmond Agitation Sedation Scale (RASS) score of −1 to 0 (i.e. alert and calm or minimally drowsy). His fluid overload was managed with a daily negative fluid balance target of −750 to −1000 mL. When sedation, analgesia, and diuresis led to relative hypotension, vasopressor support was commenced. Lorazepam 0.5 mg 8-hourly was added, enabling gradual reduction of propofol dose and negating the requirement for vasopressor support.

The weaning strategy led to a decrease in ventilatory support (Table 16.2).

Table 16.2 Observation chart demonstrating weaning of ventilator pressures over 4 days

	Day 7		Day 8		Day 9		Day 10	
Time	06:00	22:00	06:00	22:00	06:00	22:00	06:00	22:00
Ventilator mode	BiPAP	BiPAP	BiPAP	BiPAP	BiPAP	BiPAP	BiPAP	BiPAP
FiO_2	0.30	0.30	0.28	0.28	0.25	0.25	0.25	0.25
Pressure support (cmH_2O)	18	16	14	14	14	14	12	12
PEEP/CPAP (cmH_2O)	8	8	8	8	6	6	5	5
Ti (s)	1.0	0.9	0.9	0.8	0.7	0.7	0.7	0.7
Set respiratory rate	16	18	20	20	22	20	20	18
Minute ventilation (L/min)	7.3	7.7	8.9	8.3	10.8	9.3	10.6	8.9

BiPAP, bi-level positive airway pressure; CPAP, continuous positive airway pressure; FiO_2, fraction of inspired oxygen; PEEP, positive end-expiratory pressure; Ti, inspiratory time.

Despite clinical improvements in fluid overload, agitation, and delirium control, secretion management remained problematic and a tracheostomy was planned to facilitate weaning and respiratory physiotherapy. After family discussion, a size 9.0 mm internal diameter, non-fenestrated, cuffed percutaneous tracheostomy tube was inserted without complication on day 10 of mechanical ventilation. Insertion of the tracheostomy tube facilitated reduction in sedation with cessation of propofol and fentanyl by day 12.

> ### ⊗ Learning point   Timing of tracheostomy and weaning modes of ventilation
>
> For the majority of ICU patients, resolution of the acute illness is timely and simple weaning strategies with a protocolized approach, daily sedation holds, and SBT is successful [47]. Patients who are more complex or in whom this approach fails are likely to benefit more from a bespoke plan that addresses the underlying causes of failure to wean. The data supporting protocolized weaning are subject to debate with the control group in the landmark trials being weaned in a synchronous mandated mode of ventilation, which would not be considered standard practice today [48, 49].
>
> There is a lack of robust evidence of improved mortality and reduced ICU length of stay with early (<10 days) compared with late tracheostomy (>10 days) [50, 51]. Despite this, current practice within critical care is not to delay tracheostomy and most units perform tracheostomies within the first 2 weeks of invasive ventilation [52, 53]. Early tracheostomy facilitates withdrawal of sedation and promotes communication and bulbar function. There are no data to suggest patients, even those with high risk for prolonged mechanical ventilation, benefit from very early tracheostomy [54]. In these high-risk patients, thought should be given to early aggressive management of the disease process that precipitated critical care admission with a view to early extubation to NIV to avoid the complications of prolonged mechanical ventilation.
>
> Ventilator settings have a significant impact on ability to wean patients from mechanical ventilation and need to be actively managed both during and between weaning trials. Settings need to alleviate work of breathing and provide rest for respiratory muscles while avoiding iatrogenic injury. Thought is commonly given to pressure support, PEEP, and back-up rate settings to provide the patient with adequate tidal volume (6–8 mL/kg ideal body weight) and ventilation (6–12 L/min) and to control arterial CO_2. However, attention also needs to be given to settings such as inspiratory time, ventilator mode, trigger method, and trigger sensitivity which all influence efficacy of ventilation. The use of flow triggering (rather than pressure triggering) is associated with reduced work of breathing in both pressure support and intermittent mandatory modes of ventilation. In patients with expiratory flow limitation (e.g. COPD, asthma), settings should enable sufficient expiratory time and applied PEEP should be optimized to offset intrinsic PEEP and improve respiratory mechanics (see Case 8).
>
> Weaning trials should initially involve a staged reduction in pressure support during daytime with return to full respiratory support at night. Care is taken to provide an appropriate stimulus to the respiratory muscles for training while avoiding respiratory muscle fatigue, recovery from which can take longer than 24 hours. When the patient can tolerate larger reductions in respiratory support, CPAP trials can be considered. In some patients with good ventilatory reserve but difficulty with oxygenation, high-flow, humidified oxygen can be considered via tracheostomy, although little data is available on its effectiveness.

Mechanical insufflation–exsufflation (MIE), using a cough assist device attached to a tracheostomy tube catheter mount, was used to assist secretion clearance. The tracheostomy tube was downsized on day 18 to a size 8.0 mm internal diameter tracheostomy tube.

At this point, the patient was transferred from the ICU to the weaning, rehabilitation, and home mechanical ventilation centre. Cuff down trials facilitated weaning and communication, which demonstrated persistent delirium that required regular re-orientation therapy and ongoing use of low-dose lorazepam (0.5 mg three times daily). During cuff down trials, bulbar function was fully assessed by the multidisciplinary team, including speech and language therapists, allowing sensitization of the larynx and pharynx, which facilitated both upper and lower airway secretion management by improving swallow and cough function. The weaning process was delayed by an intercurrent ventilator-associated pneumonia, during which weaning was suspended. Once cuff deflation was tolerated for greater than 24 hours without problems, the

> ### ⊕ Clinical tip
> **Assisting phonation**
>
> The reduction in the external diameter of the tube facilitates airflow around the tube assisting phonation during cuff down trials. Standard critical care dual-limb ventilators are often intolerant of this 'unintentional' leak and so the use of a single-limb circuit ventilator with leak compensation is preferred.

tracheostomy was changed to a size 7.5 mm internal diameter, non-fenestrated cuffless tube. Weaning progressed from day 18 to day 25 with stepwise daytime reduction in pressure support (1–2 cmH$_2$O per day as tolerated) with a speaking valve in circuit (Passy-Muir Valve) to promote phonation and self-management of secretion clearance. Independence and self-management was encouraged and the patient was able to cough his secretions to his mouth and remove with suction. From day 25, the patient progressed to daytime CPAP trials at 8 cmH$_2$O with a speaking valve in circuit, initially intermittently and then for the duration of the day. From day 30, the patient started daytime self-ventilation trials with the speaking valve attached to the tracheostomy tube and heated humidification provided by the tracheostomy mask.

In conjunction with daytime respiratory weaning, daily goal-directed physical rehabilitation sessions were performed with a specialist multidisciplinary team including respiratory, rehabilitative, and post-polio physiotherapy, occupational therapy, dietetic therapy, and speech and language therapy. The aim of rehabilitation was to direct full recovery and return the patient to his baseline physical function.

By day 36, he had progressed to self-ventilation during the daytime and invasive ventilatory support at night (Table 16.3).

Daytime trials of NIV were started with the aim of establishing nocturnal NIV to manage rapid eye movement sleep alveolar hypoventilation (a consequence of the patient's restrictive ventilatory defect secondary to previous poliomyelitis and chest wall deformity). By day 42, the patient was established on nocturnal NIV, with the tracheostomy tube capped off at night and speaking valve applied during the daytime. To manage persistent, high-volume secretions, the tracheostomy tube was replaced with a size 4.0 mm internal diameter mini-tracheostomy tube.

> **🎓 Expert comment**
>
> The use of a speaking valve adds to the respiratory load and therefore the patient's work of breathing. However, the use of speaking valves facilitates communication and enables improved goal setting and patient motivation during prolonged weaning. The additional load can be used for a training effect on the respiratory muscles. Training should emulate the desired effect on muscle function (i.e. patients require an endurance method for training during weaning with duration of weaning interventions of >20 min) .

> **🎓 Expert comment**
>
> Following tracheostomy insertion, the use of NIV can be limited by excessive leak from the tracheostomy stoma making the use of 'bridging' NIV more complex with the need to accept high levels of leak. Downsizing of tracheostomies during weaning facilitates bulbar function and communication. Once patients can self-ventilate during the day and are tolerating NIV with adequate control of nocturnal hypoventilation at night then decannulation can be considered. However, frequently patients still have excessive secretions that are not fully mobilized by MIE alone and require suction to clear. Movement of secretions from the lower airway into the mouth for clearance is partly impeded by a large tracheostomy. The use of a mini-tracheostomy enables ongoing access to the lower respiratory tract but reduces the size of obstruction in the trachea and although not evaluated in randomized controlled trials improves secretion management in high-risk patient groups [7]. Ventilator support cannot be provided by the mini-tracheostomy; therefore, the team need to be confident that the respiratory requirements can be met non-invasively.

> **✪ Learning point Cough augmentation**
>
> Sputum retention and airway plugging can cause significant respiratory distress with associated morbidity and should be avoided by proactive chest physiotherapy. A tracheostomy facilitates airway toileting. In patients with neuromuscular disorders and ineffective cough, secretion clearance can be a barrier to decannulation. Cough function requires several steps, with lung inflation, closure of the glottis, and forced expiration against the closed glottis followed by rapid glottic opening resulting in an explosive expiratory effort. This complex process requires adequate inspiratory and expiratory muscle strength as well as bulbar function [55]. Measurement of a cough peak expiratory flow rate (PEFR) while ventilated, along with clinical assessment of respiratory muscle function and cough
>
> *(continued)*

Table 16.3 Observation chart demonstrating weaning of daytime support from daytime CPAP to intermittent daytime CPAP with interspersed self-ventilating periods over 3 days with return to invasive bi-level ventilation via tracheostomy during night-time

	Day 33							Day 34						Day 35						Day 36			
Time	06:00	10:00	14:00	18:00	22:00	02:00	06:00	10:00	14:00	18:00	22:00	02:00	06:00	10:00	14:00	18:00	22:00	02:00	06:00	10:00	14:00	18:00	22:00
Ventilator mode	PCV	CPAP	CPAP	CPAP	PCV	PCV	PCV	CPAP	SV	CPAP	PCV	PCV	PCV	SV	CPAP	SV	PCV	PCV	PCV	SV	SV	SV	PCV
FIO$_2$	0.21	0.21	0.21	0.21	0.21	0.21	0.21	0.21	0.21	0.21	0.21	0.21	0.21	0.21	0.21	0.21	0.21	0.21	0.21	0.21	0.21	0.21	0.21
Pressure support (cmH$_2$O)	13				13	13	13				13	13	13				13	13	13				13
CPAP (cmH$_2$O)	5	10	10	10	5	5	5	10		10	5	5	5		10		5	5	5				5
Set respiratory rate	16				16	16	16				16	16	16				16	16	16				16
Ti (S)	1.3				1.3	1.3	1.3				1.3	1.3	1.3				1.3	1.3	1.3				1.3

CPAP, continuous positive airway pressure; FIO$_2$, fraction of inspired oxygen; PCV, pressure control ventilation; SV, self-ventilation; Ti, inspiratory time.

adequacy, may identify patients in whom secretion clearance is a barrier to weaning. Cough PEFR may be difficult to measure but a value of less than 160 L/min indicates the need for additional support for effective secretion management [56].

The use of MIE devices, often referred to as cough assist devices, provides additional support to the respiratory muscles and aids secretion clearance [57]. MIE devices can be used during weaning via a tracheostomy or via a face mask following decannulation. The optimal settings for an individual patient vary greatly: pressure swings from +40 to −40 cmH$_2$O have traditionally been used but both larger and smaller pressure swings may be effective [57, 58]. In the acutely unwell patient, care needs to be taken to avoid lung derecruitment caused by the large negative intrathoracic pressure. Although MIE devices improve cough force and flow, there are no data showing improvement in hard clinical outcomes. Although an MIE device can assist in secretion mobilization it cannot compensate for poor bulbar function which may still prevent adequate secretion clearance following extubation or decannulation.

Nocturnal NIV was delivered by a full facemask, with circuit humidification and an FiO$_2$ of 0.21 (room air).

> **✪ Learning point Success of transition from invasive to non-invasive ventilation**
>
> Many patients with chronic respiratory disease can wean from daytime ventilatory support but may not have sufficient respiratory reserve to tolerate the challenges posed to the respiratory system during sleep. Patients with established or presumptive diagnoses of sleep-disordered breathing and chronic respiratory failure often require long-term NIV following successful weaning [33]. The transition from invasive ventilation to NIV requires careful management, as the reinstitution of invasive respiratory support following decannulation can be traumatic and is associated with significant morbidity. Once suitable patients have been established as self-ventilating via tracheostomy during daytime they can be introduced to NIV with a capped tracheostomy. This should occur after they have been taught the rationale for the transition to NIV, as understanding of the importance of this step towards decannulation and return to home maintains motivation. Patients can often find the pressure and interfaces used for NIV uncomfortable and so a period of daytime acclimatization at low pressures may be required. The choice of interface depends on patient preference, underlying diagnosis, and estimated final NIV pressures but can include nasal pillows, nasal mask, oronasal mask, total face mask, or hood. Although nasal masks can be used to provide adequate ventilation in patients with NMD they are unsuitable for higher inflation pressures and excessive mouth leak can cause sleep disruption during use [59]. When patients are able to tolerate periods of NIV overnight, limited sleep studies are performed with transcutaneous carbon dioxide monitoring to ensure adequate control of sleep hypoventilation [60]. Progression can be made towards decannulation if the results of the respiratory sleep study demonstrate satisfactory control.

Over the next 10 days, discharge plans were made alongside ongoing multidisciplinary rehabilitation and secretion management. Nocturnal NIV was optimized with overnight oximetry and capnometry. A mechanical cough assist device was used three times daily. This enabled clearing of lower airway secretions to the large airways and cough assist directing secretions to the mouth for suctioning. This facilitated removal of the mini-tracheostomy tube. The patient was discharged home on day 60, with a reinstatement of his original home care package as he had returned to his premorbid level of function.

Discussion

Approximately 5–10% of ICU patients will require prolonged mechanical ventilation (> 21 days) and these patients account for a disproportionate number of ICU bed days [61]. Although protocolized weaning strategies, with daily SBTs or a gradual reduction in pressure support ventilation, have been adopted by many centres to prevent delayed extubation and subsequent tracheostomy formation [62, 63], these protocolized strategies have limited utility with the patient requiring prolonged mechanical ventilation. The heterogeneous nature of patients with delayed weaning and prolonged mechanical ventilation requires a more bespoke plan that addresses the underlying causes of failure to wean.

The goal of weaning and rehabilitation is to achieve prompt recovery of independent function and minimize the development of acute skeletal muscle wasting [64] and other long-term complications of mechanical ventilation. For this reason, weaning and rehabilitation should start early, when the patient is in the recovery stage of their illness and is progressing towards clinical stability.

Patients who are unable to wean despite correction of the initial physiological insult will require prolonged mechanical ventilation and the development of a dynamic and bespoke weaning plan involving multiple disciplines [65]. This is achieved by goal-directed physical, respiratory, speech and language, and occupational therapy rehabilitation combined with nutritional support.

Such complex patients also require psychological and cognitive support as these are common contributors to weaning delay and failure in patients undergoing prolonged mechanical ventilation. Communication of the weaning strategy to the patient and caregivers is essential as part of a holistic approach to care. This approach also includes focusing on areas such as sleep quantity, quality, and timing as well as stimulation and motivation of the patient [66].

While many patients will be liberated from mechanical ventilation, up to 25% of patients undergoing prolonged mechanical ventilation will require transition to NIV and around 20% will require intermediate or long-term tracheostomy ventilation due to irreversible, progressive, or slowly reversible neurological conditions, chronic lung disease, or obesity-related respiratory failure [67].

As these long-term tracheostomy-ventilated patients progress to clinical stability, they will be suitable for transfer to specialized community nursing facilities and a small proportion will be suitable for discharge home, with a comprehensive care package. This is usually not an option for patients with COPD because they tend to have frequent exacerbations.

A final word from the expert

The provision of long-term acute care for long-term ventilated patients (an established strategy in the US driven principally by economic pressures to move patients out of acute care facilities) is wholly distinct from cost-effective specialist weaning centres [33, 68]. Facilities accommodating long-term tracheostomy-ventilated patients in the community need ongoing multidisciplinary support from the weaning centre to enable clinical stability in the community. A competency-based process of education and training of the community care team is essential for the management of these complex patients.

As most of these patients have a high level of comorbidity in addition to their respiratory needs, decisions about escalation of care during future hospitalization should be considered and discussed when appropriate. Patients and their relatives may have unrealistic expectations of the potential for long-term survival, and consideration should be given to all aspects of the patient's outcome which will include both their quality of life and functional ability.

References

1. Bourke SC, Tomlinson M, Williams TL, et al. Effects of non-invasive ventilation on survival and quality of life in patients with amyotrophic lateral sclerosis: a randomised controlled trial. *Lancet Neurol.* 2006;5:140–7.
2. Buyse B, Meersseman W, Demedts M. Treatment of chronic respiratory failure in kyphoscoliosis: oxygen or ventilation? *Eur Respir J.* 2003;22:525–8.
3. Lyall RA, Donaldson N, Polkey MI. Respiratory muscle strength and ventilatory failure in amyotrophic lateral sclerosis. *Brain.* 2001;124:2000–13.
4. Douglas NJ, White DP, Pickett CK, Weil JV, Zwillich CW. Respiration during sleep in normal man. *Thorax.* 1982;37:840–4.
5. Hukins CA, Hillman DR. Daytime predictors of sleep hypoventilation in Duchenne muscular dystrophy. *Am J Respir Crit Care Med.* 2000;161:166–70.
6. Ward S, Chatwin M, Heather S, Simonds AK. Randomised controlled trial of non-invasive ventilation (NIV) for nocturnal hypoventilation in neuromuscular and chest wall disease patients with daytime normocapnia. *Thorax.* 2005;60:1019–24.
7. Davidson AC, Banham S, Elliott M, et al. BTS/ICS guideline for the ventilatory management of acute hypercapnic respiratory failure in adults. *Thorax.* 2016;71 Suppl 2:ii1–35.
8. Brochard L, Mancebo J, Wysocki M, et al. Noninvasive ventilation for acute exacerbations of chronic obstructive pulmonary disease. *N Engl J Med.* 1995;333:817–22.
9. Bott J, Carroll MP, Conway JH, et al. Randomised controlled trial of nasal ventilation in acute ventilatory failure due to chronic obstructive airways disease. *Lancet.* 1993;341:1555–7.
10. Carrillo A, Ferrer M, Gonzalez-Diaz G, et al. Noninvasive ventilation in acute hypercapnic respiratory failure caused by obesity hypoventilation syndrome and chronic obstructive pulmonary disease. *Am J Respir Crit Care Med.* 2012;186:1279–85.
11. Lemyze M, Taufour P, Duhamel A, et al. Determinants of noninvasive ventilation success or failure in morbidly obese patients in acute respiratory failure. *PLoS One.* 2014;9:e97563.
12. Duarte AG, Justino E, Bigler T, Grady J. Outcomes of morbidly obese patients requiring mechanical ventilation for acute respiratory failure. *Crit Care Med.* 2007;35:732–7.
13. Carrillo A, Gonzalez-Diaz G, Ferrer M, et al. Non-invasive ventilation in community-acquired pneumonia and severe acute respiratory failure. *Intensive Care Med.* 2012;38:458–66.
14. Honrubia T, Garcia Lopez FJ, Franco N, et al. Noninvasive vs conventional mechanical ventilation in acute respiratory failure: a multicenter, randomized controlled trial. *Chest.* 2005;128:3916–24.
15. Ballard E, McDonnell L, Keilty S, Davidson AC, Hart N. Survey of knowledge of health care professionals managing patients with acute hypercapnic exacerbation of COPD requiring non-invasive ventilation. *Thorax.* 2007;62:A90.

16. Confalonieri M, Gorini M, Ambrosino N, Mollica C, Corrado A. Respiratory intensive care units in Italy: a national census and prospective cohort study. *Thorax*. 2001;56:373–8.

17. Yang KL, Tobin MJ. A prospective study of indexes predicting the outcome of trials of weaning from mechanical ventilation. *N Engl J Med*. 1991;324:1445–50.

18. Tanios MA, Nevins ML, Hendra KP, et al. A randomized, controlled trial of the role of weaning predictors in clinical decision making. *Crit Care Med*. 2006;34:2530–5.

19. Krieger BP, Ershowsky PF, Becker DA, Gazeroglu HB. Evaluation of conventional criteria for predicting successful weaning from mechanical ventilatory support in elderly patients. *Crit Care Med*. 1989;17:858–61.

20. Meade M, Guyatt G, Cook D, et al. Predicting success in weaning from mechanical ventilation. *Chest*. 2001;120:400S–24S.

21. Montgomery AB, Holle RH, Neagley SR, Pierson DJ, Schoene RB. Prediction of successful ventilator weaning using airway occlusion pressure and hypercapnic challenge. *Chest*. 1987;91:496–9.

22. Levy MM, Miyasaki A, Langston D. Work of breathing as a weaning parameter in mechanically ventilated patients. *Chest*. 1995;108:1018–20.

23. Delisle S, Francoeur M, Albert M, et al. Preliminary evaluation of a new index to predict the outcome of a spontaneous breathing trial. *Respir Care*. 2011;56:1500–5.

24. Burns KE, Meade MO, Premji A, Adhikari NK. Noninvasive positive-pressure ventilation as a weaning strategy for intubated adults with respiratory failure. *Cochrane Database Syst Rev*. 2013;12:CD004127.

25. Hernandez G, Vaquero C, Colinas L, et al. Effect of postextubation high-flow nasal cannula vs noninvasive ventilation on reintubation and postextubation respiratory failure in high-risk patients: a randomized clinical trial. *JAMA*. 2016;316:1565–74.

26. Boles JM, Bion J, Connors A, et al. Weaning from mechanical ventilation. *Eur Respir J*. 2007;29:1033–56.

27. MacIntyre NR, Epstein SK, Carson S, et al. Management of patients requiring prolonged mechanical ventilation: report of a NAMDRC consensus conference. *Chest*. 2005;128:3937–54.

28. Seneff MG, Zimmerman JE, Knaus WA, Wagner DP, Draper EA. Predicting the duration of mechanical ventilation. The importance of disease and patient characteristics. *Chest*. 1996;110:469–79.

29. Garnacho-Montero J, Amaya-Villar R, Garcia-Garmendia JL, Madrazo-Osuna J, Ortiz-Leyba C. Effect of critical illness polyneuropathy on the withdrawal from mechanical ventilation and the length of stay in septic patients. *Crit Care Med*. 2005;33:349–54.

30. De Jonghe B, Bastuji-Garin S, Durand MC, et al. Respiratory weakness is associated with limb weakness and delayed weaning in critical illness. *Crit Care Med*. 2007;35:2007–15.

31. Connolly BA, Jones GD, Curtis AA, et al. Clinical predictive value of manual muscle strength testing during critical illness: an observational cohort study. *Crit Care*. 2013;17:R229.

32. Scheinhorn DJ, Hassenpflug MS, Votto JJ, et al. Ventilator-dependent survivors of catastrophic illness transferred to 23 long-term care hospitals for weaning from prolonged mechanical ventilation. *Chest*. 2007;131:76–84.

33. Pilcher DV, Bailey MJ, Treacher DF, et al. Outcomes, cost and long term survival of patients referred to a regional weaning centre. *Thorax*. 2005;60:187–92.

34. Chatila W, Kreimer DT, Criner GJ. Quality of life in survivors of prolonged mechanical ventilatory support. *Crit Care Med*. 2001;29:737–42.

35. Steier J, Jolley CJ, Seymour J, et al. Neural respiratory drive in obesity. *Thorax*. 2009;64:719–25.

36. Steier J, Lunt A, Hart N, Polkey MI, Moxham J. Observational study of the effect of obesity on lung volumes. *Thorax*. 2014;69:752–9.

37. Sharp JT, Henry JP, Sweany SK, Meadows WR, Pietras RJ. The total work of breathing in normal and obese men. *J Clin Invest*. 1964;43:728–39.

38. Johnson D, Gallagher C, Cavanaugh M, Yip R, Mayers I. The lack of effect of routine magnesium administration on respiratory function in mechanically ventilated patients. *Chest*. 1993;104:536–41.

39. Marik PE, Desai H. Characteristics of patients with the 'malignant obesity hypoventilation syndrome' admitted to an ICU. *J Intensive Care Med*. 2013;28:124–30.

40. Hollier CA, Harmer AR, Maxwell LJ, et al. Moderate concentrations of supplemental oxygen worsen hypercapnia in obesity hypoventilation syndrome: a randomised crossover study. *Thorax*. 2014;69:346–53.

41. Lemaire F, Teboul JL, Cinotti L, et al. Acute left ventricular dysfunction during unsuccessful weaning from mechanical ventilation. *Anesthesiology*. 1988;69:171–9.

42. Chatila W, Ani S, Guaglianone D, et al. Cardiac ischemia during weaning from mechanical ventilation. *Chest*. 1996;109:1577–83.

43. Jubran A, Mathru M, Dries D, Tobin MJ. Continuous recordings of mixed venous oxygen saturation during weaning from mechanical ventilation and the ramifications thereof. *Am J Respir Crit Care Med*. 1998;158:1763–9.

44. Demoule A, Lefort Y, Lopes ME, Lemaire F. Successful weaning from mechanical ventilation after coronary angioplasty. *Br J Anaesth*. 2004;93:295–7.

45. Doorduin J, Sinderby CA, Beck J, et al. The calcium sensitizer levosimendan improves human diaphragm function. *Am J Respir Crit Care Med*. 2012;185:90–5.

46. Gordon AC, Perkins GD, Singer M, et al. Levosimendan for the prevention of acute organ dysfunction in sepsis. *N Engl J Med*. 2016;375:1638–48.

47. Scheinhorn DJ, Chao DC, Stearn-Hassenpflug M, Wallace WA. Outcomes in post-ICU mechanical ventilation: a therapist-implemented weaning protocol. *Chest*. 2001;119:236–42.

48. Esteban A, Frutos F, Tobin MJ, et al. A comparison of four methods of weaning patients from mechanical ventilation. Spanish Lung Failure Collaborative Group. *N Engl J Med*. 1995;332:345–50.

49. Brochard L, Rauss A, Benito S, et al. Comparison of three methods of gradual withdrawal from ventilatory support during weaning from mechanical ventilation. *Am J Respir Crit Care Med*. 1994;150:896–903.

50. Gomes Silva BN, Andriolo RB, Saconato H, Atallah AN, Valente O. Early versus late tracheostomy for critically ill patients. *Cochrane Database Syst Rev*. 2012;3:CD007271.

51. Siempos II, Ntaidou TK, Filippidis FT, Choi AM. Effect of early versus late or no tracheostomy on mortality and pneumonia of critically ill patients receiving mechanical ventilation: a systematic review and meta-analysis. *Lancet Respir Med*. 2015;3:150–8.

52. Krishnan K, Elliot SC, Mallick A. The current practice of tracheostomy in the United Kingdom: a postal survey. *Anaesthesia*. 2005;60:360–4.

53. Kluge S, Baumann HJ, Maier C, et al. Tracheostomy in the intensive care unit: a nationwide survey. *Anesth Analg*. 2008;107:1639–43.

54. Young D, Harrison DA, Cuthbertson BH, Rowan K. Effect of early vs late tracheostomy placement on survival in patients receiving mechanical ventilation: the TracMan randomized trial. *JAMA*. 2013;309:2121–9.

55. Bach JR. Amyotrophic lateral sclerosis: predictors for prolongation of life by noninvasive respiratory aids. *Arch Phys Med Rehabil*. 1995;76:828–32.

56. Bach JR, Saporito LR. Criteria for extubation and tracheostomy tube removal for patients with ventilatory failure. A different approach to weaning. *Chest*. 1996;110:1566–71.

57. Bach JR. Mechanical insufflation-exsufflation. Comparison of peak expiratory flows with manually assisted and unassisted coughing techniques. *Chest*. 1993;104:1553–62.

58. Chatwin M, Ross E, Hart N, et al. Cough augmentation with mechanical insufflation/exsufflation in patients with neuromuscular weakness. *Eur Respir J*. 2003;21:502–8.

59. Teschler H, Stampa J, Ragette R, Konietzko N, Berthon-Jones M. Effect of mouth leak on effectiveness of nasal bilevel ventilatory assistance and sleep architecture. *Eur Respir J*. 1999;14:1251–7.

60. Storre JH, Magnet FS, Dreher M, Windisch W. Transcutaneous monitoring as a replacement for arterial PCO(2) monitoring during nocturnal non-invasive ventilation. *Respir Med*. 2011;105:143–50.

61. Esteban A, Alia I, Ibanez J, Benito S, Tobin MJ. Modes of mechanical ventilation and weaning. A national survey of Spanish hospitals. The Spanish Lung Failure Collaborative Group. *Chest.* 1994;106:1188–93.

62. Girard TD, Kress JP, Fuchs BD, et al. Efficacy and safety of a paired sedation and ventilator weaning protocol for mechanically ventilated patients in intensive care (Awakening and Breathing Controlled trial): a randomised controlled trial. *Lancet.* 2008;371:126–34.

63. Kollef MH, Shapiro SD, Silver P, et al. A randomized, controlled trial of protocol-directed versus physician-directed weaning from mechanical ventilation. *Crit Care Med.* 1997;25:567–74.

64. Puthucheary ZA, Rawal J, McPhail M, et al. Acute skeletal muscle wasting in critical illness. *JAMA.* 2013;310:1591–600.

65. Creagh-Brown B, Steier J, Hart N. Prolonged weaning. In: Stevens RD, Hart N, Herridge M (eds) *Textbook of Post-ICU Medicine.* Oxford: Oxford University Press; 2014, pp. 559–71.

66. Jubran A, Lawm G, Kelly J, et al. Depressive disorders during weaning from prolonged mechanical ventilation. *Intensive Care Med.* 2010;36:828–35.

67. Mifsud Bonnici D, Sanctuary T, Warren A, et al. Prospective observational cohort study of patients with weaning failure admitted to a specialist weaning, rehabilitation and home mechanical ventilation centre. *BMJ Open.* 2016;6:e010025.

68. Kahn JM, Benson NM, Appleby D, Carson SS, Iwashyna TJ. Long-term acute care hospital utilization after critical illness. *JAMA.* 2010;303:2253–9.

Pandemic planning and critical care

Lucinda Gabriel

Expert Commentary Jeremy Farrar

Case history

A 46-year-old Caucasian man with a body mass index (BMI) of 40 kg/m^2 and a history of asthma was admitted to the medical unit following an unintentional paracetamol overdose. He provided a 5-day history of flu-like symptoms: generalized myalgia, fatigue, cough, and sore throat. He had a raised creatinine kinase and was lymphopenic on admission. The initial chest X-ray was unremarkable.

On day 2 of his hospital admission, he developed right-sided abdominal pain and became acutely hypoxaemic with a partial pressure of oxygen of 5.6 kPa on 15 L/min oxygen by facemask necessitating admission to the intensive care unit (ICU) for respiratory support. Based on his presentation, and a history of flu-like illness in his close contacts, he was transferred to an isolation room and droplet precautions were instituted.

✪ Learning point Variability of presentation/risk factors

There is much concern about the appearance of new influenza A virus subtypes (H5N1 in 1997, H1N1 in 2009, and H7N9 in 2013), and novel corona viruses (severe acute respiratory syndrome (SARS) in 2002 and Middle Eastern respiratory syndrome (MERS) in 2012). These outbreaks of pandemic influenza have varied widely in pathogenicity and potential for transmission [1] with major implications for how pandemic planning is approached. While there has been considerable learning from each of these episodes, there is a fundamental error in drawing learning directly from past events.

The case history illustrates that the clinical picture in severe cases of pandemic influenza is markedly different from that seen during epidemics of seasonal influenza (Table 17.1). Often there is a protracted period of illness prior to patients presenting to hospital, followed by a short period of acute respiratory deterioration. Patients with H1N1 experienced symptoms for an average of 6 days prior to hospital presentation, but rapidly worsened after hospital admission and generally required ICU admission within 1–2 days. Moreover, the clinical presentation of each pandemic influenza subtype also varies. Measures taken between pandemics to improve preparedness (inter-pandemic planning) are vital but require flexibility to enable responses that are appropriate to the variables of disease aetiology and local clinical context.

(continued)

Table 17.1 Characteristics and underlying conditions of reported hospitalized patients with 2009 pandemic influenza A (H1N1)

Patient details	Risk factors
General characteristics	Median age (37–41)
	Current smoker
	Female
Underlying conditions	Any chronic respiratory disease (e.g. asthma, chronic obstructive pulmonary disease)
	Morbid obesity
	Diabetes
	Other metabolic disease
	Pregnancy
	Cancer
	Immunodeficiency
	Cardiovascular disease
	Chronic hepatic disease or renal insufficiency
	Haemoglobinopathy or anaemia
	Cognitive dysfunction or seizures
	Asplenia
	Neuromuscular disease
	Treatment with aspirin

✪ Learning point Infection control and patient cohorting

In the initial stages of infection, pandemic influenza closely resembles that of seasonal influenza. Poor specificity of presenting features inevitably contributes to overdiagnosis and overloading of isolation facilities, especially where such facilities have competing demands [2]. Moreover, many infected individuals (including healthcare workers) are largely asymptomatic: during seasonal influenza epidemics, 10–40% of healthcare workers have been shown to have asymptomatic infection [1]. While prompt diagnosis is essential for effective and safe cohorting, rapid diagnostic testing tools have poor sensitivity and specificity, which limits their utility for identifying and excluding potentially infected patients. The potential for acquisition of infection by staff who care for patients in the ICU and by patient visitors, is therefore of great concern.

Infection control decisions are often made with limited evidence, perhaps largely extrapolated from experience of seasonal influenza in ambulant patients. The duration of patient isolation and use of personal protective equipment (PPE), and the risks associated with cohorting of patients with suspected/confirmed infection (or solely confirmed cases where isolation capacity has been exceeded), are often unknown, particularly in the early phase of an emerging epidemic.

The use of non-invasive ventilation is a risk factor for transmission of infectious disease by droplet/aerosol spread [2, 3]. Inadvertent disconnection of ventilator circuits and open tracheal suction pose a similar infection threat. However, experience of the 2009 H1N1 pandemic showed staff infection to be rare. Whether this reflected the widespread and effective use of PPE or indicated that the virus had low transmissibility within an ICU environment is unclear.

Importantly, the implications for appropriate infection control extend beyond the confines of the ICU. During epidemic surges, clinicians need to engage with infection control specialists, microbiology staff, public health experts, and other stakeholders to maintain quality of care and to receive and respond to rapidly evolving infection control advice. Local and more widespread education programmes should be implemented on appropriate use of PPE, decontamination, and disposal procedures. As the pandemic becomes recognized, public awareness campaigns should target the wider community to encourage home quarantine where appropriate, clear personal hygiene, and social distancing advice to reduce household and community transmission.

On admission to the ICU he was given a trial of high-flow nasal cannula (HFNC) oxygen at 50 L/min and a fraction of inspired oxygen of 0.8–1.0. Despite this, he continued to deteriorate rapidly. Three hours after ICU admission he underwent tracheal intubation for worsening hypoxaemia. Nasopharyngeal viral swabs were taken following intubation. He was eventually stabilized using a tidal volume-guaranteed pressure control mode of ventilation. A pre-intubation chest radiograph showed generalized lung field shadowing but no gross consolidation (Figure 17.1a).

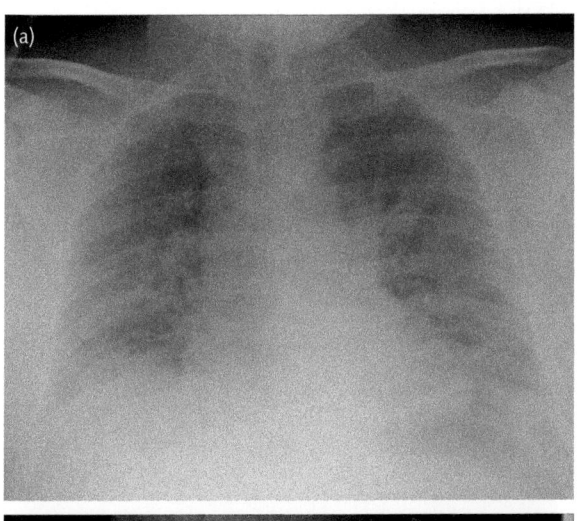

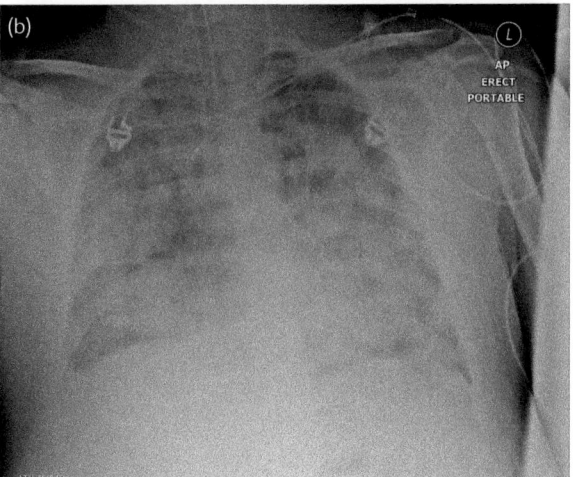

Figure 17.1 Chest X-ray (a) on admission to the ICU, (b) 3 days after ICU admission.

⊕ Learning point Presentation of pandemic influenza

The clinical features of the illness associated with different infective agents will vary with each pandemic. However, a major lesson from the 2009 H1N1 pandemic was the widespread variation in presenting features of critically ill patients with H1N1. In addition to a typical viral pneumonitis and acute respiratory distress syndrome (ARDS) (approximately 50% of ICU admissions), critically ill patients with H1N1 also presented with primary lobar pneumonia and pleural effusions. Pulmonary embolus was a common finding, being a frequent finding at postmortem. Secondary infection with bacteria (20–30%) and fungi was also common. Finally, patients, particularly children, also presented more atypically with acute abdomen, acute kidney injury, myocarditis, encephalitis, diabetic ketoacidosis, multiorgan failure, or septic shock. A high level of clinical suspicion is required to detect relevant cases in view of the multiplicity of possible presentations.

He was started on co-amoxiclav, clarithromycin, and a 5-day course of 75 mg oseltamivir twice daily. A beta-glucan assay was sent to exclude a fungal coinfection.

> ⭐ **Learning point** Guidelines for the treatment of confirmed or suspected influenza
>
> While vaccination remains the mainstay of influenza prevention, antiviral medications can provide a useful second-line defence in the treatment of illness when indicated.
>
> Empiric antiviral treatment, when indicated, should be started as early as possible and ideally within 48 hours of symptom onset (Table 17.2). However, treatment may still provide some benefit in hospitalized patients when started later. Data obtained from randomized controlled trials and observational studies show that early antiviral treatment in people with influenza can lessen illness severity, shorten time of illness, *and* reduce serious flu-related complications such as pneumonia in outpatients and death in hospitalized patients [4].
>
> **Table 17.2** Indications for antiviral treatment in influenza
>
> | Indications for starting empiric antiviral treatment of patients with influenza |
> | --- |
>
> | | |
> | --- | --- |
> | 1 | Illness requiring hospitalization |
> | 2 | Children <2 years of age |
> | 3 | Persons ≥65 years of age |
> | 4 | Pregnant women and up to 2 weeks post partum (including after miscarriage) |
> | 5 | Chronic pulmonary, cardiovascular, renal, hepatic, haematological, and metabolic disorders, neurological and neurodevelopmental conditions |
> | 6 | Immunosuppressive conditions, including secondary to medication or HIV infection |
> | 7 | Persons <19 years receiving long-term aspirin therapy |
> | 8 | Morbid obesity (BMI >40 kg/m^2) |
> | 9 | Residents of nursing home or long-term care facilities |
> | 10 | Progressive, severe, or complicated illness, irrespective of previous health status |
>
> Source: data from Centers for Disease Control and Prevention (CDC). (2016) 2016-2017 Influenza Antiviral Recommendations. Copyright ©2016 CDC. Available at https://www.cdc.gov/h1n1flu/recommendations.htm.
>
> When a definitive diagnosis is indicated, request definitive diagnostic tests (real-time reverse transcriptase polymerase chain reaction (PCR) and viral culture) rather than rapid tests (rapid influenza diagnostic test and direct immunofluorescence assay). However, treatment should not be delayed while waiting for laboratory confirmation of influenza.
>
> It may be prudent to extend the duration of treatment in those patients who remain critically unwell (Table 17.3). Oseltamivir resistance can arise from a change in the neuraminidase (NA) proteins of the virus which prevent the drug binding to and inhibiting the function of the NA protein. Antiviral resistance patterns did not change significantly in 2015–2016 compared with the previous season. In both seasons, oseltamivir resistance was found in only a few H1N1 viruses as per the US Centers for Disease Control and Prevention and the Advisory Committee on Immunization Practices. Resultantly, the 2016–2017 guidance on the use of influenza antiviral drugs remained unchanged.
>
> Dose adjustment of oseltamivir is recommended for patients with chronic kidney disease stages 3–5.
>
> **Table 17.3** Antiviral agent recommendations; dose and frequency of administration
>
> | | Dominant circulating strain has a <u>lower risk</u> of oseltamivir resistance, eg A(H3N2), influenza B* | Dominant circulating strain has a <u>higher risk</u> of oseltamivir resistance, eg A(H1N1)pdm09* |
> | --- | --- | --- |
> | Uncomplicated influenza | oseltamivir PO and clinical follow up. Commence therapy within 48 hours of onset (or later at clinical discretion) | zanamivir INH (Diskhaler®) Commence therapy within 48 hours of onset (36 for children) or later at clinical discretion OR if unable to take inhaled preparation use oseltamivir PO and clinical follow up. Commence therapy within 48 hours of onset (or later at clinical discretion) |
>
> *(continued)*

	Dominant circulating strain has a lower risk of oseltamivir resistance, eg A(H3N2), influenza B*	Dominant circulating strain has a higher risk of oseltamivir resistance, eg A(H1N1)pdm09*
Complicated influenza	*1st line:* oseltamivir PO/NG *2nd line:* zanamivir INH++ Consider switching to zanamivir if: • Poor clinical response • evidence of gastrointestinal dysfunction • Subtype testing confirms a strain with potential oseltamivir resistance, eg A(H1N1)pdm09 (see right)	zanamivir INH++ Commence therapy within 48 hours of onset (36 for children) or later at clinical discretion ++Consider Zanamivir IV if patients: • cannot use inhaled Zanamivir • have severe complicated illness such as multi-organ failure • note: commence as soon as possible and usually within 6 days.

* = also applicable if this is the strain known to be infecting patient; treatment however, should not be delayed while waiting for test results.
PHE guidance on use of antiviral agents for the treatment and prophylaxis of influenza (2019–20). Version 10.0 Public Health England. September 2019. © Crown copyright 2019. Contains public sector information licensed under the Open Government Licence v3.0. http://www.nationalarchives.gov.uk/doc/open-government-licence/version/3/

Treatment	Premature (less than 36 weeks post conceptional age)	0–12 months (36 weeks post conceptional age or greater)	>1–12 years: Does according to weight below				Adults (13 years and over)[1]
			10–15 kg	>15–23 kg	>23–40 kg	>40 kg	
Oseltamivir PO (treatment course: 5 days)	1 mg/kg/dose BD Unlicensed	3 mg/kg/dose BD	30 mg BD	45 mg BD	60 mg BD	75 mg BD	75 mg BD
Zanamivir INH (treatment course: 5 days)	Not licensed for children <5 years old. Children >5 years: 10 mg BD						10 mg BD

[1]If a person in this age group weighs 40 kg or less, it is suggested that the >23–40 kg dose for those aged >1–12 years, is used.
PHE guidance on use of antiviral agents for the treatment and prophylaxis of influenza (2019–20). Version 10.0 Public Health England. September 2019. © Crown copyright 2019. Contains public sector information licensed under the Open Government Licence v3.0. http://www.nationalarchives.gov.uk/doc/open-government-licence/version/3/

At 48 hours after admission to ICU, the results of the viral swabs confirmed influenza infection. Beta-glucan results provided no indication of fungal coinfection. On day 3 of the patient's admission, two other patients were admitted to ICU with respiratory failure and a similar history of flu-like symptoms. The first, a 35-year-old woman with asthma and type 2 diabetes presented with a 2-day history. The other, a 30-year-old pregnant woman at 20 weeks' gestation, had a 4-day history of a mild respiratory illness, now worsening. These patients occupied the remaining two isolation rooms in the ICU.

On day 4, intermittent decreases in arterial oxygen saturation down to 60% occurred in the index patient. Neuromuscular blockade, recruitment manoeuvres (inflation to 40 cmH$_2$O for 40 seconds), and increases in positive end-expiratory pressure only improved arterial oxygen saturation to 80% breathing 100% oxygen. His chest X-ray showed extensive consolidation and widespread alveolar shadowing (Figure 17.1b). He was taken for a computed tomography scan of his chest which showed consolidation, ground-glass shadowing, and several small pulmonary emboli

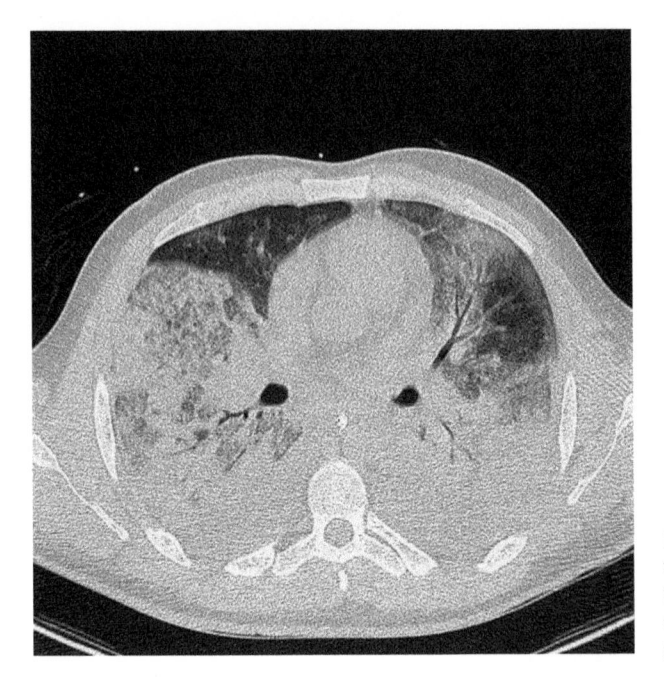

Figure 17.2 Computed tomography scan of the chest showing consolidation, and ground-glass shadowing.

(Figure 17.2). On return to the ICU he was anticoagulated, and he was turned prone for 18-hour periods in an attempt to improve oxygenation.

On day 5, a nurse who had been a primary carer for the patient during his ward admission became unwell and was admitted to the high dependency unit for observation and HFNC oxygen. PPE had not been implemented when the index patient was admitted because an infective cause of his illness was not initially considered.

In the ICU, stocks of N95 masks and protective gloves and gowns were rapidly being exhausted and suppliers had been notified urgently.

> ✪ **Learning point** **Personal protective equipment**
>
> PPE should be used for all aerosol/droplet-generating procedures in the ICU. PPE includes not only face masks but also gowns, visors or goggles, and gloves (Table 17.4). In most influenza epidemics PPE use is not burdensome and particular attention is focused only on aerosol/droplet-generating procedures (Figure 17.3). Safe donning, removal, and disposal of PPE, and staff decontamination is an essential component of infection control. In the setting of epidemics of high virulence (e.g. SARS, MERS, avian influenza, and Ebola), these requirements may include double gloving, double gowning, and meticulous disinfection. Staff may have to work in pairs to achieve this and it may have a significant impact on staffing requirements, ability to provide timely and immediate care, and unit workload (Figure 17.4).
>
> **Table 17.4** Personal protective equipment requirements
>
> | Clinical activity | Mask | Protective eyewear | Gown | Gloves |
> | --- | --- | --- | --- | --- |
> | No direct patient contact | No | | | |
> | Entering patient room | Surgical mask | Yes | As per standard precautions | |
> | Respiratory sampling | Surgical mask | Yes | | |
> | Aerosol-generating procedures | P2 or N95 | Yes | | |

(continued)

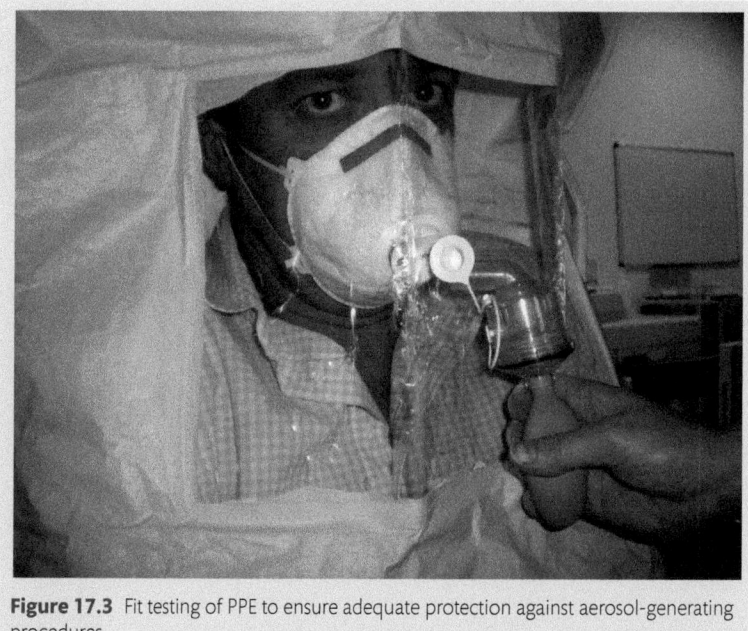

Figure 17.3 Fit testing of PPE to ensure adequate protection against aerosol-generating procedures.
Reproduced courtesy of Professor Tim Cook.

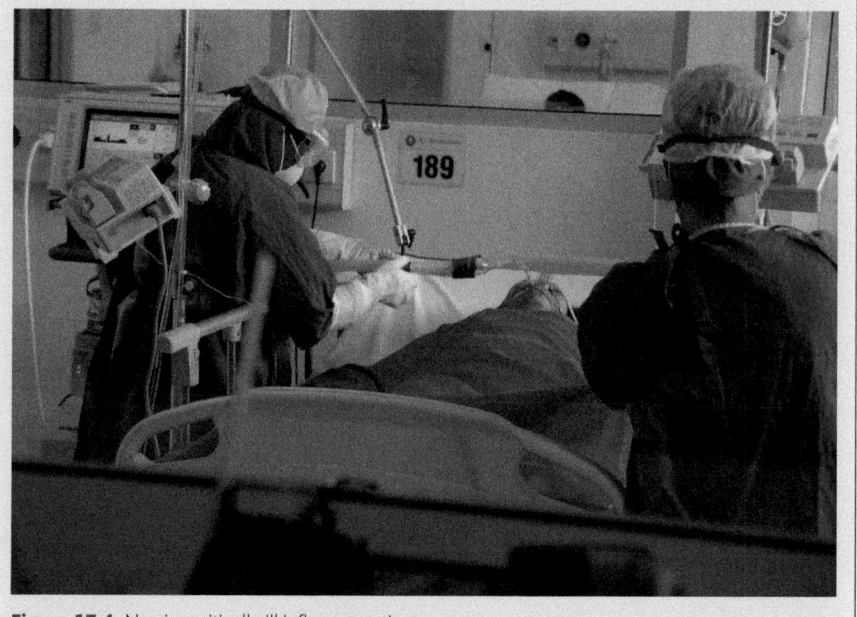

Figure 17.4 Nursing critically ill influenza patients.

Over the course of the week, five further patients had been admitted to the ICU with flu-like symptoms and subsequent respiratory compromise. This surge in admissions stretched resources immediately and rapidly overwhelmed available space, exhausted supplies, required provision of additional staffing, and created challenges in preventing cross contamination and isolation of potentially highly contagious patients. A decision was made to use the ICU exclusively for confirmed and suspected influenza patients. This facilitated use of the high dependency unit and operating theatre recovery room for non-infectious patients requiring critical care. Staffing was a significant challenge and required diversion of anaesthesia and nursing staff from other clinical areas to assist in management of the increased critical care workload. The additional level 3 ICU patients and the expansion into other clinical areas necessitated cancellation of most elective surgery in the hospital.

> ✪ **Learning point Surge capacity: the 4 S's**
>
> There are four key elements which limit surge capacity. These are availability of staff, consumables and essential equipment, bed-spaces, and management systems ('staff, stuff, space, and systems') [5]. Historically, hospital surge capacity has focused on mass casualty events characterized by many cases presenting over a relatively short period followed by the prevalence declining rapidly over the ensuing days. In contrast, pandemics occur in waves (surges), with the increase in numbers of cases persisting for weeks to months and many patients requiring prolonged ICU care. Critical care units often operate at nearly 100% of capacity and are therefore at particularly high risk of being impacted by a pandemic surge. Importantly, the normal requirement for critical care also continues and the only part of the workload that can be controlled is by deferring non-urgent surgery where postoperative ICU care was planned. A relatively small surge in ICU demand soon creates a crisis in ICU capacity and this rapidly progresses from a local to a regional and then national problem. The crisis requires increasing capacity or a significant deviation from usual care, with the implementation of tiered staffing models and rationalization of equipment, which may adversely impact on morbidity and mortality [6] (Table 17.5). The proportion of ICU beds occupied by H1N1 patients peaked at 9% in Australia and 19% in New Zealand [7]. Elsewhere services exceeded surge capacity requiring ventilation of patients outside the ICU [8]. A severe pandemic would vastly exceed ICU capacity in all countries [5, 9].
>
> As surge increases, the demand–resource imbalance worsens. With an increasing magnitude of pandemic surge, response strategies increasingly depart from the usual standard of care until patient mortality increases and effective delivery of critical care is no longer possible.

Table 17.5 Spectrum of surge capacity

	Conventional	Contingency	Crisis
Magnitude	Minor	Moderate	Major
% Increase capacity	20%	100%	200%
Staff	Regular staff plus on call to cover scheduled leave	Reallocation of staff, deferred leave, modified tasks/responsibilities	Trained staff unavailable or too few to adequately care for volume of patients, reliance on upskilling and retraining or supervision of less trained staff
Stuff	Normal stocked inventory of supplies, conserve and substitute	Conservation, adaptation, substitution of supplies, and occasional reuse	Critical supplies increasingly unavailable leading to reuse and reallocation
Space	Use of normal patient care space	Other monitored locations repurposed for patient care (e.g. critical care unit, theatre recovery, theatres)	Low acuity and non-patient care areas used. Triage in place.
Systems	Usual care	Equivalent care	Crisis standards

(continued)

Staff

The availability of nursing and medical staff trained in the care of critically ill patients can be a key limitation to managing surge capacity. Simple solutions, including amendments to rostering, cancellation of leave, increasing effective full-time quotas, altering nurse–patient ratios, and implementing overtime to meet demands can alleviate staff shortages (Table 17.6). Nurses with prior ICU experience and those working in anaesthesia, surgery, and emergency departments may have the skills to manage the ventilated critically ill patient temporarily and can potentially be reallocated. However, this usually requires structured refresher training, retraining, or upskilling and necessitates significant support of less skilled staff by regular ICU staff. Efforts must be made to ensure appropriate isolation and care of suspected and proven cases, and staff reassured that this will occur.

Staff shortages may be compounded by a desire to be available to care for affected relatives. The low virulence of H1N1, in contrast to SARS and Ebola virus, mitigated against this being a major problem [10]. The risk of community-acquired infection is universal; however, staff at high risk of occupational infection (e.g. pregnancy, medical comorbidities) should be reassigned to other clinical duties. In a severe surge, staff illness and fear of infection is likely to increase absenteeism. Antivirals and vaccines should be made readily available. In some settings, it may be desirable or necessary to provide additional remuneration to staff at significant risk, including compensation for death or disability. The provision of counselling should not be overlooked during the planning phase [11]. The psychological well-being of healthcare workers has implications both for current and any future pandemic waves, so there may be benefit in continuing this support beyond the pandemic surge.

Stuff: consumable and equipment availability

Pharmaceutical stockpiling of antivirals by health facilities may be advantageous and an early increase in production is essential to the pandemic response. Nevertheless, adequate supplies of routine medications used in ICU care may also become exhausted [12].

PPE should be rationalized. Simple surgical masks can be used where patients' lungs are ventilated using closed circuits, but N95 masks are required for aerosol-generating procedures.

Oxygen, suction, clean water, electricity, and reliable emergency generators are integral to patient care. There are many potential points of failure within these systems and while lower-income countries are more susceptible, equipment capacity can be rapidly overwhelmed even in higher-income settings.

Table 17.6 Strategies to augment surge capacity in staffing

Phase	Management strategy
Preparation (inter-pandemic phase)	Model staffing needs for staged surge conditions and formulate a plan to meet this need
	Define required skill sets
	Map critical-care staff competencies against required skillsets
	Maintain an up-to-date database of staff
	Allocate staff according to clinical need and appropriate skillset
	Refresh, cross-train, and upskill remaining staff
	Refresh standard operating procedures
	Promote use of incident reporting systems to improve practice
Acute (early surge)	Recall staff on leave/rostered off
	Stop non-essential activities (e.g. elective procedures)
	Redeploy staff to support critical care services
	Consider extending working hours
Chronic (prolonged or subsequent surges)	Provide accommodation to staff
	Mitigate fatigue (rotating rosters)
	Provide transport
	Mental health support services
	Maintain a safe working environment
	Encourage collaboration and team work

(continued)

Many hospitals have numerous older or unused ICU ventilators, and ventilators used for anaesthetic care may be suitable for ICU care in a surge situation. Identification of this resource and a staged plan for escalation should take place in the inter-pandemic period. Should demand exceed resource capacity (e.g. ventilators), with no transfer possible, pre-identified triage processes should be implemented while trying to maintain acceptable standards of care. Where lack of equipment necessitates triage, inclusion and exclusion criteria should be based on incremental probability of survival. The threshold for excluding patients will vary depending on the scale of the incident and severity of disease and may vary over time [13].

In the inter-pandemic period, equipment, such as monitors and ventilators, may be standardized and stockpiled where feasible. Preventative measures should not be overlooked; currently the annual capacity of influenza vaccine production is barely sufficient to cover one-third of the global population [14].

Space: bed space availability

In developed countries, the availability of beds to care for critically ill patients is least likely to be the major limiting factor in surge capacity, at least initially [5, 9]. A 300% expansion target for bed capacity has been suggested, but in practice few facilities would reach this goal. Recommissioning of closed bed spaces, converting high dependency beds into ICU beds, and using anaesthesia recovery units, coronary care units, and operation rooms to care for patients are effective means of creating additional space.

Cohorting of patients with confirmed infection in a single location isolates infectious patients and helps to concentrate resources and appropriately trained staff. When considering an appropriate location, factors such as the availability of antechambers to enable staff to don and doff PPE, and provision of ventilation exhaust outputs should be considered.

It is essential not to overlook that patients requiring ICU care for reasons unrelated to the surge will continue to present during the pandemic phase. Planning must accommodate these patients too.

Systems—standards of care

Each organization should ensure that it is able to respond to a pandemic in a scalable manner [5]. ICU resources vary in quantity and complexity and in the setting of a pandemic surge the necessary stringent infection control measures inevitably contribute to an increased workload. As individual hospitals and organizations can be rapidly overwhelmed, there is a need for responsiveness on a much larger scale.

Surveillance centres have a role in early detection of a pandemic, coordination of an early response, and networking with appropriate stakeholders to determine a wider strategic response based on the severity of the incident. Regional coordinating centres should be established which align with patterns of disease transmissibility rather than local geography. This may be difficult given variations in surveillance and testing strategies between countries, and the prevalence of subclinical infection. Effective communication between a hospital-based incident reporting system and a wider local, regional, and national framework is essential. This should be supported by regular communication between regulatory bodies and national and inter-regional health agencies. Critical care clinicians around the world have been heavily involved with developing operational protocols, supported by standard operating procedures, to support this. This enables rapid and efficient communication of clinical and logistical information and facilitates contingency planning.

❝ Expert comment

In the H1N1 pandemic of 2009, after some delay, international collaboration rapidly brought together a network of frontline clinicians (particularly intensivists), clinical and laboratory microbiologists and virologists, epidemiologists, pharmacologists, public health experts, researchers, health policy experts, and non-governmental senior administrators. This group shared early clinical, laboratory, and epidemiological experience of the pandemic leading to shared understanding about the nature and size of the surge and enabling identification of key problems and potential solutions. Local, national, and international strategic responses were informed by this information sharing, enabling dramatically accelerated development and cascading of clinical and governmental responses. Such coordinated global responses are now an integral response to emerging pandemic threats.

(continued)

The inter-pandemic period is of particular importance with respect to optimizing management systems. A coordinated global effort is required to establish superior surveillance, agreements on virus and vaccine sharing, to develop improved antiviral agents, more effective vaccines, greater production capacity, and faster throughput [14].

The opportunities for applying mobile technologies have yet to be fully explored. The literature suggests that implementing emergency medical systems using mobile technology is often given a low priority. However, in the future these will undoubtedly enhance communication, facilitate strategic mapping, coordinate logistics, and improve local and international responses in a timely and cost-effective manner. To date, low-income and lower middle-income countries have shown the highest uptake of surveillance activities using mobile technologies. For example, a coalition of partners in eastern Pakistan—the Indus Hospital Research Centre, a national mobile phone provider, and the Massachusetts Institute of Technology Media Lab—enables a pneumonia surveillance programme in Karachi [15].

On day 7, the patient became febrile and nasopharyngeal swabs and blood cultures were repeated as part of a complete septic workup at that time. Viral swabs showed no evidence of persisting infection; however, blood cultures grew *Staphylococcus aureus* and antibiotic cover was rationalized, to vancomycin, after consultation with the microbiologists.

> **⊕ Clinical tip Limitations of diagnostic testing during a surge**
>
> The significant increase in the number of tests performed during a surge can create major logistical problems for laboratories, compounded by increased demand for refrigeration and appropriate storage of specimens. Turnaround times may become prolonged, limiting clinical decision-making. This can lead to extended isolation for some patients and increase the risk of cross infection. In addition, accuracy of diagnosis can be difficult. Nasopharyngeal aspirates (NPA) are superior to nose–throat swabs, and the speed of rapid antigen tests is appealing. However, the utility of these tests is limited in the clinical setting due to logistical practicalities relating to transport and storage for NPAs, and poor assay characteristics for nose–throat swabs [1, 16, 17]. During the H1N1 pandemic, NPA swabs often returned negative results while tracheal aspirate samples were positive in many cases with pneumonia. It became routine for paired specimens to be sent and subsequent patient surveillance to be performed using the specimen that had yielded the positive result [12]. In many regions, nucleic acid testing was unavailable and rapid point-of-care tests had insufficient sensitivity to reliably diagnose and inform isolation decisions [1]. As the laboratory demands of the H1N1 pandemic increased, in many jurisdictions, only the seriously ill and healthcare workers were subjected to investigation. In most patients, treatment was commenced empirically and patients were tested only based on clinical suspicion [1].

In addition to activating the hospital surge capacity plan, local and regional authorities and neighbouring health facilities were notified. National and international consultation between networks became critical in limiting the spread of disease. National responses included various decisions around travel restrictions in consultation with expert stakeholders.

On a local level, patients remained cohorted according to illness severity in designated departments within healthcare facilities. Of the patients admitted to the local hospital one patient developed resistant hypoxaemia and was considered a candidate for extracorporeal membrane oxygenation (ECMO) at a nearby tertiary centre. A pregnant patient required urgent transfer to the maternity unit and subsequent caesarean section further complicating patient cohorting.

> **✪ Learning point** Extracorporeal membrane oxygenation and severe influenza
>
> ECMO can support gas exchange in patients with severe ARDS, as is characteristic of severe influenza infection. The therapy, which is independent of mechanical ventilation, may provide a rescue intervention or minimize ventilator-associated lung injury and its associated multiple organ dysfunction, both crucial determinants of survival for patients. A cohort study was conducted of all ECMO-referred patients with H1N1-related ARDS referred, accepted, and transferred to one of the four adult ECMO centres in the UK during the H1N1 2009 pandemic [18]. The ECMO-referred patients were matched with non-ECMO-referred patients using data from a concurrent, longitudinal cohort study (Swine Flu Triage study) of critically ill patients with suspected or confirmed H1N1. Transfer to an ECMO centre for patients with H1N1-related ARDS was associated with lower hospital mortality compared with matched non-ECMO-referred patients. However, limited ECMO capacity and significant associated costs, which are estimated to be double the routine ICU costs, would preclude widespread use in the event of a pandemic.

> **❻ Expert comment**
>
> Experience with previous pandemics shows the critical role leadership plays in addressing the challenges in delivering critical care. Leadership involves using existing infrastructures and strengthening the capacity of national and international surveillance systems, in ways that ensure accurate detection of suspected human cases, reliable laboratory confirmation, effective field investigation, and complete reporting in a timely manner. The ICU generates information about the evolving pandemic and has the potential to communicate this in real time. Open and active lines of communication between the ICU, the hospital, and the wider health system enable partnerships to be established with governmental organizations and governments, regulatory authorities, agriculturalists, academic institutes, and industry. Decisions can then be made about containment of the outbreak, maximizing surge capacity and accelerating research and development.
>
> Once a pandemic has been declared, national health authorities collaborate with the World Health Organization's Global Outbreak Alert and Response Network. Various research consortia (e.g. the International Severe Acute Respiratory and Emerging Infection Consortium (https://isaric.tghn.org/about/) and the International Forum for Acute Care Trialists (http://www.infactglobal.org/About.aspx)) have been established during the inter-pandemic period to facilitate collaboration and preparedness [19].
>
> Leadership extends beyond the boundaries of the healthcare system. Leaders must provide guidance to all stakeholders, especially the media, to deliver accurate information about the pandemic. The media play a crucial role in communicating important health information. During the H1N1 pandemic, it proved difficult for the media to develop messages that incorporated both the mild nature of the illness in most patients and the potential for severe disease in only a minority. As a result, community doctors' offices and hospital emergency departments were crowded with anxious, minimally unwell individuals, at times impairing the assessment and management of more seriously ill patients and potentially increasing the risk of transmission [8]. At the same time the 'mild disease' message proved inappropriate for particular high-risk populations, such as the obese and pregnant women [5].

Over the course of the patient's admission he developed multiorgan dysfunction, including worsening ARDS, acute kidney injury, hypernatraemia, elevated liver enzymes, and international normalized ratio values. He was commenced on continuous venovenous haemofiltration. This reduced his serum sodium concentration and achieved a negative fluid balance which helped to optimize his respiratory function.

At this point his family were approached to consent the patient for participation in a clinical trial. The hospital's ethics committee had expedited ethical approval of a trial of convalescent serum; approval of trials involving treatment algorithms remained pending. Given the patient remained intubated and sedated, and unable to provide consent, surrogate consent was attained.

A case report is often the first document describing an atypical infection and highlighting unique clinical or epidemiological features of the disease. However, publication of such cases will lag temporally. While considered weak evidence, these case reports may have a role in drawing attention to abnormal clusters of severe cases in specific patient groups and alerting health authorities [20].

Role of clinical research

Clinical research conducted during a pandemic has the potential to positively impact the pandemic trajectory (Figure 17.5). Hospitals and critical care units are in a unique position to generate information about incidence, case presentation, infection control, resource utilization, optimal care, and outcomes. This crucial information can inform clinical and public health decision-making [14] but there are multiple challenges in performing such research.

When planning research related to a pandemic, time is critical because if research is not initiated rapidly the opportunity will be lost, and future patients may come to avoidable harm. Research questions should focus on the most important and impactful projects. The type of study will depend on the local context. For confined outbreaks where the data set is complete, cohort studies may be ideal. Whereas for larger outbreaks, a case series of those patients exhibiting clinical symptoms may be more appropriate. Case–control studies can help identify patients and environments associated with disease and thus risk factors associated with poor outcomes.

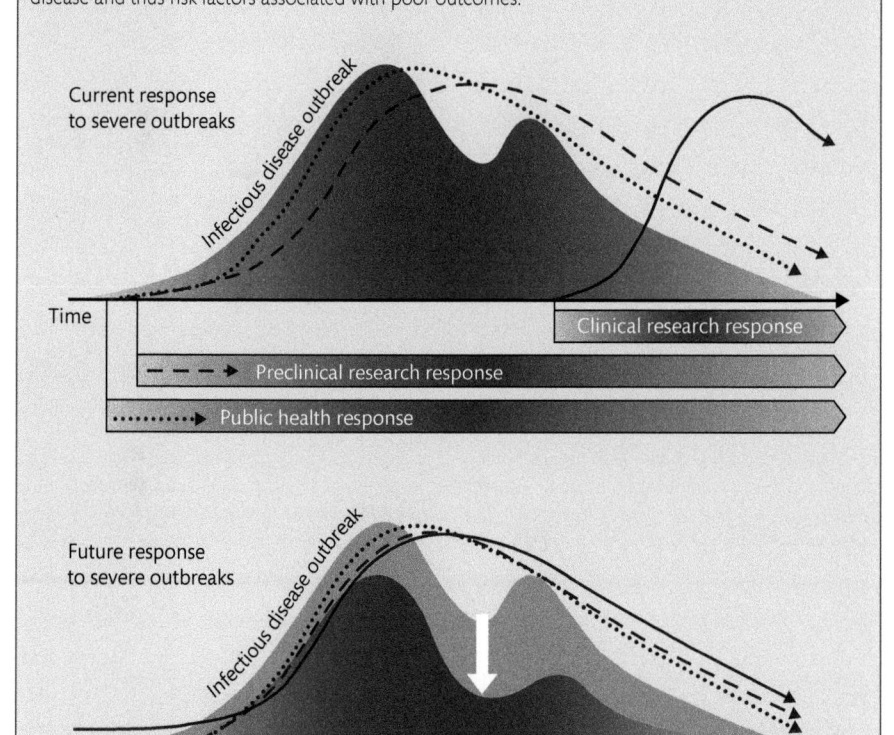

Figure 17.5 Conceptual time course of public health severity of a major outbreak without (upper panel) and with (lower panel) an early effective clinical research response that provides information to clinicians on optimal diagnosis and management as well as information to public health authorities.

Reproduced with permission from Gabriel, L. and Webb, S. Preparing ICUs for pandemics. *Current Opinion in Critical Care.* 19(5), 467–473. Copyright © 2013 Wolters Kluwer Health, Inc.

(continued)

Creation of generic case report forms that can be tailored to local requirements and easily translated into other languages may facilitate early data collection. Appropriate case definitions and careful categorization of patients into confirmed, probable, or suspected disease enables greater accuracy in defining clinical cases retrospectively.

The availability of research personnel is also critical to conducting research during a pandemic. This will be affected by similar constraints as the availability of other healthcare workers. There will be pressure on clinicians who usually participate in research to increase clinical workload and research staff, particularly nurses, may be required to return to clinical duties. However, it is important that research is prioritized as well as clinical care.

ⓘ Expert comment

Research conducted during a pandemic should be held to the same scientific and ethical standards as that conducted at non-emergent times. It should aim to advance knowledge or improve health, be methodologically sound, scientifically valid, and the benefits to both society and the individual should outweigh any harm. The 2015 West African Ebola epidemic provided vital lessons in the challenges of delivering ethical research practices during a pandemic where mortality rates are high and no cure exists [21]. The challenges included balancing the randomization of patients to untested interventions with unknown risk–benefit profiles and navigating the moral hazard of reconciling collective interests with those of the individual. Novel vaccine trials have highlighted a collective international multidisciplinary endeavour to conduct accelerated clinical trials, testing unproven potentially lifesaving interventions and challenging the existing principles of therapeutic research. There must be appropriate oversight and timely ethics approval. Historically, these approvals have been delayed until after the initial wave of the pandemic has passed, thus precluding data collection. While the ethics application and study protocol routinely take 2–3 months to be prepared and approved, ideally the response should take hours or days.

ⓘ Expert comment

Critically ill patients are vulnerable, and the ethical integrity of informed consent is challenging even in those who have the capacity to provide prospective permissions [22–24]. Critical illness by its very nature diminishes a patient's capacity to provide informed consent. With this in mind, several models are used to facilitate the ethical conduct of emergency or critical care research, namely deferred consent, third-party consent, and waived consent [25, 26]. Observational studies, involving the collation of de-identified data obtained during routine clinical care, should not require patient or surrogate consent. In fact, such consent processes can be associated with authorization bias and invalid results [27]. Interventional designs and even the collection of patient samples external to routine care, may involve negligible risk to the patient and a 'no consent' or 'deferred model' may be suitable. Hybrid models that proportionate to the level of risk, that take account of the patient's condition and the availability of surrogate decision makers are essential.

Finally, all the usual challenges to conducting clinical research remain [28].

On day 8, as his condition improved, the patient was weaned to a spontaneous mode of ventilation. Hepatic and renal function began to improve. He was extubated at day 11, was free of renal support by day 14, and was discharged from ICU on day 17. In the longer term he made a good recovery without any major sequelae.

Of the seven other patients with suspected pandemic influenza admitted to the ICU during the patient's stay, three were confirmed using PCR and two were positive for the viral antigen. All seven patients required invasive ventilation. Two were without risk factors while those with risk factors included one pregnant woman, two patients with asthma, one with a raised BMI, and one who was also an insulin-dependent diabetic.

These patients spent a cumulative 67 days in the ICU; two died, while the others made a good recovery with minimal long-term morbidity.

With the pandemic in its infancy and the virulence of the organism unknown, there were efforts made to provide a prophylactic course of oseltamivir to contacts of the patient, hospital staff, and family members. Initially these people were then followed for onset of symptoms, but this soon became unrealistic given the magnitude of the task and instead regional health authorities instituted educational campaigns.

Discussion

A pandemic represents the global spread of a new, or re-emergent, disease. Pandemics arise because of the emergence of an antigenically novel virus (i.e. for which there is no prior immunity), usually with a mixture (reassortment) of previously human and animal viral genomes. These viruses often arise in developing countries where animal and human contact is close.

Animal reservoirs, particularly birds and pigs, are a genetic mixing bowl for antigenic variation. Presumably, the number and proximity of animals drive the amount of genetic mixing. In this regard, it is notable that over the past 45 years, the population of farmed pigs in China has increased from 5.2 million to at least 500 million, and the number of domestic poultry has increased from 5.2 million to 6 billion. The 2009 influenza pandemic was a new strain of H1N1 resulting when a previous triple reassortment of bird, swine, and human flu viruses further combined with a Eurasian pig flu virus. Now, with the popularity of global airline travel, a new strain will spread within days to weeks. Arguably, the capacity to form new strains to which humanity is immunologically naïve, which have pandemic potential, is greater than ever in history.

The critical feature of all pandemics is uncertainty [1, 2]; uncertainty surrounding pathogenicity, age-specific incidence of critical illness, mortality rate, risk factors, and transmissibility. Historically, the predominant form of critical illness associated with pandemics has been pneumonia, either primary viral influenza, or secondary bacterial [3]. During an influenza pandemic it has been shown that 12–30% of the population will develop clinical illness (compared with 5–15% for seasonal influenza), with approximately 4% of those patients requiring hospital admissions and at least one in five of those requiring critical care [4]. With more patients with atypical aetiology requiring intubation and mechanical ventilation, the ICU becomes a satellite surveillance centre, the so-called canary in the coal mine. The ICU therefore has the potential to play a unique role in mapping the impact of the pandemic and disseminating that information outwards.

When a large portion of the population is infected, even if the proportion that goes on to develop severe disease is small, the total number of severe cases can overwhelm the healthcare system. As a result, the provision of critical care poses many challenges in terms of preparedness, encompassing surge capacity, management systems, infection control, and clinical leadership. ICU admissions of H1N1 influenza in Australia were 15 times greater than for viral pneumonitis in recent seasonal influenza outbreaks with one in seven of those admitted dying [5]. Preparedness to rapidly conduct high-quality clinical research to guide effective and efficient care is also critical and highlights existing barriers to conducting research in the acute care environment.

A final word from the expert

Pandemics will continue to challenge clinicians, policymakers, and public health leaders in critical care. They are unexpected but inevitable events and are characterized only by their uncertain scope, duration, and effect. Any preparedness plan should encompass both local and international coordination in order to function more efficiently with the finite resources available.

Vulnerabilities in global, national, and local public health capacities; limitations of scientific knowledge; difficulties in decision-making under conditions of uncertainty; complexities in cooperation between relevant stakeholders; and challenges in communication among experts, policymakers, and the public need to be addressed now (6). Deaths resulting from a new pandemic will be regrettable. Those that result from insufficient planning, inequitable allocation of resources, and inadequate preparation will be especially tragic [7].

References

1. Kotsimbos T, Waterer G, Jenkins C, et al. Influenza A/H1N1_09: Australia and New Zealand's winter of discontent. *Am J Respir Crit Care Med.* 2010;181:300–6.
2. Fowler RA, Lapinsky SE, Hallett D, et al. Critically ill patients with severe acute respiratory syndrome. *JAMA.* 2003;290:367–73.
3. Hui DS, Hall SD, Chan MT, et al. Non-invasive positive pressure ventilation: an experimental model to assess air and particle dispersion. *Chest.* 2006;130:730–40.
4. Muthuri SG, Venkatesan S, Myles PR, et al. Effectiveness of neuraminidase inhibitors in reducing mortality in patients admitted to hospital with influenza A H1N1pdm09 virus infection: a meta-analysis of individual participant data. *Lancet Respir Med.* 2014;2:395–404.
5. Hota S, Fried E, Burry L, et al. Preparing your intensive care unit for the second wave of H1N1 and future surges. *Crit Care Med.* 2010;38;e110–19.
6. Hick JL, Christian MD, Sprung CL. Chapter 2. Surge capacity and infrastructure considerations for mass critical care. *Intensive Care Med.* 2010;36:S11–20.
7. The ANZIC Influenza Investigators. Critical care services and 2009 H1N1 Influenza in Australia and New Zealand. *N Engl J Med.* 2009;361:1925–34.
8. Dominguez-Cherit G, Lapinsky SE, Macias AE, et al. Critically ill patients with 2009 influenza A(H1N1) in Mexico. *JAMA.* 2009:302:1880–7.
9. Gabriel LE, Webb SA. Preparing ICUs for pandemics. *Curr Opin Crit Care.* 2013;19:467–73.
10. Wise ME, De Perio M, Halpin J, et al. Transmission of pandemic H1N1 (2009) influenza to healthcare personnel in the United States. *Clin Infect Dis.* 2011;52:S198–204.
11. Gomersall CD, Joynt JM, Ho OM, et al. Transmission of SARS to healthcare workers. The experience of a Hong Kong ICU. *Intensive Care Med.* 2006;32:564–9.
12. Funk DJ, Siddiqui F, Wiebe K, et al. Practical lessons from the first outbreaks; clinical presentation, obstacles, and management strategies for severe pandemic (pH1N1) 2009 influenza pneumonitis. *Crit Care Med.* 2010;38;e30–7.
13. Christian MD, Sprung CL, King MA, et al. Triage: care of the critically ill and injured during pandemics and disasters: CHEST consensus statement. *Chest.* 2014;146:e61S–74S.
14. Fineberg H. Pandemic preparedness and response—lessons from the H1N1 influenza of 2009. *N Engl J Med.* 2014;370:1335–42.
15. World Health Organization (WHO). *mHealth: New Horizons for Health in Mobile Technologies.* Global Observatory for eHealth Series, Volume 3. Geneva: WHO; 2011. Available from: http://www.WHO.int/goe/publications/goe_mhealth_web.pdf.

16. Cheng AC, Dwyer DE, Kotsimbos ATC, et al. Summary of the Australian Society for Infectious Diseases and the Thoracic Society of Australia and New Zealand guidelines: treatment and prevention of H1N1 09 (human swine influenza) with antiviral agents. *MJA*. 2009;191:142–5.

17. Faix DJ, Sherman SS, Waterman SH. Rapid-test sensitivity for novel swine-origin influenza A (H1N1) virus in humans. *N Engl J Med*. 2009;361:728–9.

18. Noah MA, Peek GJ, Finney SJ, et al. Referral to an extracorporeal membrane oxygenation center and mortality among patients with severe 2009 influenza A(H1N1). *JAMA*. 2011;306:1659–68.

19. The ANZIC Influenza Investigators. Critical care services and 2009 H1N1 influenza in Australia and New Zealand. *N Engl J Med*. 2009;361:1925–34.

20. Wiwanitkit V. The usefulness of case reports in managing emerging infectious disease. *J Med Case Rep*. 2011;5:194.

21. Calain, P. The Ebola clinical trials: a precedent for research ethics in disasters. *J Med Ethics*. 2018;44:3–8.

22. Gobat NH, Gal M, Francis NA, et al. Key stakeholder perceptions about consent to participate in acute illness research: a rapid, systematic review to inform epi/pandemic research preparedness. *Trials*. 2015;16:591.

23. Annane D, Outin H, Fisch C, et al. The effect of waiving consent on enrollment in a sepsis trial. *Intensive Care Med*. 2004;30:321–4.

24. Davies H, Shakur H, Padkin A, et al. Guide to the design and review of emergency research when it is proposed that consent and consultation be waived. *Emerg Med J*. 2014;31:794–5.

25. The NICE-SUGAR Study Investigators. Intensive versus conventional glucose control in critically ill patients. *N Engl J Med*. 2009;360:1283–97.

26. Tu JV, Willison DJ, Silver FL, et al. Impracticability of informed consent in the registry of the Canadian Stroke Network. *N Engl J Med*. 2004; 350:1414–21.

27. Fowler RA, Webb SA, Rowan KM, et al. Early observational research and registries during the 2009–2010 influenza A pandemic. *Crit Care Med*. 2010;38:e120–32.

28. Schuchat A, Bell BP, Redd SC. The science behind preparing and responding to pandemic influenza: the lessons and limits of science. *Clin Infect Dis*. 2011;52:S8–12.

18 Organ donation and transplantation

Andrew Ray

⊕ **Expert Commentary** Alex Manara

This case discussion is based on a patient admitted to an intensive care unit (ICU) in the UK and much of the discussions relating to professional, ethical, and legal issues are based on UK law and guidance from UK professional and regulatory bodies. While many other countries practising deceased donation will have broadly similar guidance, there may be significant differences in some aspects of practice. The reader should not necessarily extrapolate these interpretations of legal, ethical, and professional guidance to what is acceptable in their own country.

Case history

An 81-year-old man was admitted to hospital following a collapse on the golf course at 12:45. A medical emergency response team was dispatched along with a paramedic crew. On initial assessment, the man had a patent airway and was self-ventilating with a respiratory rate of 14 breaths/min and arterial blood oxygen saturation of 95% breathing air. His blood pressure was 182/94 mmHg, his heart rate was 76 beats/min, and he was in atrial fibrillation. His Glasgow Coma Scale score was 4/15 (E1, V1, M2) and he had a fixed, dilated right pupil. His trachea was intubated at the scene and he was transferred to the nearest emergency department (ED). On arrival, he underwent an urgent computed tomography scan of his brain. This demonstrated a large, right-sided parietal intraparenchymal haemorrhage extending into the subdural space, subarachnoid space, and ventricular system (Figure 18.1). By this time, his wife had been contacted and had arrived in the hospital. She confirmed that he was usually fit and active with a relatively minimal past medical history. He was a treated hypertensive and had chronic atrial fibrillation for which he was taking apixaban for stroke prophylaxis.

The patient was discussed with the neurosurgical team who reviewed his scans and concluded that this was an unsurvivable brain injury and that withdrawal of life-sustaining treatment (WLST) should be considered. The ED team and the ICU team who were managing the patient had two possible options for ongoing management. The first was to undertake WLST in the ED with a plan to transfer to a medical ward for continued end of life care. Organ donation would not have been a possibility as the patient did not meet the criteria for the determination of death using neurological criteria. The other option was for the patient to be transferred to ICU and follow a devastating brain injury pathway (Figure 18.2) [1] providing time for better prognostication and to facilitate optimization of his end of life care. After a frank and honest discussion with his wife regarding the expected outcomes and the high likelihood that

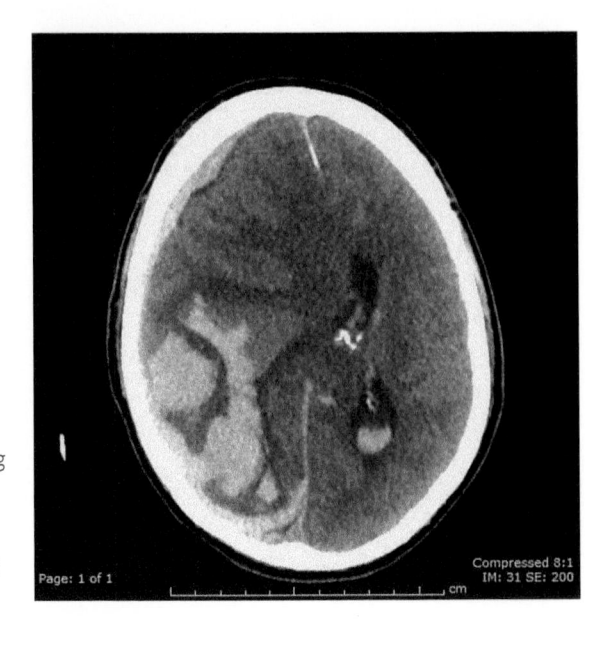

Figure 18.1 Computed tomography scan of head showing right parietal intraparenchymal haemorrhage extending into the subdural space, subarachnoid space, and ventricular system with a significant midline shift.

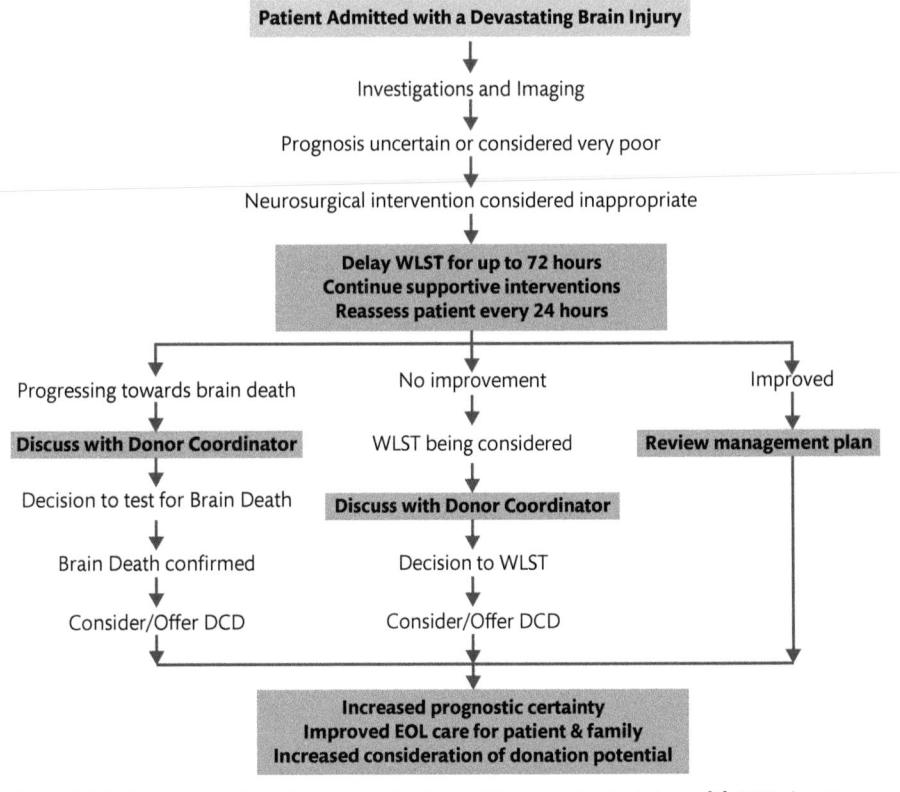

Figure 18.2 Suggested pathway for intubated patients with devastating brain injury [1]. DBD, donation after brain death; DCD, death after cardiovascular death; EOL end of life; WLST, withdrawal of life-sustaining treatment.

Reproduced with permission from Manara, AR., et al. A Case for Stopping the Early Withdrawal of Life Sustaining Therapies in Patients with Devastating Brain Injuries. *Journal of Intensive Care Society.* 17(4), 295–301. Copyright © 2016 SAGE.

he would continue to deteriorate and die, it was agreed to admit him to ICU for continued observation and end of life care. This allowed time for the patient's three children to travel from elsewhere in the UK and abroad to see their father and to support their mother at this difficult time. It also enabled further exploration of the patient's preferences and values, with his family, including the option of WLST in view of the hopeless prognosis. The specialist nurse in organ donation (SN-OD, commonly known as a donor coordinator in many countries) was notified of the patient's admission to consider whether organ donation could be a possible component of his end of life care.

✪ Learning point Devastating brain injury pathways

Recommendations for the critical care management of devastating brain injury have been published recently by the Neurocritical Care Society [2]. Devastating brain injury pathways are being introduced in some hospitals for patients admitted with life-threatening brain insults (subarachnoid haemorrhage, trauma, intracerebral haemorrhage) and where an early decision to undertake WLST is being considered. The primary intervention is to delay the WLST to provide more time for physiological stabilization and continued observation of the patient. This has the benefits of increasing prognostic certainty, allowing more time to explore the patient's preferences and wishes which can then be incorporated into a bespoke end of life care plan. Finally, it allows more time for the consideration of organ donation.

✪ Learning point Background of organ donation and transplantation

There are currently nearly 7000 patients on an organ transplant waiting list in the UK. Approximately 3400 organs are transplanted in the UK each year. The demand for organs for transplantation continues to outstrip the supply in virtually every country practising organ transplantation, including all those in the developed world. Since the first successful kidney transplant in 1954, surgical techniques, immunosuppressant therapies, and intensive care have advanced significantly to enable transplantation of other solid organs such as the liver, lungs, heart, pancreas, and small bowel. Until more recently, all deceased organ donors were patients confirmed as dead using neurological criteria (donation after brain death (DBD)), However the first heart transplant performed by Christian Barnard was retrieved from a donor whose death was confirmed using circulatory criteria (donation after circulatory death (DCD)). The continued demand for organs for transplantation has led to the reintroduction of DCD programmes in many countries including Australia, the Netherlands, the US, Spain, and the UK.

While more than 500,000 people die each year in the UK, only around 1% (i.e. approximately 5000) of them do so in circumstances where organ donation could be possible. There has been an increase of almost 70% in the number of deceased organ donors (from 809 to 1364) between the publication of the Organ Donation Taskforce Report [3] in 2008 (whose purpose was to address all barriers to organ donation and transplantation) and 2016. This increase in donor numbers was primarily due to increased identification and referral of potential donors from ICUs and EDs. DCD accounted for approximately 75% of the increase in organ donors so that DCD now accounts for just over 40% of all deceased donors and 35% of all transplants in the UK. The transplant programmes of other countries, particularly the Netherlands and Australia, also rely on a large proportion of DCD donors. There has been little change in the consent versus refusal rate. However there remains a substantial shortfall in the number of organs available for transplantation, the number of patients dying on the transplant waiting list has not decreased, and access to the transplant waiting list is restricted by stringent criteria.

Efforts to ensure that all potential donors are given the best opportunity to donate their organs after death is a cornerstone of the National Health Service (NHS) Blood and Transplant and the UK Health Departments' strategy 'Taking Organ Transplantation to 2020 [4].

❝ Expert comment

Devastating brain injury pathways already exist for the management of hypoxic-ischaemic brain injuries following out-of-hospital cardiac arrest, and are associated with improved outcomes. It is likely that professional guidance will be provided on the development of similar pathways for other causes of devastating brain injury.

❝ Expert comment

The increase in donors over the past 8 years has been primarily driven by staff in ICUs and EDs identifying and referring more potential donors and thus more families being approached for donation. The current 2020 strategy [4] recognizes that further increases in donors requires further contributions from NHS commissioners, society, and individuals as well as from hospital donation and transplantation teams.

ⓘ Expert comment

The guidance from the GMC, NICE, and the Donation Ethics Committee tells doctors what can and should be done. Strategy documents such as 'Timely identification and referral of potential organ donors: A strategy for implementation of best practice' [8] can be more helpful in telling doctors how to implement these recommendations in practice.

❂ Learning point   Identifying and referring potential donors

The General Medical Council's (GMC) guidance states that, when a patient is close to death, doctors should explore the patient's donation wishes with the relatives and that they should follow any national recommendations on the identification and referral of potential donors [5]. The UK National Institute for Health and Care Excellence (NICE) published guidance on the referral and identification of potential donors to SN-ODs [6] and recommends that early referral is based upon three easily applied clinical triggers:

• An intention to diagnose death using neurological criteria (brainstem death) *or*
• A decision to withdraw life-sustaining treatments *or*
• Admission of a patient with a severe brain injury of such severity that one or more brainstem reflexes have been lost and the Glasgow Coma Scale score is 3 or 4.

The guidance also emphasizes the need to avoid premature treatment limitation/withdrawal decisions until the possibility of donation and the wishes of the patient have been explored. It is important that the referral is timely since this may reduce distressing delays for the family while awaiting organ recovery. The UK Donation Ethics Committee states that there is no ethical dilemma in discussing a patient with a SN-OD before a formal decision to WLST has been discussed with the relatives [7]. Despite this advice, individual clinicians continue to feel conflicted if they contact a SN-OD to discuss the suitability for organ donation before they have discussed the WLST with the family.

The SN-OD confirmed that the patient's age was a contraindication to DCD, but also recognized that the severity of the brain injury was such that the clinical condition could progress to the point where confirmation of death using neurological criteria may be possible, in which case the patient would be suitable for DBD. By the following morning, the patient had not received any further sedation, had fixed pupils, no responses, and was not making respiratory efforts. The patient met all the preconditions for confirming the diagnosis of death using neurological criteria. The family were now all present, and were told that the ICU team suspected that the patient had already died but that further clinical tests were needed to confirm this. The family were invited to observe the testing and accepted this offer. The tests were performed twice by two ICU consultants and the patient was declared dead using neurological criteria.

ⓘ Expert comment

The transition from a devastating brain injury to brain death increases over time after admission to hospital. Only 20% of those who progress to brain death do so in the first 24 hours after admission compared to 70% by 72–96 hours [9].

❂ Learning point   Diagnosing death using neurological criteria (brainstem death testing)

Death is defined as irreversible loss of the capacity for consciousness and the capacity to breathe and can occur due to cessation of brainstem function or cessation of cardiorespiratory function [10]. When brain death is suspected, the patient should be formally tested by two medical practitioners who are competent in making the diagnosis. Both must have been registered for more than 5 years and one must be a consultant. Two sets of tests must be completed. This is usually achieved with the two doctors working together: the first doctor conducting the first set of tests while the second doctor observes; and the second doctor conducts the second set of tests with the first doctor observing. There is no prescribed time interval between the tests. Some prefer to conduct the second set of tests immediately after the first set, while others prefer to allow various time intervals between tests.

The following criteria must be satisfied before undertaking the clinical tests:

• The patient must be deeply comatose, unresponsive, apnoeic, and dependent on mechanical ventilation.
• There should be no doubt that brain damage is irreversible and the underlying aetiology must be known.
• Reversible causes of coma must be excluded:
  ○ Residual effects of sedative drugs.
  ○ Hypothermia—the core temperature must be greater than 34°C.

- o Residual neuromuscular blockade.
- o Cervical spinal cord injury.
- o Reversible metabolic, endocrine, and circulatory disturbances. The Academy of Medical Royal Colleges' report 'A code of practice for the diagnosis and confirmation of death' recommends testing within the following parameters:
  - Mean arterial pressure greater than 60 mmHg
  - Partial pressure of carbon dioxide ($PaCO_2$) less than 6.0 kPa
  - Partial pressure of oxygen (PaO_2) greater than 10 kPa
  - pH 7.35–7.45
  - Na^+ 115–160 mmol/L
  - K^+ greater than 2 mmol/L
  - Mg^{2+} and PO_4 0.5–3.0 mmol/L
  - Serum glucose 3.0–20 mmol/L.

> ✚ **Clinical tip Practicalities of testing**
>
> Ensuring that the preconditions are fully satisfied is the crucial and occasionally more challenging part of diagnosing death using neurological criteria. When this is done and the clinicians proceed to the clinical test, the criteria are then satisfied in 98.5% of patients.
>
> The diagnosis of death using neurological criteria is only made approximately 1500 times a year in the UK—that is, fewer than six per year per ICU and considerably fewer in non-neurosurgical ICUs—meaning that this is an unusual procedure for many individual consultants. Forms endorsed by the UK's Faculty of Intensive Care Medicine and the Intensive Care Society are available to guide doctors to undertake the tests in accordance with national guidance and help standardize the procedure [11].

Once the preconditions have been met, the clinical tests can be undertaken to confirm death:

- Pupils bilaterally fixed and unresponsive to light (direct and consensual responses).
- Absent corneal reflexes bilaterally.
- Absent oculovestibular reflexes—no eye movements in response to 50 mL of ice cold water being injected in each ear in turn (confirm that the ear canals are clear before testing).
- No cranial nerve motor response to the application of supraorbital pressure.
- Absent cough reflex on tracheal suctioning.
- Absent gag reflex on stimulation of the posterior pharynx.
- No respiratory movement on disconnection from mechanical ventilation. This test takes place last and only after demonstrating the absence of all other reflexes. It is conducted as follows:
  - o Increase the patient's fraction of inspired oxygen to 1.0.
  - o Reduce minute ventilation to achieve a $PaCO_2$ greater than 6.0 kPa and a pH lower than 7.40.
  - o Ensure an adequate blood pressure is maintained throughout.
  - o Next, disconnect the patient from the ventilator.
  - o Maintain oxygenation by delivering oxygen at 5 L/min via a tracheal catheter or a Mapleson C breathing system. Monitor oxygen saturation by pulse oximetry throughout.
  - o Confirm the absence of respiratory effort for a minimum of 5 min.
  - o Repeat an arterial blood gas analysis to demonstrate an increase in $PaCO_2$ of greater than 0.5 kPa from the starting value.
  - o Perform a recruitment manoeuvre on completion of the apnoea test, reconnect the ventilator, and adjust ventilation to achieve a normal $PaCO_2$ and pH.

> **❝ Expert comment**
>
> The diagnosis of death using neurological criteria should ideally be made whenever it is a possibility, as suggested by the UK Donation Ethics Committee [12] rather than simply as a means of facilitating organ donation. As in this case, the diagnosis of death can provide the family with the certainty they need. The diagnosis of death using neurological criteria is accepted by the law courts and protects doctors from any potential criticism about the more subjective decisions regarding the WLST (a diagnosis versus a prognosis).

Once the second set of tests were completed, a further discussion was had with the relatives to inform them that the patient had died and to confirm their understanding of the diagnosis. The family was grateful for the certainty of a diagnosis of death rather than a decision to WLST based on prognostication. The relatives were then offered a short break before meeting again to discuss what happens next. In the meantime, the

SN-OD had established that the patient was not on the organ donor register, but that he should be considered for DBD since the abdominal organs would be suitable for transplantation. The approach to the relatives for organ donation was planned and conducted collaboratively with the SN-OD present. Further discussions of a medical nature were led by the ICU consultant. The discussions leading to an approach for organ donation was led by the SN-OD. The family were firmly of the opinion that organ donation was consistent with the patient's values and preferences. After further information was given to the relatives they consented to organ donation.

✪ Learning point Suitability for donation

Absolute exclusion criteria for donation of solid organs in the UK include:

- age greater than 80 for DCD
- age greater than 85 for DBD
- known or suspected Creutzfeldt–Jakob disease
- disseminated malignancy
- known patient refusal.

Most transplant organizations no longer provide lists of relative contraindications as these are unhelpful, ever changing, and often organ specific, which does not preclude donation of other organs. All donors are considered individually and potential donors with conditions that were absolute or relative contraindications may now be accepted on a case-by-case basis, for example, in the past, HIV-positive patients were not considered for donation but now they may be able to donate their organs to an HIV-positive recipient. The SN-OD will request several investigations to assess the suitability of an individual to donate their organs, and others to determine the suitability of individual organs for transplantation. These generally include tissue typing, tests to exclude the presence of transmissible disease, blood urea and electrolytes, estimated glomerular filtration rate, liver function tests, chest radiography, electrocardiography, echocardiography, and imaging to exclude damage to organs being considered for donation.

Once consent has been obtained from the family, the individual organs are offered to transplant centres to assess suitability for transplantation in any of the centre's potential recipients. The kidney offering system is undertaken centrally by the organ procurement organization. All other organs are offered by the SN-ODs sequentially to transplant centres.

❛❛ Expert comment

Whether organs are considered suitable for transplantation depends on recipient factors and circumstances as well as donor factors. While intensivists have an obvious role in informing SN-ODs if they are concerned about the suitability of any potential donor, the decision to accept organs for transplantation can be made only by the transplant teams who hold information on potential recipients. The best approach is to discuss with a SN-OD all patients meeting the referral triggers.

✪ Learning point Approaching organ donation with families

Approaching a family for organ donation should be planned, and undertaken only after they have understood and accepted the determination of death using neurological criteria or the reasons for WLST and the inevitability of death. It is good practice to separate the approach for organ donation from the conversations about prognosis and potential WLST [13]. The coroner needs to be informed of many patients before donation can proceed since the causes of death that that are most commonly associated with organ donation are reportable to a coroner. These include causes of sudden death such as subarachnoid and intracerebral haemorrhage and death following trauma including severe head injury. While coroners are generally supportive of organ donation, there are occasions when they may only allow certain organs to be donated, and other occasions when they will not allow donation to proceed at all. These situations most commonly occur when the patient's death is likely to be followed by a criminal investigation by the police and forensic pathologists.

While the wish of a patient to be an organ donor after death is occasionally known, it is more common to have to explore their preferences and wishes regarding organ donation with their relatives. Opinion polls have suggested that around 90% of the UK population support organ donation, yet only 62% of families approached for donation will give their consent or authorization for organ donation to proceed. Efforts should be made to support families by providing appropriate information in a suitable environment and enabling them to understand the potential benefit of organ donation. It is good practice to use a collaborative approach between the SN-OD and the ICU team when approaching families (Figure 18.3). SN-ODs are specifically trained in supporting families

(continued)

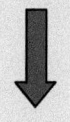

Planning

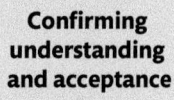

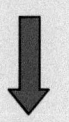

Confirming understanding and acceptance

Discussing donation

- **Who:** Consultant, SN-OD and nurse
- **Why:**
  - Clarify clinical situation
  - Seek evidence of prior consent/authorisation (eg ODR or other)
  - Identify key family members by name
  - Define key family issues
  - Agree a process of approach and who will be involved
  - Agree timing and setting, ensuring these are appropriate to family needs
  - Involve others as required, eg faith leaders
- **When and where:** in private and before meeting the family to confirm understanding and acceptance of loss

For a potential DBD donor, ensure the family understand that death has occurred. Spend time with the concept, using diagrams or scans if necessary.

In the DCD setting, ensure the family understand and accept the reasons for treatment withdrawal and the inevitability of death thereafter.

Donation should only be raised at this point if it is clear that a family has understood and accepted their loss. If this is not the case, suggest a break. The key is to ensure that the family have accepted and understood the clinical situation before donation is raised.

- Re-confirm the family's understanding of the clinical situation.
- Provide specific information on the process before expecting a response
- Avoid negative or apologetic language
- Avoid manipulative or coercive language
- Emphasise the benefits of transplantation – the ability to save and transform several lives
- Sensitively explore an initial 'No,' some causes of which can be addressed or are a result of misconceptions about donation.

Recognising their training and experience, wherever possible utilise the SN-OD throughout the family approach to:

- Provide knowledge and expertise
- Discuss options
- Help recognise modifiable factors and challenge misconceptions
- Support and spend time with the family.

Figure 18.3 The three stages recommended in approaching a family for organ donation. ODR, organ donation register; SN-OD, specialist nurse in organ donation.
Reproduced from NHS Blood and Transplant (2013). *Approaching the families of potential organ donors. Best practice guidance.* Copyright © 2013 NHS. Contains public sector information licensed under the Open Government Licence v3.0. Available at: http://www.odt.nhs.uk/pdf/family_approach_best_practice_guide.pdf.

(*continued*)

through this decision-making process and can provide all the detailed and accurate information required by families. Also, the involvement of a SN-OD in the family approach is associated with significantly higher rates of consent to organ donation [14].

> **❻ Expert comment**
>
> While various factors are associated with increased consent rates for organ donation, the one that is most easily modifiable by the ICU and ED staff is how they plan and execute the approach to the family. This means involving a trained requestor in the family approach. This is almost always the SN-OD. The SN-OD can also provide more up-to-date information, answer all the family's questions on donation, and almost invariably has more time to support the family through the process than the busy clinical team.

Apart from the involvement of the SN-OD in the family approach, the other factors significantly associated with consent are the patient's ethnicity and a prior knowledge of a patient's wish to donate after death (Figure 18.4) [14]. When a patient's wish to donate is already known, some 90% of families will agree to organ donation. The other 10% will, however, override the wish of their relative and will not consent to donation. While it is common practice to accept the wishes of the family, it is also important to explore their reasons for not respecting that individual's wishes, as it is possible they may regret their decision in the future.

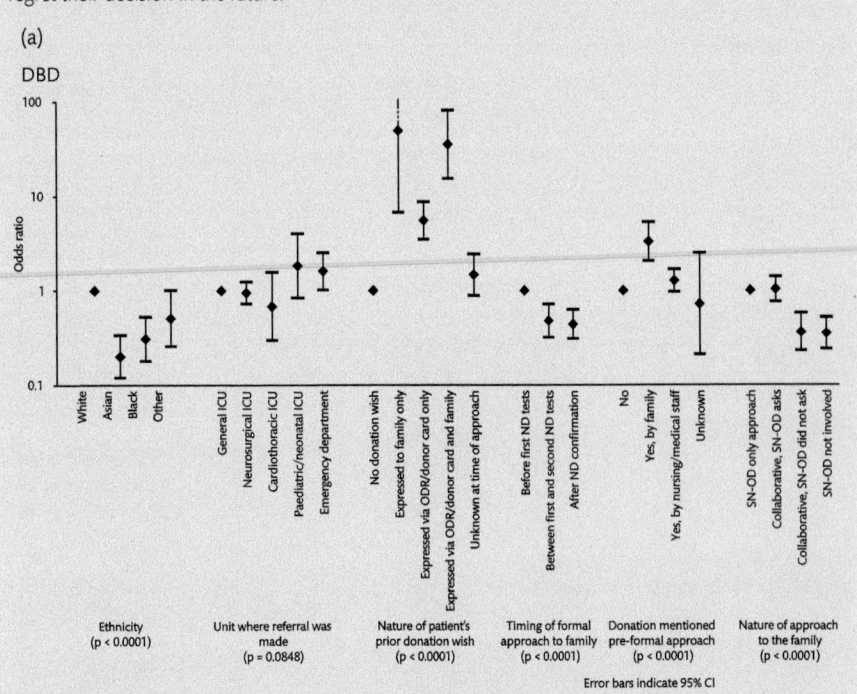

Figure 18.4 Odds ratio for the effect of various factors on the consent rate in donation after brain death (DBD) and donation after circulatory death (DCD). White ethnicity, general ICU, no known donation wish, approach before the first set of brain death tests, no mention of donation before family approach, presence of a specialist nurse in organ donation (SN-OD) and a SN-OD-only approach was used as the baseline for comparison (odds ratio 1). Error bars indicate 95% confidence intervals (CIs). Reproduced with permission from Hulme, W., et al. Factors influencing the family consent rate for organ donation in the UK. *Anaesthesia.* 2016(71), 1053–1063. Copyright © 2016 The Association of Anaesthetists of Great Britain and Ireland.

(continued)

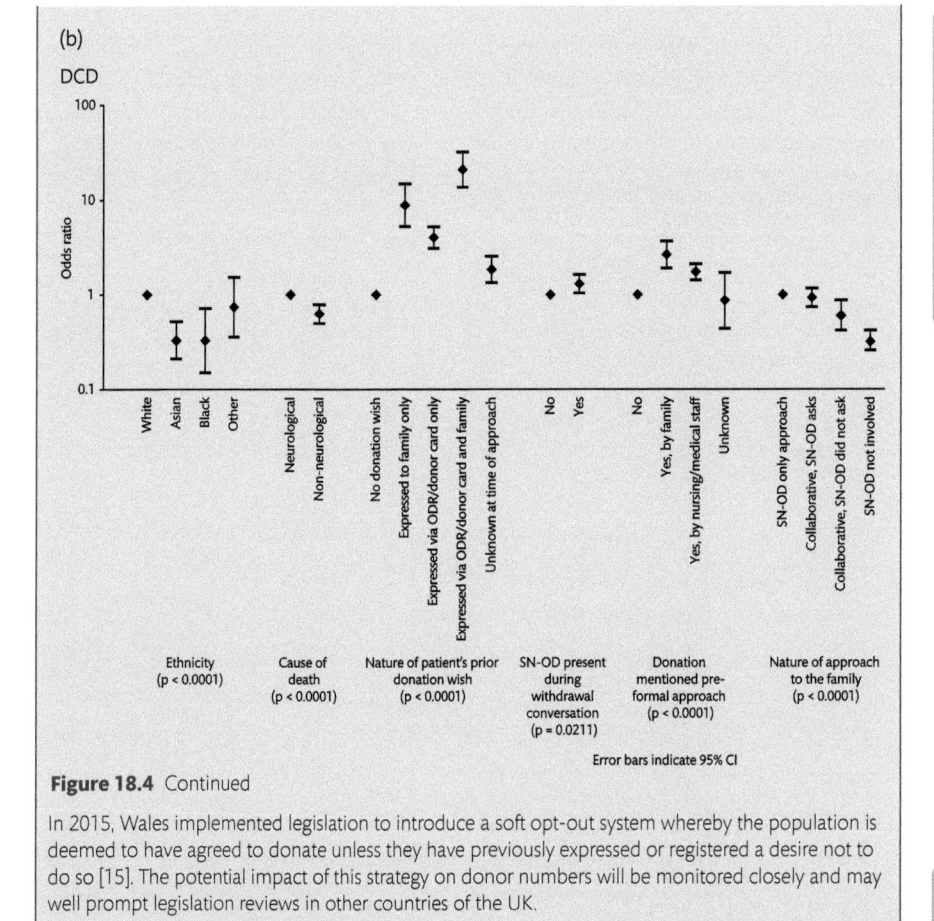

Figure 18.4 Continued

In 2015, Wales implemented legislation to introduce a soft opt-out system whereby the population is deemed to have agreed to donate unless they have previously expressed or registered a desire not to do so [15]. The potential impact of this strategy on donor numbers will be monitored closely and may well prompt legislation reviews in other countries of the UK.

Expert comment

When a potential donor is on the organ donor register or subject to the Welsh opt-out legislation and deemed to have given consent, then it is appropriate that a presumptive approach is made to the family. The approach assumes that consent has already been given by the patient and the conversation is primarily about how to make their wish a reality.

Expert comment

Vasopressin was used instead of noradrenaline as the vasoconstrictor of choice because it improves the outcomes of transplanted kidneys and also treats the diabetes insipidus the patient had developed.

Expert comment

The results of transplantation are not only dependent on the number of organs available but more importantly on the quality of the organs recovered. Management of a potential DBD donor is in effect the provision of high-quality intensive care management. Intensivist-led management of potential DBD donors can increase the number of organs successfully recovered and transplanted, particularly lungs [17].

The SN-OD offered the organs to the transplant teams who accepted the kidneys, liver, and pancreas for transplantation. While awaiting the arrival of the organ retrieval team, the patient's further management changed to a strategy to optimize the function of the organs to be transplanted and avoid any damage that can result from the physiological changes that accompany brainstem death [16]. Initially the patient developed diabetes insipidus which was manged with intermittent doses of intravenous desmopressin. The patient's hypotension was managed with fluids and an infusion of vasopressin to maintain mean arterial pressure.

He was actively warmed to maintain normothermia and insulin was infused to manage hyperglycaemia. A lung protective ventilation strategy was continued. The patient was transferred to the operating theatre where he was manged by a senior anaesthetist who continued the vasopressin infusion, fluids, and ventilatory strategy used on the ICU but also administered neuromuscular blocking drugs and opioids during the 3-hour retrieval procedure. This was carried out by a single abdominal surgical retrieval team. On this occasion, a second thoracic retrieval team was not required as the heart and lungs were not suitable for transplantation. The kidneys and liver were successfully transplanted into three recipients, while the pancreas was used for research. The use of retrieved organs for research purposes when they are not transplanted is a routine component of the consent process. The SN-ODs later wrote to the patient's relatives to thank them for the gift the patient had made and to provide them with anonymized details of the patients who had benefited from the organ transplants.

★ Learning point Physiological support of the donor

There are several physiological changes that occur following brain death. Many can cause damage to organs being considered for transplantation. The incidence of these changes is:

- hypotension 80%
- diabetes insipidus 65%
- disseminated intravascular coagulation 30%
- cardia arrhythmias 30%
- pulmonary oedema 20%
- metabolic acidosis 10%.

Managing these physiological changes appropriately can increase the chances of organs being transplanted successfully [16]. Donor care bundles are increasingly used to guide the optimization of potential DBD donors and to set appropriate physiological targets to aim for. A donor care bundle in common use in the UK is provided by NHS Blood and Transplant (Figure 18.5) [18].

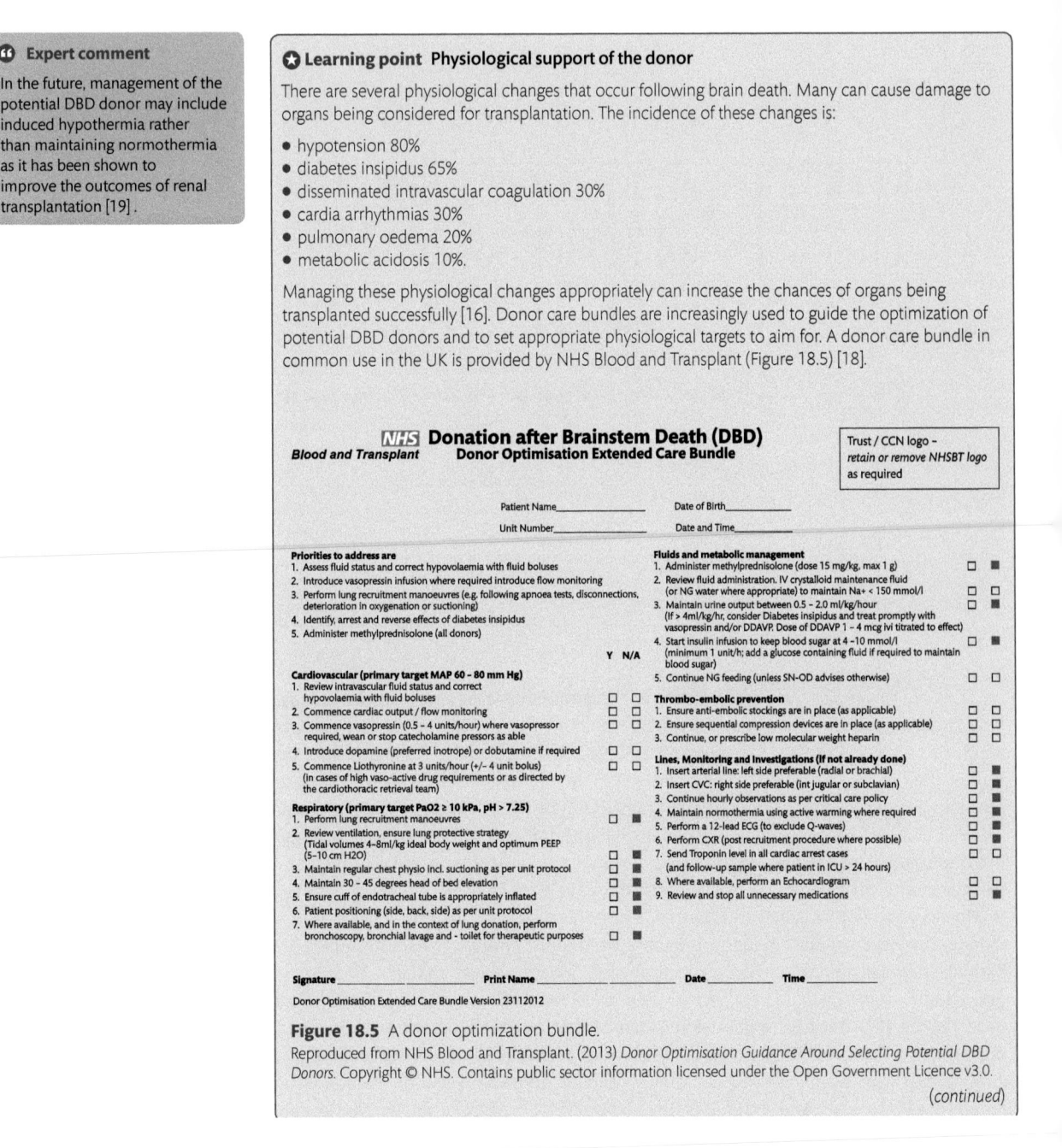

Figure 18.5 A donor optimization bundle.

Reproduced from NHS Blood and Transplant. (2013) *Donor Optimisation Guidance Around Selecting Potential DBD Donors.* Copyright © NHS. Contains public sector information licensed under the Open Government Licence v3.0.

(continued)

Figure 18.5 Continued

⊕ Learning point Donation after circulatory death

DCD describes recovery of organs after death has been confirmed using circulatory criteria. In the US, Australia, the Netherlands, and the UK, controlled DCD is the DCD pathway practised. It is the only deceased donation pathway where the patient is still alive and awaiting the WLST when donation decisions are made and antemortem interventions to maintain donation potential are applied. All aspects of this form of donation and many of its ethical, legal, and professional challenges have been reviewed in detail [22]. DCD was primarily a kidney-only recovery pathway with data showing that transplanted DCD kidneys had the same long-term outcome as DBD kidneys. Today, DCD is a multiorgan recovery pathway enabling successful transplantation of kidneys, liver, pancreas, lungs, and recently also the heart.

Patients suitable for controlled DCD are generally those with devastating brain injuries who do not meet the criteria for testing for brain death and a decision to undertake WLST has been reached once ongoing treatment is no longer deemed to be in the patient's best interests. In these circumstances, the suitability of the patient for donation is discussed with a SN-OD, and then the family are approached for consent to donation before the WLST. If the family agree to donation, the WLST is delayed and physiological stability is maintained until the retrieval team is on site and prepared in the operating theatre. The WLST is undertaken in a location close to or within the theatre complex to reduce the warm ischaemic damage to organs after asystole. Death is confirmed in a timely manner after 5 min of continuous coma, apnoea, and absence of the circulation as recommended by national guidance [10]. The patient is then rapidly transferred to the operating theatre for the organ recovery procedure. In general, the donation process is stopped if the time from WLST to death exceeds 2–3 hours. The main concern from the transplantation perspective is the damage caused by the warm ischaemic time. This is the time that the organ remains at body temperature without adequate perfusion. It is measured as the period between a sustained drop in systolic blood pressure to less

(continued)

than 50 mmHg until the start of cold perfusion and must be kept to a minimum to maximize the chance of successful organ transplantation. Development of new technologies such as normothermic regional perfusion, to reduce warm ischaemic damage, will continue to improve the outcomes of transplanted organs recovered from DCD donors (Figure 18.6). Normothermic regional perfusion involves the insertion of catheters with balloons to isolate the circulation of organs to be transplanted. The organs are reperfused with warm oxygenated blood for, usually, 2 hours after the cardiac arrest before cold perfusion is commenced, although the optimal duration remains to be defined. Normothermic regional perfusion does not reduce the functional warm ischaemia time but reverses some of the damage done, allows further evaluation of donor organs before a decision to transplant is made, and appears to improve transplant outcomes.

Despite the success of DCD programmes, the gold standard pathway for deceased donation remains DBD since more organs are retrieved and transplanted from DBDs than DCDs and the outcomes are often considered better. Also, DBD is the more efficient deceased donation pathway as 45% of potential DBD donors become actual donors compared to only 10% of potential DCD donors who become actual donors. Potential DBD donors are patients whose clinical condition is suspected to fulfil the criteria for confirming death using neurological criteria. Potential DCD donors are patients in whom cardiorespiratory arrest is anticipated to occur after the WLST within a time frame that will enable organ recovery.

Overall, DBD is the preferred model for organ donation—because it increases rates of organ retrieval and successful transplantation. As the number of DCD donors in the UK has increased each year since 2002 (and now accounts for 42% of all deceased organ donors), there has been concern that this increase is at the expense of DBD because of WLST in patients who might otherwise be DBD donors. However, the evidence indicates that DCD donors are an additional pool of organ donors, and the

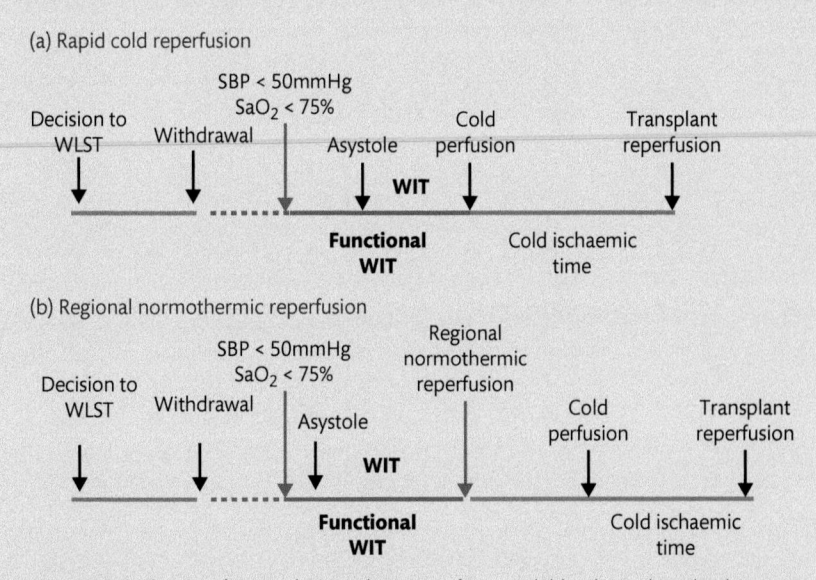

Figure 18.6 The use of regional normothermic perfusion with blood to reduce the damage caused by the warm ischaemic time (WIT) before the onset of organ perfusion with cold solutions. The acceptable functional WIT varies for different organs and ranges from 30 min for the liver and pancreas to 60 min for kidneys and lungs. SaO_2, oxygen saturation of arterial blood; SBP, systolic blood pressure.

(continued)

pool of DBD donors has not decreased. Despite this, it is estimated that the common practice of early WLST decisions in the UK and other northern European countries prevents around a quarter of DCD donors progressing to brainstem death and the potential for DBD donation [23]. Modification of end of life practices has the possibility of increasing the chances of meeting the stated wishes of patients who will not survive, to donate their organs after their death.

Discussion

Organ donation may not be a common occurrence in many hospitals, but should always be considered as a routine part of end of life care for all patients dying in the ICU or ED. The deceased donation pathway that a patient follows will depend on the circumstances (Figure 18.7) [20]. Only DBD and controlled DCD are routinely practised in the UK and the Netherlands, which is a reflection of the greater frequency with which WLST is practised in northern Europe compared with southern European countries such as Spain, Italy, and Portugal. In these southern European counties, WLST is much less frequent and thus the incidence of brain death is about four times more common, while uncontrolled DCD is more common. While not all patients will be suitable for organ donation and not all families will consent to or authorize organs, any potential for organ donation is lost immediately if potential organ donors are not identified and referred by the ICU or ED team.

In the case described in this chapter, routine practice in many hospitals would have been to explore the option of organ donation in the ED when a decision to WLST had been reached. Since the patient was older than 80 years, which excludes DCD, and because he still had brainstem reflexes excluding consideration of DBD, it is likely that he would have been extubated in the ED, and end of life care continued there or on a general medical ward. However, by transferring him to the ICU as part of a devastating brain injury pathway, it enabled his family members to attend the hospital, giving them more time to come to terms with his diagnosis and to explore the patient's preferences and values to create a bespoke end of life care plan [21], which on this occasion included the potential for organ donation. It also provided the opportunity for the family to witness the clinical tests to confirm death, helping them understand the absolute futility of ongoing organ support. In doing so, the patient was also able to become a DBD and donated his kidneys, pancreas, and liver. Furthermore, the likelihood of his wife agreeing to authorize DCD without her family being present and without the support of a SN-OD is significantly less than the prospect of her authorizing DBD. Finally, admitting the patient to ICU also enabled best practice to be followed in the key steps of the organ donation pathway including timely referral, approaching the family, confirming death using neurological criteria, and optimizing the donor's physiology.

	Donation after brain death (DBD)	Controlled donation after cardiac death (cDCD)	Uncontrolled donation after cardiac death (uDCD)
Donor population	Devastating brain injury	85% Devastating brain injury 15 % Non-neurological diagnosis	Unexpected cardiac arrest
Location	ICU	ICU Occasionally emergency department	Community followed by emergency department
Trigger for referral to donor coordinator Antemortem interventions	Coma and loss of several brainstem reflexes and no planned medical or surgical intervention A decision to test for brain death Maintenance of physiological stability in devastating brain injury before neurological testing	A decision to withdraw life-sustainin gtreatments being considered in ICU or emergency department To reduce warm ischemic time Need legal frameowrk to define interventions considered acceptable	Unsuccessful resuscitation after cardiac arrest CPR withour drugs or fluids continued until in-hospital declaration of death
Recommended timing of family approach	After family understand and accept brain death diagnosis	After family understand and accept withdrawal of life-sustaining treatments and inevitability of death Decopule withdrawal of life-sustaining treatments conversation from approach for donation	Possibility of uDCD often raised by out of hospital emergency services. After explanation of the sudden death of the patient
Recommended approach Professional diagnosing death Postmortem interventions	Trained requestor Collaborative approach Trained in brain death testing Independent of donation and transplantation teams Application of donor management protocol Intensivist-led management	Trained requestor Collaborative approach Trained individual Independent of donation and transplantion teams To reduce warm ischemic damage increase organ viability None that may restore cerebral perfusion	Trained requestor Collaborative approach Trained individual Independent of donation and transplantation teams To reduce warm ischemic damage and increase organ viability
Retrieval team	Time of retrieval agreed between retrieval team and donor hospital	On site and prepared in theater at time of withdrawal of life-sustaining treatments Retrieval starts immediately after death	Only in transplantaino centers with an in-house retrieval team available
Organs possibly suitable for transplantation	Kidneys, heart, lungs, liver, pancreas	kidneys, heart, lungs, liver, pancreas	Mainly kidneys. Occasionally liver and lungs

Figure 18.7 A comparison of the three-principle deceased donation pathways.

Reproduced with permission from Citerio, G., et al. Organ donation: a critical care perspective. *Intensive Care Medicine*. 2016;42:305–315. Copyright © Springer-Verlag Berlin Heidelberg and ESICM 2015.

A final word from the expert

This case demonstrates best practice applied to each step of the donation pathway, particularly those where donation potential is most likely to be lost. There is guidance from our professional and regulatory bodies on the identification and referral of potential donors using clinical triggers, confirming death using neurological or circulatory criteria, assessing suitability for donation, approaching the relatives for organ donation, gaining consent/authorization, and optimization of the potential donor to maximize the number and quality of organs to be transplanted. All this best practice is endorsed by the Intensive Care Society and Faculty of Intensive Care Medicine in the section on organ donation in their Guidelines for the Provision of Intensive Care Services [24]. While in the past some may have perceived many of these recommendations as being in the best interests of the recipient rather than the donor, those views are based on a narrow interpretation of only the patient's medical best interests and are inconsistent with the more current interpretation of best interests as enshrined within the UK's Mental Capacity Act 2005 [25]. This requires those making decisions on behalf of an adult lacking competence to consider the person's past and present wishes and feelings, the beliefs and values that would be likely to influence that person's decision if they had capacity, and the other factors that they would be likely to consider if they were able to do so. A patient's wish to donate should therefore be considered when making decisions on their behalf. This case is possibly even more challenging because the patient was admitted to the ICU as part of a devastating brain injury pathway despite a very poor prognosis and before establishing the patient's wishes about organ donation. The ambitions of such pathways (which include improving accurate prognostication, improving end of life care for the patient and their relatives, and enabling exploration and facilitation of their end of life choices, including organ donation) can also be interpreted as being in that individual patient's best interests.

References

1. Manara AR, Thomas I, Harding R. A case for stopping the early withdrawal of life sustaining therapies in patients with devastating brain injuries. *J Intensive Care Soc.* 2016;17:295–301.
2. Souter MJ, Blissitt PA, Blosser S, et al. Recommendations for the critical care management of devastating brain injury: prognostication, psychosocial, and ethical management. A position statement for healthcare professionals from the neurocritical care society. *Neurocrit Care.* 2015;23:4–13.
3. Department of Health. *Organs for Transplants: A Report from the Organ Donation Taskforce.* London: Department of Health; 2008. Available from: https://webarchive.nationalarchives. gov.uk/20130105051141/http://www.dh.gov.uk/en/Publicationsandstatistics/Publications/ PublicationsPolicyAndGuidance/DH_082122.
4. NHS Blood and Transplant and the UK Departments of Heath. Taking Organ Transplantation to 2020. A UK Strategy [Internet]. Available from: https://www.nhsbt.nhs.uk/tot2020/the-strategy/ (accessed 29 November 2016).
5. General Medical Council. *Treatment and Care Towards the End of Life: Good Practice in Decision Making.* London: General Medical Council; 2010. Available from: http://www.gmc-uk.org/ static/documents/content/Treatment_and_care_towards_the_end_of_life_-_English_1015.pdf.
6. National Institute for Health and Care Excellence. *Organ Donation for Transplantation: Improving Donor Identification and Consent Rates for Deceased Organ Donation.* Clinical guideline [CG135]. London: National Institute for Health and Care Excellence; 2011. Available from: https://www.nice.org.uk/guidance/cg135.
7. Academy of Medical Royal Colleges Donation Ethics Committee Consultation Document. An Ethical Framework for Controlled Donation after Circulatory Death [Internet]. 2011.

Available from: http://www.aomrc.org.uk/wp-content/uploads/2016/05/Controlled_dona-tion_circulatory_death_consultation_0111.pdf (accessed 29 November 2016).

8. NHS Blood and Transplant. Timely Identification and Referral of Potential Organ Donors: A Strategy for Implementation of Best Practice [Internet]. 2012. Available at: http://www.odt.nhs.uk/pdf/timely-identification-and-referral-potential-donors.pdf (accessed 29 November 2016).

9. Sanchez-Ibanez J. Potential and evolution of organ donation in Galicia (Spain) 2006–2012. *Transplant.* 2013;96:S165–280.

10. Academy of Medical Royal Colleges. A Code of Practice for the Diagnosis and Confirmation Death [Internet]. 2008. Available from: http://www.odt.nhs.uk/pdf/code-of-practice-for-the-diagnosis-and-confirmation-of-death.pdf (accessed 29 November 2016).

11. Faculty of Intensive Care Medicine. Form for the Diagnosis of Death using Neurological Criteria (abbreviated guidance version) [Internet]. 2016. Available from: https://www.ficm.ac.uk/sites/default/files/Form%20for%20the%20Diagnosis%20of%20Death%20using%20Neurological%20Criteria%20-%20Abbreviated%20Version%20%282015%29_0.pdf (accessed 29 November 2016).

12. Academy of Medical Royal Colleges Donation Ethics Committee. An ethical framework for do-nation after confirmation of death using neurological criteria (DBD) [Internet]. 2016. Available from: http://www.aomrc.org.uk/wp-content/uploads/2016/07/Ethical_framework_donation_after_confirmation_death_using_neurological_criteria-2.pdf (accessed 29 November 2016).

13. NHS Blood and Transplant. Approaching the Families of Potential Organ Donors: Best Practise Guidance [Internet]. 2013. Available from: http://www.odt.nhs.uk/pdf/family_approach_best_practice_guide.pdf (accessed 29 November 2016).

14. Hulme W, Allen J, Manara AR, et al. Factors influencing the family consent rate for organ donation in the UK. *Anaesth.* 2016;71:1053–63.

15. Human Transplantation (Wales) Act 2013 [Internet]. Available from: http://www.legislation.gov.uk/anaw/2013/5/pdfs/anaw_20130005_en.pdf (accessed 29 November 2016).

16. McKeown DW, Bonser RS, Kellum JA. Management of the heartbeating brain-dead organ donor. *Br J Anaesth.* 2012;108:i96–107.

17. Singbartl K, Murugan R, Kaynar AM, et al. Intensivist-led management of brain-dead donors is associated with an increase in organ recovery for transplantation. *Am J Transplant.* 2011;11:1517–21.

18. NHS Blood and Transplant. Donor Optimisation Guideline for Management of the Brain-Stem Dead Donor [Internet]. 2012. Available from: http://odt.nhs.uk/pdf/donor_optimisa-tion_guideline.pdf (accessed 29 November 2016).

19. Niemann CU, Feiner J, Swain S, et al. Therapeutic hypothermia in deceased organ donors and kidney-graft function. *N Engl J Med.* 2015;373:405–14.

20. Citerio G, Cypel M, Dobb GJ, et al. Organ donation: a critical care perspective. *Intensive Care Med.* 2016;42:305–15.

21. Manara A. Bespoke end-of-life decision making in ICU: has the tailor got the right measure-ments? *Crit Care Med.* 2015;43:909–10.

22. Manara AR, Murphy PG, O'Callaghan GO. Donation after circulatory death. *Br J Anaesth.* 2012;108:i108–21.

23. Broderick AR, Manara A, Bramhall S, Cartmill M, Gardiner D, Neuberger J. A donation after circulatory death program has the potential to increase the number of donors after brain death. *Crit Care Med.* 2016;44:352–9.

24. Manara A, Gardiner D. Specialised critical care: organ donation. In: Faculty of Intensive Care Medicine and The Intensive Care Society (eds) *Guidelines for the Provision of Intensive Care Services.* London: Faculty of Intensive Care Medicine and The Intensive Care Society; 2015, pp. 138–41. Available from: https://www.ficm.ac.uk/sites/default/files/gpics_ed.1.1_-_2016_-_final_with_covers.pdf.

25. UK Parliament. Mental Capacity Act 2005 [Internet]. 2005. Available from: http://www.legislation.gov.uk/ukpga/2005/9/pdfs/ukpga_20050009_en.pdf (accessed 29 November 2016).

INDEX

Tables, figures and boxes are indicated by *t*, *f* and *b* following the page number